Ernst Schering Research Foundation Workshop
Supplement 3
Testicular Function:
From Gene Expression to Genetic Manipulation

Springer-Verlag Berlin Heidelberg GmbH

Ernst Schering Research Foundation Workshop
Supplement 3

Testicular Function: From Gene Expression to Genetic Manipulation

M. Stefanini, C. Boitani, M. Galdieri, R. Geremia,
F. Palombi
Editors

With 59 Figures and 8 Tables

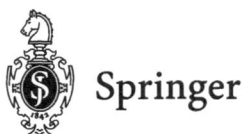

Springer

Series Editors: G. Stock and U.-F. Habenicht

CIP data applied for

Die Deutsche Bibliothek – CIP-Einheitsaufnahme
Testicular function : from gene expression to genetic manipulation ; with 8 tables / M. Stefanini ... ed.
- Berlin ; Heidelberg ; New York ; Barcelona ; Budapest ; Hongkong ; London ; Milan ; Paris ; Santa
Clara ; Singapore ; Tokyo : Springer 1998
(Ernst Schering Research Foundation Workshop : Supplement ; 3)

Schering-Forschungsgesellschaft <Berlin>: [Ernst Schering Research Foundation Workshop / Supple-
ment] Ernst Schering Research Foundation Workshop. Supplement. - Berlin ; Heidelberg ; New
York ; Barcelona ; Budapest ; Hongkong ; London ; Milan ; Paris ; Santa Clara ; Singapore ; Tokyo :
Springer
Reihe Supplemnt zu: Schering-Forschungsgesellschaft <Berlin>: Ernst Schering Research Foundation
Workshop
3. Testicular function. - 1998

ISBN 978-3-662-03673-0   ISBN 978-3-662-03671-6 (eBook)
DOI 10.1007/978-3-662-03671-6

© Springer-Verlag Berlin Heidelberg 1998
Originally published by Springer-Verlag Berlin Heidelberg New York in 1998
Softcover reprint of the hardcover 1st edition 1998

Production: PROEDIT GmbH, D-69126 Heidelberg
Typesetting: Data Conversion by Springer-Verlag

SPIN: 10665852   13/3135–5 4 3 2 1 0 – Printed on acid-free paper

Preface

This volume contains the text of the main lectures given by internationally recognized scientists at the Tenth European Workshop on Molecular and Cellular Endocrinology of the Testis, held in Capri, Italy, from 28 March to 1 April 1998.

Topics include spermatogonial transplantation, germ stem cell biology, regulation of meiosis and spermiogenesis, growth factors, cell signaling and transduction, steroidogenesis, androgen-regulated genes, sperm activation and sperm factors active at fertilization and the molecular basis of specific pathologies of the testis. Looking back at the previous "Capri edition" (1986), the lectures of which were published by Elsevier, it is perhaps not surprising to notice that many of the topics addressed at that time are basically the same now. On the other hand, it appears evident that the search for experimental models of significant physiological value to study testicular function has advanced greatly. In this connection, the use of genetically manipulated animal models in the study of the regulation of spermatogenesis and of the endocrine role of the testis represents a core part of the present volume.

The authors deserve our special thanks not only for delivering excellent state-of-the-art lectures, but also for providing their manuscripts well before the meeting.

The Workshop was supported by funds from the Ares Serono Foundation, the Ernst Schering Research Foundation, the European Academy of Andrology, the Merck Sharp & Dohme Company, the University of Rome "La Sapienza," and the University of Rome "Tor Vergata." We acknowledge the support and assistance provided by the members of the Permanent Scientific Committee of the European

Study Group for Molecular and Cellular Endocrinology of the Testis, as well as by the members of the local organizing committee as listed below. Finally, we are grateful to the Ernst Schering Research Foundation for publishing the present volume in its workshop series.

The book will be of great interest to biologists, endocrinologists, urologists, and medical students who want to improve their knowledge in male reproduction.

M. Stefanini, C. Boitani, M. Galdieri, R. Geremia, F. Palombi

Permanent Scientific Committee of the European Study Group for Molecular and Cellular Endocrinology of the Testis
Brian A. Cooke, London; Vidar Hansson, Oslo, Ilpo Huhtaniemi, Turku; Eberhard Nieschlag, Münster; Focko F.G. Rommerts, Rotterdam; José Saez, Lyon; Olle Söder, Stockholm; Mario Stefanini, Rome; Guido Verhoeven, Leuven.
Local Organizing Committee of the 10th European Workshop on Molecular and Cellular Endocrinology of the Testis
Mario Stefanini; Carla Boitani; Angela D'Agostino; Paolo De Cesaris; Michaela Galdieri; Antonio Filippini; Andrea Fabbri; Gianni Forti; Raffaele Geremia; Andrea Lenzi; Fioretta Palombi; Pellegrino Rossi; Mario A. Russo; Claudio Sette; Elena Vicini; Elio Ziparo.

Table of Contents

List of Editors and Contributors

Editors

M. Stefanini
Department of Histology and Medical Embryology, University of Rome
"La Sapienza", Via Antonio Scarpa 14, 00161 Rome, Italy

C. Boitani
Department of Histology and Medical Embryology, University of Rome
"La Sapienza", Via Antonio Scarpa 14, 00161 Rome, Italy

M. Galdieri
Institute of Histology and General Embryology, Second University of Naples,
Via Luciano Armanni 5, 80138 Naples, Italy

R. Geremia
Department of Public Health and Cell Biology, Section of Anatomy,
University of Rome "Tor Vergata", Via Orazio Raimondo, 00173 Rome, Italy

F. Palombi
Department of Histology and Medical Embryology, University of Rome
"La Sapienza", Via Antonio Scarpa 14, 00161 Rome, Italy

Contributors

K. Aittomäki
Department of Clinical Genetics, Helsinki University Central Hospital,
00290 Oulu, Finland

W.M. Baarends
Department of Endocrinology and Reproduction, Faculty of Medicine and
Health Sciences, Erasmus University Rotterdam, PO Box 1738,
3000 DR Rotterdam, The Netherlands

E. Bernstein
Department of Pathology, Emory University, Room 7107A WMB,
1639 Pierce Drive, Atlanta, GA 30322, USA

K.E. Bernstein
Department of Pathology, Emory University, Room 7107A WMB,
1639 Pierce Drive, Atlanta, GA 30322, USA

A. Bevilacqua
Departments of Psychology and Institute of Histology and Medical
Embryology, University of Rome "La Sapienza", Via Antonio Scarpa 14,
00161 Rome, Italy

R.L. Brinster
Department of Animal Biology, University of Pennsylvania School
of Veterinary Medicine, Philadelphia, PA 19104-6009, USA

M. De Felici
Department of Public Health and Cell Biology, Section of Histology
and Embryology, University of Rome "Tor Vergata", Via Orazio Raimondo,
00173 Rome, Italy

A. Di Carlo
Department of Public Health and Cell Biology, Section of Histology
and Embryology, University of Rome "Tor Vergata", Via Orazio Raimondo,
00173 Rome, Italy

S. Dolci
Department of Public Health and Cell Biology, Section of Anatomy,
University of Rome "Tor Vergata", Via Orazio Raimondo, 00173 Rome, Italy

M.T. Fuller
Departments of Developmental Biology and Genetics, Stanford University
School of Medicine, Beckman Center B-300, Stanford, CA 94305, USA

A. Galione
University Department of Pharmacology, Oxford University, Mansfield Road,
Oxford OX1 3QT, UK

R. Geremia
Department of Public Health and Cell Biology, Section of Anatomy,
University of Rome "Tor Vergata", Via Orazio Raimondo, 00173 Rome, Italy

N.B. Gilula
Department of Cell Biology, The Scripps Research Institute, 10550 N. Torrey
Pines Road, La Jolla, CA 92037-1092, USA

J. Gromoll
Institute of Reproductive Medicine of the University, Domagkstraße 11,
48129 Münster, Germany

J.A. Grootegoed
Department of Endocrinology and Reproduction, Faculty of Medicine
and Health Sciences, Erasmus University Rotterdam, PO Box 1738,
3000 DR Rotterdam, The Netherlands

P.J.M. Hendriksen
Department of Endocrinology and Reproduction, Faculty of Medicine and
Health Sciences, Erasmus University Rotterdam, PO Box 1738,
3000 DR Rotterdam, The Netherlands

O. Hirsch Pescovitz
Section of Pediatric Endocrinology and Diabetology and Herman B. Wells
Center for Pediatric Research, Department of Pediatrics, Indiana University,
James Whitcomb Riley Hospital for Children, 702 Barnhill Drive,
Room 5984, Indianapolis, IN 46202-5225, USA

J.H.J. Hoeijmakers
Department of Cell Biology and Genetics, Faculty of Medicine and Health
Sciences, Erasmus University Rotterdam, PO Box 1738, 3000 DR Rotterdam,
The Netherlands

J.W. Hoogerbrugge
Department of Endocrinology and Reproduction, Faculty of Medicine
and Health Sciences, Erasmus University Rotterdam, PO Box 1738,
3000 DR Rotterdam, The Netherlands

A.J.W. Hsueh
Division of Reproductive Biology, Department of Gynecology and Obstetrics,
Stanford University Medical Center, Stanford, CA 94305-5317, USA

I.T. Huhtaniemi
Department of Physiology, Institute of Biomedicine, University of Turku,
20520 Turku, Finland

M. Ikawa
Department of Science for Laboratory Animal Experimentation,
Research Institute for Microbial Diseases, Osaka University, Yamadaoka 3-1,
Suita Osaka 565, Japan

M. Kudo
Division of Reproductive Biology, Department of Gynecology and Obstetrics,
Stanford University Medical Center, Stanford, CA 94305-5317, USA

N.M. Kumar
Department of Cell Biology, The Scripps Research Institute,
10550 N. Torrey Pines Road, La Jolla, CA 92037, USA

F. Mangia
Departments of Psychology and Institute of Histology and Medical
Embryology, University of Rome "La Sapienza", Via Antonio Scarpa 14,
00161 Rome Rome, Italy

M. Nagano
Department of Animal Biology, University of Pennsylvania School
of Veterinary Medicine, Philadelphia, PA 19104-6009, USA

E. Nieschlag
Institute of Reproductive Medicine of the University, Domagkstraße 11,
48129 Münster, Germany

Y. Nishimune
Department of Science for Laboratory Animal Experimentation,
Research Institute for Microbial Diseases, Osaka University, Yamadaoka 3-1,
Suita Osaka 565, Japan

M. Okabe
Department of Science for Laboratory Animal Experimentation,
Research Institute for Microbial Diseases, Osaka University, Yamadaoka 3-1,
Suita Osaka 565, Japan

Y. Osuga
Division of Reproductive Biology, Department of Gynecology and Obstetrics,
Stanford University Medical Center, Stanford, CA 94305-5317, USA

M. Pesce
European Molecular Biology Laboratory, Meyerhofstraße 1,
69117 Heidelberg, Germany

H.P. Roest
Department of Endocrinology and Reproduction, Faculty of Medicine
and Health Sciences, Erasmus University Rotterdam, PO Box 1738,
3000 DR Rotterdam, The Netherlands

P. Rossi
Department of Public Health and Cell Biology, Section of Anatomy,
University of Rome "Tor Vergata", Via Orazio Raimondo, 00173 Rome, Italy

L.D. Russell
Department of Physiology, Southern Illinois University School of Medicine,
Carbondale, IL 62901-6512, USA

K.K. Samaddar
Department of Physiology and Biophysics, Indiana University Medical
Center, 702 Barnhill Drive, Indianapolis, IN 46202, USA

C. Sette
Department of Public Health and Cell Biology, Section of Anatomy,
University of Rome "Tor Vergata", Via Orazio Raimondo, 00173 Rome, Italy

M. Simoni
Institute of Reproductive Medicine of the University, Domagkstraße 11,
48129 Münster, Germany

D.M. Stocco
Department of Cell Biology and Biochemistry, Health Sciences Center, Texas
Technical University, 3601 4th Street, Lubbock, TX 79430, USA

H. Tanaka
Department of Science for Laboratory Animal Experimentation,
Research Institute for Microbial Diseases, Osaka University, Yamadaoka 3-1,
Suita Osaka 565, Japan

J.S. Tapanainen
Department of Obstetrics and Gynecology, University of Oulu, 90220 Oulu,
Finland

T.M. Todoran
Department of Physiology and Biophysics, Indiana University Medical
Center, 702 Barnhill Drive, Indianapolis, IN 46202, USA

J. Tsuchida
Department of Science for Laboratory Animal Experimentation,
Research Institute for Microbial Diseases, Osaka University, Yamadaoka 3-1,
Suita Osaka 565, Japan

T. Vaskivuo
Department of Obstetrics and Gynecology, University of Oulu, 90220 Oulu,
Finland

C.M. Wayne
Department of Immunology, Smith Research Building, M.D. Anderson
Cancer Center, University of Texas, Houston, TX 77030, USA

G.F. Weinbauer
Institute of Reproductive Medicine of the University, Domagkstraße 11,
48129 Münster, Germany

H. White-Cooper
Departments of Developmental Biology and Genetics, Beckman Center
B-300, Stanford University School of Medicine, Stanford, CA 94305, USA

M.F. Wilkinson
Department of Immunology, Smith Research Building, M.D. Anderson
Cancer Center, University of Texas, Houston, TX 77030, USA

H.L. Wilson
University Department of Pharmacology, Mansfield Road, Oxford OX1 3QT,
Oxford, UK

K. Yomogida
Department of Science for Laboratory Animal Experimentation,
Research Institute for Microbial Diseases, Osaka University, Yamadaoka 3-1,
Suita Osaka 565, Japan

Y. Yoshimura
Department of Science for Laboratory Animal Experimentation,
Research Institute for Microbial Diseases, Osaka University, Yamadaoka 3-1,
Suita Osaka 565, Japan

1 Gap Junctional Communication and the Regulation of Multicellular Functions

N.B. Gilula and N.M. Kumar

1.1 Introduction

Gap junctional communication between cells via gap junctions is a fundamental mechanism that is used to regulate the activities of multicellular systems in virtually all animal organisms. Although cells in higher plants also communicate with one another, this occurs via structures termed plasmadesmata (McLean et al. 1997).

Our present appreciation for the relationship between gap junctional structures and communication pathways was established 30 years ago by studies that integrated electron microscopy with electrophysiological observations, and the use of mammalian genetics to study the metabolic cooperation properties between cells (Loewenstein 1981). One of these studies provided evidence for a direct relationship between the expression of gap junction structures between cells and the acquisition of pathways for both electrical coupling and metabolic cooperation between cells (Gilula et al. 1972). Since that time the appearance of gap junction structures between cells and the detection of low-resistance pathways between cells have been used as the criteria to document the presence of this property between almost all cell types in mammalian organisms. There are still a few cell types, such as erythroid cells, lymphoid cells, skeletal muscle fibers, and most neurons where it has been difficult to document the existence of communication pathways. Once the structure/function relationship was established for the gap junction structures and communication pathways, numerous studies were published documenting the widespread distribution and expression of this property between cells in mammalian organisms (Loewenstein 1981). A number of more comprehensive reviews have been published that contain an extensive discussion of the progress in the gap junction field (Paul 1995; Bruzzone et al. 1996; Kumar and Gilula 1996; Munari-Silem and Rousset 1996).

1.2 Gap Junction Multigene Family

In 1986 the first sequence for a gap junction protein was deduced from the cDNA analysis of transcripts obtained from mammalian liver (Kumar and Gilula 1986; Paul 1986). The product was predicted to be 32 kDa in size, and this protein product was not found exclusively in liver. After the first gap junction gene product was identified, it was referred to as a connexin. Subsequently an entire multigene family of connexins was described (Bruzzone et al. 1996; Kumar and Gilula 1996). In this multigene family there are two broad classes, one termed α and the other termed β (Kumar and Gilula 1992). Currently in mammals 13 connexin genes have been reported. Of these there are 7 members of the α class and 6 members of the β class. The members of the multigene family are described either with Greek (α and β) designations or by the deduced molecular size of the gene product (Table 1).

Table 1. Connexin multigene family

Nomenclature				*Chromosome location*		
Greek letter	Molecular mass	Species	Predicted molecular mass (kDa)	Human	Mouse	Examples of organs with expression
α_1	Cx43	Human	43	6q21–q23.2	–	–
	Cx43	Bovine	43.2	–	–	–
	Cx43	Rodent	43	–	10	Heart
	Cx43	Chicken	43.2	–	–	–
	Cx43	*Xenopus*	43	–	–	–
α_2	Cx38	*Xenopus*	37.8	–	–	Embryo
α_3	Cx44	Bovine	44.4	13q11–q12	–	–
	Cx46	Rodent	46	–	14D1–E1	Lens
	Cx56	Chicken	55.9	–	–	–
α_4	Cx37	Human	37.2	1p35.1	–	–
	Cx37	Rodent	37.6	–	4	Endothelium
	Cx41	*Xenopus*	40.6	–	–	–
α_5	Cx40	Human	40.6	1q21.1	–	–
	Cx40	Canine	39.9	–	–	–
	Cx40	Rodent	40.4	–	3	Lung
	Cx42	Chicken	41.7	–	–	–
α_6	Cx45	Human	45.5	–	–	–
	Cx45	Canine	45.5	–	–	–
	Cx45	Rodent	45.7	–	11	Heart
	Cx45	Chicken	45.4	–	–	–
α_7	Cx33	Rodent	32.9	–	X	Testes
α_8	Cx50	Human	48.2	1q21.1	–	–
	Cx49	Ovine	49.2	–	–	–
	Cx50	Rodent	49.6	–	3	Lens
	Cx45.6	Chicken	45.6	–	–	–
β_1	Cx32	Human	32	Xq13.1	–	–
	Cx32	Rodent	32	–	X	Pancreas
	Cx30	*Xenopus*	30.1	–	–	–
β_2	Cx26	Human	26.2	13q11–q12	–	–
	Cx26	Rodent	26.5	–	14D1–E1	Placenta
β_3	Cx31	Rodent	31	–	4	Skin
β_4	Cx31.1	Rodent	31.1	–	4	Skin
β_5	Cx30.3	Rodent	30.3	–	4	Skin
β_6	Cx30	Rodent	30.4	–	–	Skin

All members of this family contain a basic structural motif consisting of four transmembrane domains. The linear sequence of the products in this multigene family has been modeled topologically into the membrane and studied using site-specific antibodies, protease digestions, and structural analyses (Milks et al. 1988; Tibbitts et al. 1990; Yeager and Gilula 1992). The topological analysis has provided direct evidence that the members of this family contain both amino and carboxyl termini on the cytoplasmic surface with two external loops, referred to as E1 and E2, that are directed towards the extracellular space or gap. There is a high degree of similarity between the extracellular domains of different connexins. The two extracellular loops, based on perturbation and mutagenesis studies, have been suggested to participate in the formation process that is associated with the establishment of gap junctional contact between two adjacent membranes (Dahl et al. 1992; Meyer et al. 1992; White et al. 1994). Further, it has been determined using heterologous expression systems that there is specificity as to which connexin can interact to form a functional gap junction channel (Bruzzone et al. 1993; Elfgang et al. 1995; White et al. 1995). Using chimeric connexins, it has been suggested that the specificity domain resides in the second extracellular domain (Bruzzone et al. 1994a; White et al. 1994, 1995). These studies have been extended to indicate that both extracellular domains and intracellular domains must be derived from one type of connexin to ensure formation of a functional channel (Haubrich et al. 1996).

In the transmembrane regions, one of the four transmembrane domains, transmembrane domain 3 (M3), has an organization of amino acid residues that, if present in an α helical arrangement, can provide a natural "face" for the polar or hydrophilic property that is required for the movement of ions between cells (Milks et al. 1988). These features of the gap junction channel have been recently supported by high-resolution electron microscopic analysis of a truncated, recombinant α_1 (Cx43) connexin (Unger et al. 1997). Using the relative permeability to various cations and chloride, it has been determined that the pore has a radius of 6.3 Å (Wang and Veenstra 1997).

1.3 Gap Junction Channel Properties

The diversity in protein sequence among the members of this family reflects the diversity of channel function that may be required to regulate the different types of cell-specific channel events that occur in vivo. In this context, studies in model systems have provided evidence that the various members of this family can produce channel activities with different conductance properties (Spray 1994).

Biophysical studies have provided evidence that gap junction channel permeabilities can vary in different cell types (Brissette et al. 1994; Steinberg et al. 1994). Distinct ionic and dye permeabilities of the different connexin isoforms has been experimentally determined in cells in culture (Brissette et al. 1994; Elfgang et al. 1995; Veenstra et al. 1995). In general, the channels are permeable to molecules that are on the order of cyclic nucleotides in size or smaller. Of course, this would include a whole host of inorganic ions such as sodium, potassium, and calcium. However, larger molecules such as enzymes, nucleic acids, and carbohydrates do not appear to pass readily through these gap junction channels. Consequently, it is felt that the molecular information that moves through these gap junction channels can be important for regulating and synchronizing the activities that occur between cells in multicellular systems, without directly determining the differentiation state of different cell types. The permeability of the channels is regulated by many different cellular and environmental factors. For example, channel permeability can be affected by production of ATP, by changes in calcium, by changes in pH, and by treatment with a whole host of different substances, many of which are toxic. The influence of various hormones on gap junctional communication has been described also (Meda et al. 1993; Munari-Silem and Rousset 1996).

One of the most interesting avenues for understanding the regulation of gap junction channels has been with changes in second messenger systems, particularly those systems that might influence the phosphorylation state of the gap junction proteins. There are a number of rigorous reports demonstrating that several of the gap junction proteins have residues which are the potential sites of phosphorylation by different kinases (Darrow et al. 1995; Lau et al. 1996). Further, the kinase activities are reported to have a direct consequence on the permeability of gap junction channels in certain cell types (Moreno et al. 1994; Kwak et al. 1995).

The extent of junctional coupling is dependent on both the number and the functional state of the channels. Effects that are rapid and short term result from channel gating and/or from mobilization of a preexisting pool of gap junction channel precursors. Thus changes in Ca^{2+} and H^+ ions, as well as second messengers, have been implicated in the regulation of gap junctional coupling. At least some of these effects are likely to be mediated via protein kinases that can phosphorylate connexins (Stagg and Fletcher 1990).

The same agent may have multiple effects on gap junctions. For example, cAMP has been demonstrated to gate, via protein kinases, gap junctional channels (Saez et al. 1989), influence their assembly into gap junction plaques (Wang and Rose 1995), and have an effect on the connexin gene transcription rate (Mehta et al. 1992; Civitelli et al. 1998). Furthermore, cAMP can pass through gap junctions, and it has been implicated in the transmission of hormone signals between adjacent cells via gap junctions (Lawrence et al. 1978).

Long-term effects on communication can result from alterations in the number and size of gap junctions as well as the connexin isoform that is expressed. For example, in the mammary gland the gap junction plaques, consisting of α_1 connexin, increase in size and number during pregnancy and lactation (Pozzi et al. 1995; Yamanaka et al. 1997). Another example is provided by the uterus, in which during labor the contractile activity of smooth muscle fibers is coordinated by gap junctions (Garfield et al. 1989). Just prior to parturition there is a dramatic increase in the number of gap junctions in the uterine myometrium. Analysis of α_1 connexin transcript levels during partition are consistent with the observed changes in the number of gap junctions reflecting an increased transcriptional rate of the α_1 connexin gene in this tissue (Risek et al. 1990). Furthermore, it has been demonstrated that α_1 connexin expression in the uterine myometrium is regulated by estrogen and progesterone (Petrocelli and Lye 1993). This is consistent with the presence of a putative estrogen responsive element in the promoter region of the α_1 connexin gene (Yu et al. 1994; Lefebvre et al. 1995) as well as other regulatory elements (Chen et al. 1995). The rapid disappearance of gap junctions in the uterine myometrium after delivery may be due to connexin degradation that may involve a ubiquitin-dependent proteolysis mechanism (Laing and Beyer 1995).

1.4 Assembly of Gap Junction Channels

Recent studies have indicated that individual cell types can utilize multiple connexins simultaneously, and that multiple connexins can be organized into channel oligomers to form hetero-oligomeric channel structures (Stauffer 1995; Jiang and Goodenough 1996). A heteromeric gap junction in which each hemichannel (connexon) contained two different connexins, α_1 and α_4, has been demonstrated to have different electrophysiological properties to those composed of the homotypic or heterotypic forms of these channels (Brink et al. 1997). The potential formation of heteromeric, homomeric, homotypic, and heterotypic channels may play an important role in the formation of communication compartments as well as providing a mechanism for creating channels that are selectively permeable to different signaling molecules. Currently there is a great deal of emphasis on trying to understand the rules that determine which of the connexin subunits can be associated with each other.

The gap junction channels are assembled by the synthesis of gap junction protein in the endoplasmic reticulum. Subsequently the gap junction protein is assembled into oligomers and then transported to the plasma membrane. Currently there is one published study indicating in NRK cells that the assembly of the oligomers takes place after the protein has moved through the Golgi. In contrast, another study indicated the potential for formation of gap junctions in the endoplasmic reticulum of cells overexpressing connexin (Kumar et al. 1995). Other studies that have been published using cell-free systems indicate that the oligomerization of gap junction proteins can take place in the endoplasmic reticulum (Falk et al. 1997). Clearly, more information concerning assembly and transport in different cell types will be necessary to develop a more definitive appreciation for the gap junction assembly process.

1.5 Gap Junctional Communication in Embryonic Systems

Gap junctional communication starts very early in vertebrate embryos, shortly after fertilization. A study on early frog embryos demonstrated that the perturbation of gap junctional communication pathways in the early embryo results in developmental defects that are consistent with a contribution of gap junctional communication to the patterning process that takes place to generate proper symmetries in *Xenopus* frog embryos (Warner et al. 1984). Similar patterning influences of gap junctional communication have also been observed in the coelenterate Hydra (Fraser et al. 1987). In mouse embryos the perturbation of gap junctional communication in early stages results in elimination of the communication-defective cells from the embryo proper by a process of decompaction (Lee et al. 1987). All of the early studies on gap junctional communication in development were based on perturbations using an antibody that blocks the communication pathways. The antibody presumably recognized multiple connexin isoforms, and hence it was able to affect gap junction pathways in a wide range of cells from diverse organisms. More recently, specific peptide antibodies have been used to determine the role of different connexin domains in their functional and biological properties (Becker et al. 1995; Bastide et al. 1996). Currently, antibody-independent selective perturbations can be carried out in embryonic systems using genetic approaches as discussed below.

1.6 Gap Junctional Communication in the Testis

There is a complex network of intercellular communication pathways in the testes that is mediated by growth factors. Contact-dependent communication events that are mediated by gap junctions have received less attention in defining their role in testis function.

Gap junctional communication was reported in the testis a number of years ago. Gap junctions are quite numerous between Leydig cells and also between Sertoli cells (Gilula et al. 1976; McGinley et al. 1979). Communication between the Sertoli cells has been thought to have a very important consequence on the synchronization of events that take place in the seminiferous tubule. The existence of electrical and dye coupling between Sertoli cells and between Leydig cells has been well documented (Eusebi et al. 1983; Grassi et al. 1986; Kawa et al. 1987; Risley et al. 1992; Varanda and Campos de Carvalho 1994). Gap junctional communication between Sertoli cells in culture can be influenced by many agents, including cAMP and diacylglycerol (Grassi et al. 1986). Recently it has been demonstrated that a lipophilic substance, oleamide, inhibits gap junctional communication between cells in culture (Guan et al. 1997). Other lipophilic compounds such as gossypol (Hervé et al. 1996a) and steroids, such as testosterone (Pluciennik et al. 1996) have also been reported to uncouple Sertoli cells in culture. These uncoupling effects could result from the insertion of the lipophilic substances into the membrane, which in turn promote conformational changes in gap junction channels (Hervé et al. 1996b). This selectivity in action of these different lipophilic compounds may rely on the association of cholesterol with gap junctions (Hervé et al. 1996a; Pluciennik et al. 1996; Lerner 1997).

The utilization of gap junction gene products in the testis has proved to be quite interesting. No less than three members of the connexin multigene family have been identified in the mammalian testis. Connexin α_1 has been identified with the gap junctions that are formed between Leydig cells and also with the gap junctions that connect Sertoli cells (Risley et al. 1992; Pelletier and Byers 1992; Perez-Armendariz et al. 1994). In addition to α_1, a novel connexin, α_7 (Cx33), also is utilized in the gap junctional regions between Sertoli cells (Tan et al 1996). The role of α_7 connexin in these cells has not been established, but it has been proposed to have some inhibitory function that would be beneficial for the Sertoli cell/germ cell involvement in the testis (Chang et al. 1996). This proposal, which is based on studies in a model system (paired frog oocytes), must wait further clarity from studies examining this connexin in other model systems, as well as in vivo. These analyses must also take into account the possibility of heteromeric and heterotypic channels, containing both α_1 and α_7 connexin, and how this may influence the properties of the gap junctions. A third connexin, α_4, (Cx37) is used also in the testis, principally in the endothelium that is associated with the blood vessels (Tan et al. 1996).

Northern blot analysis has indicated the presence of low levels of β_1 (Cx32) and β_2 (Cx26) connexins in rat testes (Zhang and Nicholson 1989). Immunofluorescence analysis indicated that β_1 and β_2 connexins may exist in the apical regions of the seminiferous epithelium although their precise location has not been defined (Risley et al. 1992). The connexin composition of Sertoli–germ cell gap junctions. remains undefined, and this may be due to the small size of germ cell gap junctions or the occurrence of unidentified connexin in these junctions.

The abundance and composition of gap junctions between Sertoli cells is regulated during testis maturation and the cycle of the seminiferous epithelium (Tan et al. 1996). Additionally, the α_1 and α_7 connexin are modulated independently of each other (Tan et al. 1996). This suggests that these two connexins have a functionally unique and different role in the various stages of the seminiferous epithelium.

In the adult testis Sertoli cells have unique tight junction complexes that are responsible for the formation of the blood-testis barrier (Gilula et al. 1976; Pelletier and Byers 1992). Furthermore, they divide the seminiferous epithelium into several compartments, each of which contains spermatocytes at different stages of development (Russell and Malone 1980). In the immature testis typical gap junctions are common, and there is an absence of tight junctions (Gilula et al. 1976). As development proceeds, these gap junctions become less numerous and the tight junctions become more prevalent. The correlation in appearance of tight junctions and disappearance of gap junctions suggests that these two structures have mutually exclusive roles in the function of the testis. In addition, the observation of gap junction particles interspersed between rows of tight junction fibrils suggests a potential interaction between the components of these two junctions. Recently the protein component of tight junctions, occludin (Ando-Akatsuka et al. 1996), has been identified. The availability of probes to both connexin and occludin and their application to study the development of junctions in the testis is likely to provide some fruitful insight into the assembly and disassembly of both gap and tight junctions.

1.7 Contribution of Gap Junctional Communication to Multicellular Function Using Gene Disruption Procedures in Mice

The targeted disruption of connexin genes, a procedure which is commonly called gene "knockout," has been carried out with several connexin genes in mice. Thus far β_1, β_2, α_1, α_3, α_4, and α_5 connexin genes have been disrupted by homologous recombination in mice to provide some appreciation for their function in multicellular organs in vivo. The α_1 gene was the first connexin gene to be disrupted in mice (Reaume et al. 1995). In these organisms there is a cardiac defect that contributes to lethality. Further analysis of the α_1 knockout animals, particularly in the embryonic stages, has led to an appreciation for a number of defects in several organs, in addition to the heart, which indicate a significant influence of α_1 in the development and function of multiple organs in the mouse. Thus it remains possible that the lethality in these α_1 knockout mice is due to problems in other organs that ultimately are manifested in the heart. Due to the lethality of these knockout mice shortly after birth it has not been possible to utilize these mice for studying the role of α_1 connexin in the adult mouse.

The α_1 connexin is expressed early on in mouse development prior to the compaction stage (Nishi et al. 1991). Thus it was surprising that the α_1 connexin knockout mice developed normally, at least to the time of implantation. One possibility is that embryos with the disrupted α_1 connexin utilize other connexin isoforms to support development. The recent report of the expression of other connexins and the retention of coupling in preimplantation embryos of the α_1 knockout mice supports this possibility (Davies et al. 1996; De Sousa et al. 1997).

One very interesting study in this regard has been the sequence of the α_1 connexin, which in a human genetic disease contains mutations in the coding sequence where phosphorylation normally takes place to the wild-type protein (Britz-Cunningham et al. 1995). It is very interesting from that analysis to consider the possibility that the mutated residues create a defect in the heart since the gap junction protein cannot be phosphorylated normally. However, another analysis has questioned the occurrence of these mutations in patients with visceroatrial heterotaxia (Splitt et al. 1997).

β_1 Connexin is widely expressed in many tissues, including the liver. When the β_1 connexin gene was knocked out in the mouse, there was no dramatic effect or phenotype in these animals (Nelles et al. 1996). However, there was a detectable change in the glucose metabolism in the liver of those animals. The X-linked neurodegenerative disease called Charcot-Marie-Tooth (CMTX) has been linked to mutations within the β_1 connexin locus (Bergoffen et al. 1993). Further analysis of the β_1 knockout mouse indicated detectable effects on the peripheral nervous system with features similar to those of CMTX patients (Anzini et al. 1997). The β_1 gene product is currently thought to be important for an interaction in the myelin region of Schwann cells, such that reflexive gap junction channels are formed between incisures and paranodal membranes (Paul 1995).

In an effort to directly determine the effect of mutations on β_1 connexin function, mutants of β_1 connexin have been expressed in heterologous expression systems and the resulting consequences on formation of a functional channel determined. These studies have indicated that, depending on the mutation, there are effects on trafficking (Deschênes et al. 1997), gating or assembly (Bruzzone et al. 1994b), and permeability (Oh et al. 1997) of the β_1 connexin.

Recently mutations in the β_2 connexin gene have been implicated in one form of hereditary deafness in humans (Kelsell et al. 1997; Zelante et al. 1997). Consistent with this is the immunohistochemical and ultrastructural localization of β_2 connexin in the rat cochlea (Kikuchi et al. 1995). By contrast, a knockout of $8b_2$ results in embryonic lethality in mice. A subsequent analysis of these embryos indicates that the lethality is related to an essential use for the β_2 channels in maternal/fetal interactions that take place across the placental barrier. In the absence of β_2 the proper interactions cannot take place, and the embryos subsequently die. It should be noted that gene disruptions may not have the same consequences as point mutations. Furthermore, the distribution and function of connexins may differ between the mouse and other organisms.

During follicular development gap junctions enable ovarian follicular and luteal cells to communicate with each other and with the oocyte (Anderson and Albertini 1976; Gilula et al. 1978; Grazul-Bilska et al. 1997). This extensive communication results in a structural and functional syncytium that is involved in regulation of meiotic differentiation and maturation of the cumulus-oocyte complex (Epping 1991). In addition, the gap junctions may be necessary for transfer of nutrients and metabolites to the poorly vascularized granulosa layer and developing corpora lutea.

At least five different connexin products have been identified in the ovary, α_1, α_4, α_5, β_1, and β_2, and they have been demonstrated to exist in the different cell types of the ovary (Grazul-Bilska et al. 1997). The pattern of expression of these connexins change in the ovary throughout the estrous cycle and following steroid hormone administration (Risek et al. 1995; Grazul-Bilska et al. 1997).

The role of gap junctions in follicular development has been assessed by disrupting the α_4 connexin gene (Simon et al. 1997). In these mice there was a lack of mature follicles as well as a failure to ovulate, resulting in female sterility. Immunocytochemistry indicates that α_1 connexin is found in the cumulus oophorus cells of the granulosa layer, and α_4 connexin is the predominant oocyte connexin. It appears that in the absence of this connexin the interactions between the oocyte and the cumulus cells cannot take place properly, and the oocyte subsequently fails to undergo proper meiotic maturation. Thus the sterility appears to result from an improper follicular maturation and ovulation. Disruption of communication pathways by gap junctional inhibitors, such as lindane, also support a role for gap junctions in morphogenesis of ovarian follicles (Li and Mather 1997).

The lens provides a unique system for studying metabolic cooperation between cells through gap junctions in vivo. In this tissue the cells in the lens interior do not have access to a blood supply, and hence they are able to survive only by diffusion of metabolites from the aqueous humor into the lens. This suggests a model in which fiber cells are coupled to epithelial cells (Benedetti et al. 1981; Goodenough 1992). The existence of electrical and dye communication between lens fiber cells is now well established (reviewed in Mathias et al. 1997). In addition to their role in communication, gap junctions may make an important contribution to cell-cell adhesion in the lens which is important for the transmission of light (Kuszak et al. 1980). Three connexin isoforms have been reported in the lens. The lens epithelial cells appear to express only α_1 connexin (Beyer et al. 1989). The α_3 (Cx 46) and α_8 (Cx50) connexins are most abundantly expressed in the lens fiber cells (Paul et al. 1991; White et al. 1992).

To determine the specific role of α_3 connexin in vivo the α_3 connexin gene was disrupted in mice (Gong et al. 1997). Although the absence of the α_3 connexin had no obvious influence on the early stages of lens formation and the differentiation of lens fibers, mice homozygous for the disrupted α_3 gene developed nuclear cataracts at the age of 2–3 weeks. The cataract phenotype in these mice was quite similar to the age-dependent or senile cataracts that appear in humans. Gap junctions containing α_8 connexin were found in the homozygous mice, but they could not compensate for the functional loss of α_3 connexin in the lens nucleus. The nuclear cataracts resulted from light scattering of high molecular weight aggregates formed by the lens proteins linked together via disulfide bonds. A significant amount of degraded crystallins, in particular a unique fragmentation of γ crystallin, was detected in the α_3 homozygote lenses, suggesting that proteolysis in the lens plays a critical role in the cataractogenesis of the α_3 (–/–) mice. Preliminary results indicate that it is a loss of cell coupling in the central fiber cells that is correlated to the loss of the α_3 connexin.

This study uniquely established the importance of gap junctions in maintaining the function of a normal lens. Specifically the results indicated that the α_3 connexin gene is essential for providing a cell-cell signaling pathway or structural component for maintaining the organization of lens membrane and cytoplasmic proteins that is required for normal lens transparency. Further, the results suggest that a loss of α_3 connexin initiates a process in the lens that may involve an apoptosis pathway.

1.8 Summary

Recent progress in the field of gap junctional biology has benefited from the use of selective targeted gene disruption of members of the multigene family of connexins to define the contributions that individual connexin genes make to the function of multicellular systems in the mammal. This approach has provided us with an understanding of the way in which the members of the multigene connexin family are utilized in vivo to provide a diversity of functions that are required for the diversity of cellular functions in vivo. A great challenge for research in this area has been raised by recent results which indicate that multiple connexins can be expressed by individual cells simultaneously, and these multiple connexins can associate to form individual connexin oligomers which will predictably have unique gap junctional properties. These recent factors must be applied to develop an appreciation for the utilization of multiple connexin genes to regulate the diverse multicellular functions in the testis.

References

Anderson E, Albertini PF (1976) Gap junctions between the oocyte and the companion follicle cells in the mammalian ovary. J Cell Biol 71:680–686

Ando-Akatsuka Y, Saitou M, Hirase T, Kishi M, Sakakibara A, Itoh M, Yonemura S, Furuse M, Tsukita S (1996) Interspecies diversity of the occludin sequence: cDNA cloning of human, mouse, dog, and rat-kangaroo homologues. J Cell Biol 133(1):43–47

Anzini P, Neuberg DH, Schachner M, Nelles E, Willecke K, Zielasek J, Toyka KV, Suter U, Martini R (1997) Structural abnormalities and deficient maintenance of peripheral nerve myelin in mice lacking the gap junction protein connexin 32. J Neurosci 17:4545–4551

Bastide B, Jarry-Guichard T, Briand JP, Délèze J, Gros D (1996) Effect of anti-peptide antibodies directed against three domains of connexin43 on the gap junctional permeability of cultured heart cells. J Membr Biol 150:243–253

Becker DL, Evans WH, Green CR, Warner A (1995) Functional analysis of amino acid sequences in connexin43 involved in intercellular communication through gap junctions. J Cell Sci 108:1455–1467

Benedetti EL, Dunia I, Ramaeckers FCS, Kibbelaar MA (1981) Lenticular plasma membranes and cytoskeleton. In Bloemendal H (ed) Molecular and cellular biology of the eye lens. Wiley, New York, pp 137–188

Bergoffen J, Scherer SS, Wang S, Scott MO, Bone LJ, Paul DL, Chen K, Lensch MW, Chance PF, Fischbeck KH (1993) Connexin mutations in X-linked Charcot-Marie-Tooth disease. Science 262:2039–2042

Beyer EC, Kistler J, Paul DL, Goodenough DA (1989) Antisera directed against connexin 43 peptides react with a 43-kD protein localized to gap junctions in myocardium and other tissues. J Cell Biol 108:595–605

Brink PR, Cronin K, Banach K, Peterson E, Westphale EM, Seul KH, Ramanan SV, Beyer EC (1997) Evidence for heteromeric gap junction channels formed from rat connexin43 and human connexin37. Am J Physiol 273:C1386–C1396

Brissette JL, Kumar NM, Gilula NB, Hall JE, Dotto GP (1994) Switch in gap junction protein expression is associated with selective changes in junctional permeability during keratinocyte differentiation. Proc Natl Acad Sci USA 91:6453–6457

Britz-Cunningham SH, Shah MM, Zuppan CW, Fletcher WH (1995) Mutations of the *connexin43* gap-junction gene in patients with heart malformations and defects of laterality. N Engl J Med 332:1323–1329

Bruzzone R, Haefliger J-A, Gimlich RL, Paul DL (1993) Connexin40, a component of gap junctions in vascular endothelium, is restricted in its ability to interact with other connexins. Mol Biol Cell 4:7–20

Bruzzone R, White TW, Paul DL (1994a) Expression of chimeric connexins reveals new properties of the formation and gating behavior of gap junction channels. J Cell Sci 107:955–967

Bruzzone R, White TW, Scherer SS, Fischbeck KH, Paul DL (1994b) Null mutations of connexin32 in patients with X-linked Charcot-Marie-Tooth disease. Neuron 13:1253–1260

Bruzzone R, White TW, Paul DL (1996) Connections with connexins: The molecular basis of direct intercellular signaling. Eur J Biochem 238:1–27

Chang M, Werner R, Dahl G (1996) A role for an inhibitory connexin in testis? Dev Biol 175:50–56

Chen Z-Q, Lefebvre D, Bai X-H, Reaume A, Rossant J, Lye SJ (1995) Identification of two regulatory elements within the promoter region of the mouse connexin 43 gene. J Biol Chem 270:3863–3868

Civitelli R, Konstantinos Z, Warlow PM, Lecanda F, Nelson T, Harley J, Atal N, Beyer EC, Steinberg TH (1998) Regulation of connexin43 expression and function by prostaglandin E2 (PGEs) and parathyroid hormone (PTH) in osteoblastic cells. J of Cellular Biochem 68:8–21

Dahl G, Werner R, Levine E, Rabadan-Diehl C (1992) Mutational analysis of gap junction formation. Biophys J 62:172–182

Darrow BJ, Laing JG, Lampe PD, Saffitz JE, Beyer EC (1995) Expression of multiple connexins in cultured neonatal rat ventricular myocytes. Circ Res 76:381–387

Davies TC, Barr KJ, Jones DH, Zhu DG, Kidder GM (1996) Multiple members of the connexin gene family participate in preimplantation development of the mouse. Dev Genet 18:234–243

De Sousa PA, Juneja SC, Caveney S, Houghton DF, Davies TC, Reaume AG, Rossant J, Kidder GM (1997) Normal development of preimplantation mouse embryos deficient in gap junctional coupling. J Cell Sci 110:1751–1758

Deschênes SM, Walcott JL, Wexler TL, Scherer SS, Fischbeck KH (1997) Altered trafficking of mutant connexin32. J Neurosci 17(23):9077–9084

Elfgang C, Eckert R, Lichtenberg-Fraté H, Butterweck A, Traub O, Klein RA, Hülser DF, Willecke K (1995) Specific permeability and selective formation of gap junction channels in connexin-transfected HeLa cells. J Cell Biol 129:805–817

Eppig JJ (1991) Intercommunication between mammalian oocytes and companion somatic cells. Bioessays 13:569–574

Eusebi F, Ziparo E, Fratamico G, Russo MA, Stefanini M (1983) Intercellular communication in rat seminiferous tubules. Dev Biol 100:249–255

Fraser SE, Green CR, Bode HR, Gilula NB (1987) Selective disruption of gap junctional communication interferes with a patterning process in hydra. Science 237:49–55

Falk MM, Buehler LK, Kumar NM, Gilula NB (1997) Cell-free synthesis and assembly of connexins into functional gap junction membrane channels. EMBO J 16:2703–2716

Garfield RE, Cole WC, Blennerhassett MG (1989) Gap junctions in uterine smooth muscle. In: Sperelakis N, Cole WC (eds) Cell Interactions and gap junctions. CRC, Baca Raton, pp 239–266

Gilula NB, Reeves OR, Steinbach A (1972) Metabolic coupling, ionic coupling and cell contacts. Nature (Lond) 235:262–265

Gilula NB, Fawcett DW, Aoki A (1976) The Sertoli cell occluding junctions and gap junctions in mature and developing mammalian testis. Dev Biol 50:142–168

Gilula NB, Epstein ML, Beers WH (1978) Cell communication and ovulation. J Cell Biol 78:58–75

Gong X, Li E, Klier FG, Huang Q, Wu Y, Lei H, Kumar NM, Horwitz J, and Gilula NB (1997) Disruption of α_3 connexin gene leads to proteolysis and cataractogenesis in mice. Cell 91:833–843

Goodenough DA (1992) The crystalline lens. A system networked by gap junctional intercellular communication. Semin Cell Biol 3:49–58

Grassi F, Monaco L, Fratamico G (1986) Putative second messengers affect cell coupling in the seminiferous tubules. Cell Biol Int Rep 10:631–640

Grazul-Bilska AT, Reynolds LP, Redmer DA (1997) Gap junctions in the ovaries. Biol Reprod 57:947–957

Guan X, Cravatt BF Ehring GR Hall JE Boger DL Lerner RA Gilula NB (1997) The sleep–inducing lipid oleamide deconvolutes gap junction communication and calcium wave transmission in glial cells. J Cell Biol 134:784–793

Haubrich S, Schwarz HJ, Bukauskas F, Lichtenberg-Frate H, Traub O, Weingart R, Willecke K (1996) Incompatibility of connexin 40 and 43 hemichannels in gap junctions between mammalian cells is determined by intracellular domains. Mol Biol Cell 7:1995–2006

Hervé JC, Pluciennik F, Bastide B, Cronier L, Verrecchia F, Malassiné A, Joffre M, Délèze J (1996a) Contraceptive gossypol blocks cell-to-cell communication in human and rat cells. Eur J Pharmacol 313:243–255

Hervé JC, Pluciennik F, Verrecchia F, Bastide B, Delage B, Joffre M, Délèze J (199b) Influence of the molecular structure of steroids on their ability to interrupt gap junctional communication. J Membr Biol 149:17987

Jiang JX, Goodenough DA (1996) Heteromeric connexons in lens gap junction channels. Proc Natl Acad Sci USA 93:1287–1291

Kawa K (1987) Existence of calcium channels and intercellular coupling in the testosterone-secreting cells of the mouse. J Physiol (Lond) 393:647–666

Kelsell DP, Dunlop J, Stevens HP, Lench NJ, Liang JN, Parry G, Mueller RF, Leigh IM (1997) Connexin 26 mutations in hereditary non-syndromic sensorineural deafness. Nature 387:80–83

Kikuchi T, Kimura RS, Paul DL, Adams JC (1995) Gap junctions in the rat cochlea: immunohistochemical and ultrastructural analysis. Anat Embryol (Berl) 191:101–118

Kumar NM, Gilula NB (1986) Cloning and characterization of human and rat liver cDNAs coding for a gap junction protein. J Cell Biol 103:767–776

Kumar NM, Gilula NB (1992) Molecular biology and genetics of gap junction channels. Seminars Cell Biol 3:3–16

Kumar NM, Gilula NB (1996) The gap junction communication channel. Cell 84:381–388

Kumar NM, Friend DS, Gilula NB (1995) Synthesis and assembly of human β_1 gap junctions in BHK cells by DNA transfection with the human β_1 cDNA. J Cell Sci 108:3725–3734

Kuszak JR, Alcala J, Maisel H (1980) The surface morphology of embryonic and adult chicken lens fibre cells. Exp Eye Res 33:157–166

Kwak BR, Hermans MMP, De Jonge HR, Lohmann SM, Jongsma HJ, Chanson M (1995) Differential regulation of distinct types of gap junction channels by similar phosphorylating conditions. Mol Biol Cell 6:1707–1719

Laing JG, Beyer EC (1995) The gap junction protein connexin43 is degraded via the ubiquitin proteasome pathway. J Biol Chem 270:26399–26403

Lau AF, Kurata WE, Kanemitsu MY, Loo LWM, Warn-Cramer BJ, Eckhart W, Lampe PD (1996) Regulation of connexin43 function by activated tyrosine protein kinases. J Bioenerg Biomembr 28:359–368

Lawrence TS, Beers WH, Gilula NB (1978) Transmission of hormonal stimulation by cell-to-cell communication. Nature 272:501–506

Lee S, Gilula NB, Warner AE (1987) Gap junctional communication and compaction during preimplantation stages of mouse development. Cell 51:851–860

Lefebvre DL, Piersanti M, Bai XH, Chen ZQ, Lye SJ (1995) Myometrial transcriptional regulation of the gap junction gene, Connexin-43. Reprod Fertil Dev 7:603–611

Lerner RA (1997) A hypothesis about the endogenous analogue of general anesthesia. Proc Natl Acad Sci USA 94:13375–13377

Li R, Mather JP (1997) Lindane, an inhibitor of gap junction formation, abolishes oocyte directed follicle organizing activity in vitro. Endocrinol 138:4477–4480

Loewenstein WR (1981) Junctional intercellular communication: the cell-to-cell membrane channel. Physiol Rev 61:829–913

Mathias RT, Rae JL, Baldo GJ (1997) Physiological properties of the normal lens. Physiol Rev 77:21–49

McGinley DM, Posalaky Z, Porvaznik M, Russell L (1979) Gap junctions between Sertoli and germ cells of rat seminiferous tubules. Tissue Cell 11:741–754

McLean BG, Hempel FD, Zambryski PC (1997) Plant intercellular communication via plasmodesmata. Plant Cell 9:1043–1054

Meda P, Pepper MS, Traub O, Willecke K, Gros D, Beyer E, Nicholson B, Paul D, Orci L (1993) Differential expression of gap junction connexins in endocrine and exocrine glands. Endocrinol 133:2371–2378

Mehta PP, Yamamoto M, Rose B (1992) Transcription of the gene for the gap junctional protein connexin43 and expression of functional cell-to-cell channels are regulated by cAMP. Mol Biol Cell 3(8):839–850

Meyer RA, Laird DW, Revel J-P, Johnson RG (1992) Inhibition of gap junction and adherens junction assembly by connexin and A-CAM antibodies. J Cell Biol 119(1):179–189

Milks LC, Kumar NM, Houghten N, Unwin N, Gilula NB (1988) Topology of the 32-kD liver gap junction protein determined by site-directed antibody localizations. EMBO J 2967–2975

Moreno AP, Sáez JC, Fishman GI, Spray DC (1994) Human connexin43 gap junction channels: Regulation of unitary conductances by phosphorylation. Circ Res 74:1050–1057

Munari-Silem Y, Rousset B (1996) Gap junction-mediated cell-to-cell communication in endocrine glands – molecular and functional aspects: a review. Eur J Endocrinol 135:251–264

Nelles E, Bützler C, Jung D, Temme A, Gabriel HD, Dahl U, Traub O, Stümpel F, Jungermann K, Zielasek J, Toyka KV, Dermietzel R, Willecke K (1996) Defective propagation of signals generated by sympathetic nerve stimulation in the liver of connexin32-deficient mice. Proc Natl Acad Sci USA 93:9565–9570

Nishi M, Kumar NM, Gilula NB (1991) Developmental regulation of gap junction gene expression during mouse embryonic development. Dev Biol 146(1):117–130

Oh S, Ri Y, Bennett MV, Trexler EB, Verselis VK, Bargiello TA (1997) Changes in permeability caused by connexin 32 mutations underlie X-linked Charcot-Marie-Tooth disease. Neuron 19:927–938

Paul D (1986) Molecular cloning of cDNA for rat liver gap junction protein. J Cell Biol 103:123–134

Paul DL (1995) New functions for gap junctions. Curr Opin Cell Biol 7:665–672

Paul DL, Ebihara L, Takemoto LJ, Swenson KI, Goodenough DA (1991) Connexin46, a novel lens gap junction protein, induces voltage-gated currents in nonjunctional plasma membrane of Xenopus oocytes. J Cell Biol 115(4):1077–1089

Pelletier R-M, Byers SW (1992) The blood-testis barrier and Sertoli cell junctions: structural considerations. J Microsc Res Tech 20:3–33

Perez-Armendariz EM, Romano MC, Luna J, Miranda C, Bennett MVL, Moreno AP (1994) Characterization of gap junctions between pairs of Leydig cells from mouse testis. Am J Phy 267:C570–C580

Petrocelli T, Lye SJ (1993) Regulation of transcripts encoding the myometrial gap junction protein, connexin-43, by estrogen and progesterone. Endocrinol 133:284–290

Pluciennik F, Verrecchia F, Bastide B, Hervé JC, Joffre M, Délèze J (1996) Reversible interruption of gap junctional communication by testosterone propionate in cultured Sertoli cells and cardiac myocytes. J Membr Biol 149:169–177

Pozzi A, Risek B, Kiang DT, Gilula NB, Kumar NM (1995) Analysis of multiple gap junction gene products in the rodent and human mammary gland. Exp Cell Res 220:212–219

Reaume AG, De Sousa PA, Kulkarni S, Langille BL, Zhu D, Davies TC, Juenja SC, Kidder GM, Rossant J (1995) Cardiac malformation in neonatal mice lacking connexin43. Science 267:1831–1834

Risek B, Guthrie S, Kumar N, Gilula NB (1990) Modulation of gap junction transcript and protein expression during pregnancy in the rat. J Cell Biol 110:269–282

Risek B, Klier FG, Phillips A, Hahn DW, Gilula NB (1995) Gap junction regulation in the uterus and ovaries of immature rats by estrogen and progesterone. J Cell Sci 108:1017–1032

Risley MS, Tan IP, Roy C, Saez JC (1992) Cell-, age- and stage-dependent distribution of connexin43 gap junctions in testes. J Cell Sci 103(1):81–96

Russell LD, Malone JP (1980) A study of Sertoli-spermatid tubulobulbar complexes in selected mammals. Tissue Cell 12(2):263–285

Saez JC, Gregory WA, Watanabe T, Dermietzel R, Hertzberg EL, Reid L, Bennett MVL, Spray DC (1989) cAMP delays disappearance of gap junctions between pairs of rat hepatocytes in primary culture. Am J Physiol 257:C1–C11

Simon AM, Goodenough DA, Li E, Paul DL (1997) Female infertility in mice lacking connexin 37. Nature 385:525–529

Splitt MP, Tsai MY, Burn J, Goodship JA (1997) Absence of mutations in the regulatory domain of the gap junction protein connexin 43 in patients with visceroatrial heterotaxy. Heart 77:369–370

Spray DC (1994) Physiological and pharmacological regulation of gap junction channels. In: Citi S (ed) Molecular mechanisms of epithelial cell junctions: from development to disease. Landes, Austin, pp 195–215

Stagg RB, Fletcher WH (1990) The hormone-induced regulation of contact-dependent cell-cell communication by phosphorylation. Endocr Rev 11:302–325

Stauffer KA (1995) The gap junction proteins β1-connexin (connexin-32) and β2 connexin (connexin-26) can form heteromeric hemichannels. J Biol Chem 270:6768–6772

Steinberg TH, Civitelli R, Geist ST, Robertson AJ, Hick E, Veenstra RD, Wang H-Z, Warlow PM, Westphale EM, Laing JG, Beyer EC (1994) Connexin43 and connexin45 form gap junctions with different molecular permeabilities in osteoblastic cells. EMBO J 13:744–750

Tan IP, Roy C, Sáez JC, Sáez CG, Paul DL, Risley MS (1996) Regulated assembly of connexin33 and connexin43 into rat Sertoli cell gap junctions. Biol Reprod 54:1300–1310

Tibbitts TT, Caspar DLD, Phillips WC, Goodenough DA (1990) Diffraction diagnosis of protein folding in gap junction connexons. Biophys J 57:1025–1036

Unger VM, Kumar NM, Gilula NB, Yeager M (1997) Projection structure of a gap junction membrane channel at 7 Å resolution. Nat Struct Biol 4:39–43

Varanda WA, Campos de Carvalho AC (1994) Intercellular communication between mouse Leydig cells. Am J Physiol Cell Physiol 267:C563–C569

Veenstra RD, Wang HZ, Beblo DA, Chilton MG, Harris AL, Beyer EC, Brink PR (1995) Selectivity of connexin-specific gap junctions does not correlate with channel conductance. Circ Res 77:1156–1165

Wang HZ, Veenstra RD (1997) Monovalent ion selectivity sequences of the rat connexin43 gap junction channel. J Gen Physiol 109:491–507

Warner AE, Guthrie SC, Gilula NB (1984) Antibodies to gap junctional protein selectively disrupt junctional communication in the early amphibian embryo. Nature 311:127–131

Wang YJ, Rose B (1995) Clustering of Cx43 cell-to-cell channels into gap junction plaques: Regulation by cAMP and microfilaments. J Cell Sci 108:3501–3508

White TW, Bruzzone R, Goodenough DA, Paul DL (1992) Mouse Cx50, a functional member of the connexin family of gap junction proteins, is the lens fiber protein MP70. Mol Biol Cell 3:711–720

White TW, Bruzzone R, Wolfram S, Paul DL, Goodenough DA (1994) Selective interactions among the multiple connexin proteins expressed in the vertebrate lens: the second extracellular domain is a determinant of compatibility between connexins. J Cell Biol 125:879–892

White TW, Paul DL, Goodenough DA, Bruzzone R (1995) Functional analysis of selective interactions among rodent connexins. Mol Biol Cell 6:459–470

Yamanaka I, Kuraoka A, Inai T, Ishibashi T, Shibata Y (1997) Changes in the phosphorylation states of connexin43 in myoepithelial cells of lactating rat mammary glands. Eur J Cell Biol 72:166–173

Yeager M, Gilula NB (1992) Membrane topology and quaternary structure of cardiac gap junction ion channels. J Mol Biol 223:929–948

Yu W, Dahl G, Werner R (1994) The connexin43 gene is responsive to oestro-
    gen. Proc R Soc Lond (Biol) 255:125–132
Zelante L, Gasparini P, Estivill X, Melchionda S, D'Agruma L, Govea N, Milá
    M, Della M, Lutfi J, Shohat M, Mansfield E, Delgrosso K, Rappaport E,
    Surrey S, Fortina P (1997) Connexin26 mutations associated with the most
    common form of non-syndromic neurosensory autosomal recessive deaf-
    ness (DFNB1) in Mediterraneans. Hum Mol Genet 6:1605–1609
Zhang J-T, Nicholson BJ (1989) Sequence and tissue distribution of a second
    protein of hepatic gap junctions, Cx26, as deduced from its cDNA. J Cell
    Biol 109:3391–3401

2 Experimental In Vitro Approaches to the Study of Mouse Primordial Germ Cell Development

M. De Felici, A. Di Carlo, S. Dolci, and M. Pesce

2.1 Introduction

Primordial germ cells (PGCs) are the founder cells of germ line. In all mammalian species studied, including humans, they originate extragonadally during early embryogenesis before moving toward and colonizing the gonadal ridges. Upon entering the gonads, PGCs differentiate into meiotic oocytes in the fetal ovary and prospermatogonia in the fetal testis.

Since there are several recent reviews about the biology of mouse PGCs (see, for instance, De Felici et 1992; Wylie and Heasman 1993; McLaren 1994; Donovan 1994; De Felici and Pesce 1994; Buehr 1997), this chapter focuses especially on the information about the mechanisms of PGC migration and the control of their proliferation and meiotic division that have been obtained in our laboratory using a variety of in vitro experimental approaches.

PGCs developing in their normal environment are largely inaccessible to experimental investigation. We therefore have devised various methods for PGC isolation and in vitro culture systems to approach the study of the cellular and molecular mechanisms underlying their development. Detailed technical information about these methods is presented by De Felici (1997).

Progress in such methods has been quite slow and difficult owing to inherent problems of the cellular system. For example, in the early mouse embryo germ cells are present only in small numbers, change position quickly, never exist as an independent tissue, and are always associated with somatic cells.

Although the methods currently available for purification and in vitro culture of PGCs are imperfect and need to be improved, much of the current information on the biology of mammalian PGCs has been derived over the past decade from the use of such techniques.

2.2 Isolation and Purification of Migratory and Postmigratory PGCs

To enable PGCs to be studied in vitro, the regions in which they are present (allantois and posterior primitive streak, dorsal mesentery and urogenital ridges, urogenital ridges from 8.5-, 10.5-, and 11.5- to 12.5-dpc embryos, respectively) must be dissected from the embryo and a cell suspension made from them before transfer to the appropriate culture conditions. At all stages of their development PGCs can be identified in three ways: by their morphological characteristics, by expression of the enzyme alkaline phosphatase (AP), and with antibodies that recognize antigens specific to PGCs (i.e. SSEA-1, Forssman antigen). Using a monoclonal antibody called TG-1 directed against a surface antigen of PGCs (Wylie et al. 1986), we have recently devised methods for rapid and efficient purification of PGCs from 10.5-dpc embryos onward (De Felici and Pesce 1995; Pesce and De Felici 1995). A schematic representation of the MiniMACS magnetic separation system is shown in Fig. 1. Figure 2 compares various PGC purification methods devised over the years in our laboratory.

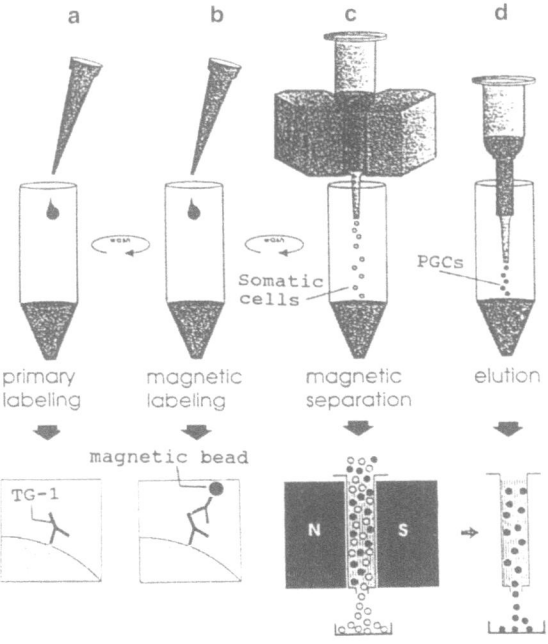

Fig. 1a–d. Schematic representation of the magnetic cell sorting of mouse PGCs using MiniMACS. The method consists of four main steps: (a) cells are labeled with the primary monoclonal antibody TG-1, (b) magnetic labeling is performed with anti-immunoglobulin coated microbeads, (c) cells are passed over a separation column placed in a magnetic field, and (d) the column is removed from the magnetic field, and the retained cells (PGCs) are eluted. (For details, see Pesce and De Felici 1995)

The ability to isolate PGCs and gonadal somatic cells in reasonable numbers and purity provides the opportunity to pursue molecular and biochemical analyses of such cells. For instance, we have used reverse-transcriptase polymerase chain reaction (RT-PCR) and immunoblotting to study the expression of genes by PGCs of various ages following their purification by the MiniMACS method (Pesce et al. 1996a, 1997). Moreover, cDNA libraries from PGCs and gonadal somatic cells of different ages and sex are currently in preparation.

M. De Felici

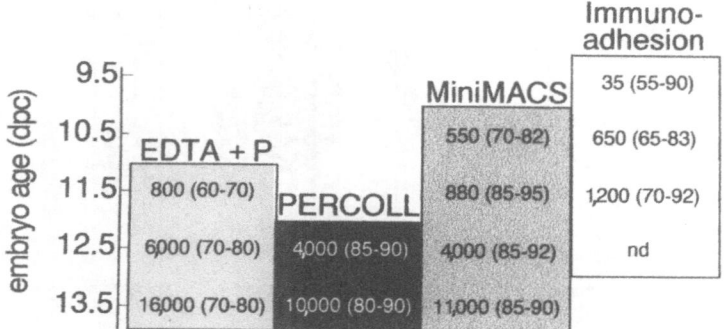

Fig. 2. Four methods devised in our laboratory for PGC purification, compared for yield and purity (*in parentheses*, percentage of PGC), and the embryonic stages in which can be used. *P*, Percoll. (For details, see De Felici and McLaren 1982; De Felici and Pesce 1995; Pesce and De Felici 1995)

Unfortunately, as shown in the next section, isolated PGCs have a limited ability to survive in the absence of suitable somatic cell support. However, they survive and proliferate on certain cell feeder layers and have been successfully used in many in vitro studies analyzing growth factor regulation of PGC development.

2.3 Culture of Isolated PGCs Without Somatic Cell Feeder Layers

PGCs can be cultured in a variety of conditions, including organ culture, feeder cell independent, and feeder cell dependent culture. Each technique has its uses and problems. A system for the culture of isolated PGCs is useful, for example, in revealing the extent to which processes such as migration, proliferation, and differentiation are autonomous properties of germ cells themselves, rather than being dependent on interactions with somatic cells. Unfortunately, our early studies have established that isolated PGCs in migratory and early gonadal phases cultured on glass, plastic, agar, or gelatin-coated substrates survive for only a few hours (De Felici and McLaren 1983). The addition of extracellular matrix components such as fibronectin (FN), laminin (LM),

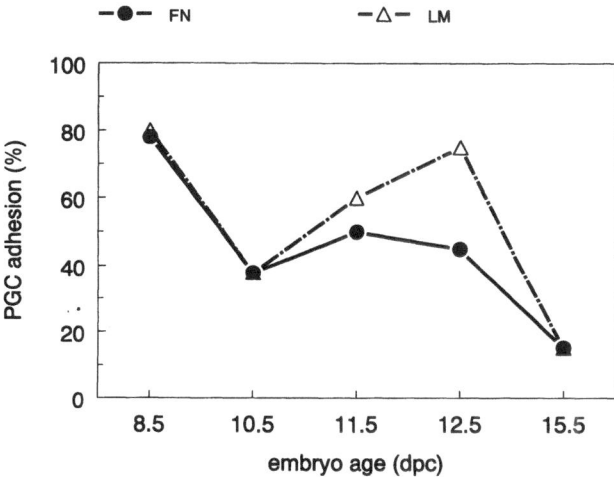

Fig. 3. Adhesiveness of PGCs of different ages to FN and LM substrata in vitro. (Values for 8.5-dpc PGCs from ffrench-Constant et al. 1991; for details see De Felici and Dolci 1989)

and type I collagen scarcely improves PGC survival (De Felici and Dolci 1989). These initial studies clearly indicated that the survival of PGCs is strictly dependent on factors produced by the surrounding somatic environment. Moreover, they yielded valuable information on certain aspects of their migration and survival. The simple approach to seed purified PGCs obtained from embryos of various ages on substrates of glycoproteins of the extracellular matrix provided the first indirect indications that PGCs possess integrin receptors and suggested a possible role of FN and LM in PGC migration. In this regard, we observed that PGCs adhere to FN and LM with different affinity, and that their adhesiveness changes over the migratory period with distinct profiles (Fig. 3; De Felici and Dolci 1989).

Subsequently the presence of some integrins such as $\alpha_3\beta_1$, $\alpha_5\beta_1$, and $\alpha_6\beta_1$ on the PGC surface was confirmed by immunohistochemical and immunoprecipitation experiments (Fig. 4), and the involvement of FN and LM in PGC migration was proved by other works (French-Constant et al. 1991; Garcia-Castro et al. 1997). Interaction with FN and/or LM is

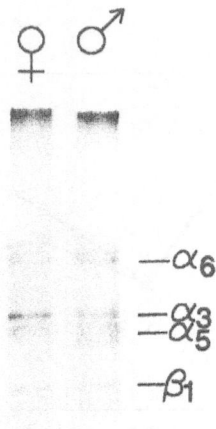

Fig. 4. Identification of integrin receptor in mouse PGCs: 12.5-dpc were isolated and labeled for 4–5 h in vitro with [^{35}S]methionine. Cells were then
lysed and the protein immunoprecipitated with a polyclonal antibody against
β_1; with β_1 also α_6, α_3, and α_5 integrins were coprecipitated

certainly only one of the factors involved in the complex process of PGC
migration. In fact, PGCs which attach to FN or LM substrates do not
show a motility behavior (Fig. 5A; De Felici and Dolci 1989). This is
shown when they are seeded onto some but not all cell monolayers. For
example, a significant number (about 20%) of PGCs show an elongated
morphology typical of motile cells after 5–6 h of culture on STO (an
embryo-derived fibroblast cell line) or TM4 (a mouse Sertoli cell-de-
rived cell line) cells (Fig. 5B–D), whereas they remain round and sta-
tionary when attached to F9 cell monolayers. This suggests that interaction with somatic cells may exert both positive and negative control on
PGC migration. Such control mechanisms are not known, but in princi-
ple they can be investigated in culture systems of PGCs seeded onto
somatic cell feeder layers. As seen in the next section, these systems
have proven useful in studying several aspects of PGC biology.

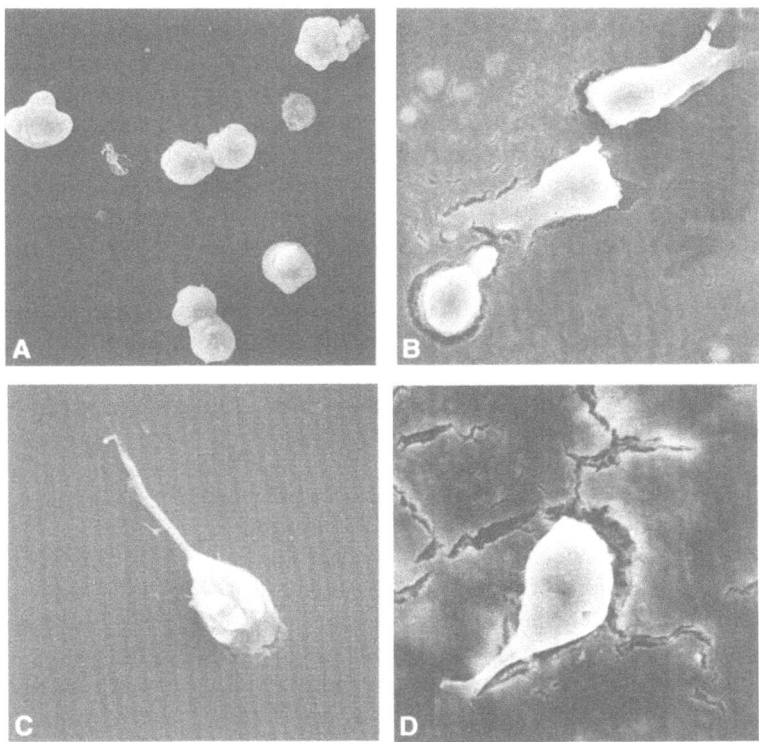

Fig. 5. Scanning electron micrographs of 11.5-dpc PGCs seeded on LM substratum (**A**) or TM4 cell feeder layers (**B–D**). Note the elongated morphologies typical of motile cells in PGCs cultured on TM4 cells

Lastly, the culture of isolated PGCs has also been helpful in elucidating the reason of the rapid loss of viability by isolated PGCs in culture and consequently in identifying one probably of the most important mechanisms that control PGC survival in the embryo. We discovered that purified PGCs undergo apoptosis after 4–5 h in culture, as demonstrated by several morphological and biochemical criteria (Pesce at al 1993; Pesce and De Felici 1994). Most importantly, we found that the addition of stem cell factor (SCF) or leukemia inhibitory factor (LIF) to the culture medium, two cytokines known to favor the survival and/or proliferation of PGCs on cell feeder layers (see below), markedly reduces apoptosis in PGCs during the first hours of culture (Pesce et al. 1993). Since it is known that SCF is produced by the somatic cells surrounding migratory and postmigratory PGCs, and that its receptor c-kit is expressed on the surface of PGCs (Matsui et al. 1990), our results suggest an elegant mechanism for controlling both PGC survival and migration. Thus PGCs that stray from their migratory pathway might be eliminated through apoptosis. Moreover, the antiapoptotic effect of SCF on PGCs can explain the germ cell deficiency that characterize the *Sl* and *W* mutations in the mouse. Several groups have recently shown that the product of the *W* gene is the transmembrane tyrosine kinase receptor c-kit, and that its ligand is SCF encoded by the *Sl* locus (for references, see De Felici and Pesce 1994).

2.4   Culture of PGCs on Somatic Cell Feeder Layers

Two experimental approaches allow PGCs to survive in culture for reasonable periods of time. PGCs cocultured on feeder layers of their own embryonic somatic cells or of established cell lines. PGCs can be easily identified and counted in such cultures by AP histochemistry (Fig. 6) or by reactivity with antibodies directed against cell surface antigens.

In the first method, the tissue-containing PGCs are dispersed with EDTA-trypsin and seeded in tissue culture wells. After 1 and 3 days of culture, despite somatic cells formed a nearly complete cell monolayer, the number of PGCs from all ages undergoes a large decrease (Dolci et al. 1993). Although these cultures do not allow long term culture of PGCs, the method is useful for a rapid screening of the effects of compounds on the survival and proliferation of PGCs and to compare the results obtained with those found employing preformed feeder layers of cell lines.

The use of preformed feeder layers of TM_4 or STO, allows culture of PGC-containing tissues or purified PGCs in conditions in which they survive and proliferate for up to 5–6 days. When isolated into culture, PGCs are initially identified as single cells growing on top of feeder layers. After a few days of culture small groups of PGCs form either by clonal division or by aggregation (Fig. 6). These groups enlarge over the

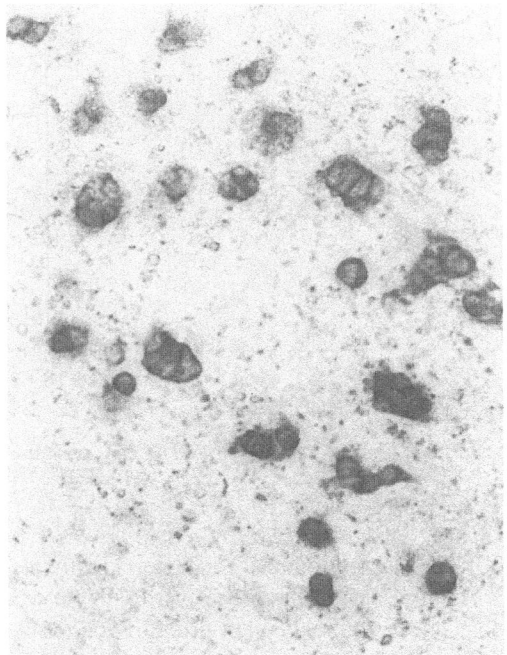

Fig. 6. Colonies of AP-positive PGCs on TM4 cell monolayers after 3 days of culture

next 3–4 days of culture, but they eventually disappear. Interestingly, we found that the proliferative behavior of PGCs cultured on TM4 or STO cell feeder layers resembles their growth pattern in vivo. For example, PGCs obtained from embryos at 8.5 dpc proliferate for 4 days before ending growth, while PGCs at 10.5 dpc proliferate for 2 days, and those at 11.5 dpc proliferate for 1 day only. There is no significant proliferation of PGCs obtained at 12.5 dpc (Fig. 7). These results suggest that in vitro as in vivo PGCs have a finite proliferative time and cease proliferating around 12.5 dpc. Comparing in vivo (Tam and Snow 1981) and in vitro (Fig. 7) PGC proliferation rates between 8.5 and 12.5 dpc shows, however, that the latter is still only a fraction of that in vivo.

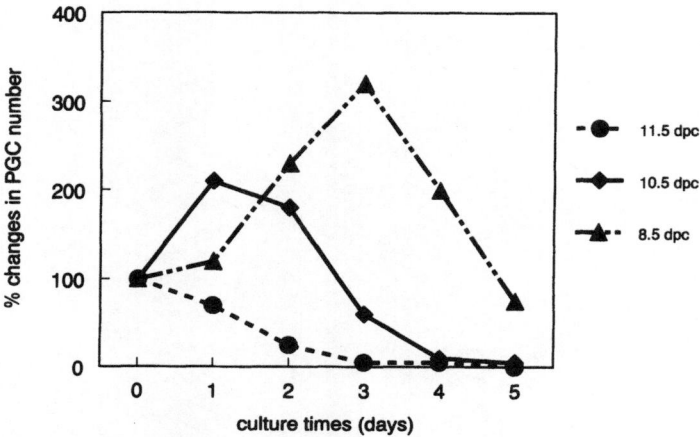

Fig. 7. Changes in the numbers of PGCs after 1–3 days of culture on TM$_4$ cell feeder layers

The use of feeder layer culture for PGCs gradually led to improvements in PGC culture and to the identification of growth factors that increase survival and/or stimulate their proliferation (Table 1). LIF was the first growth factor identified by us to increase significantly the PGC survival (De Felici and Dolci 1991). Other authors (Cheng et al. 1994; Koshimizu et al. 1996) have since shown then that the receptor complex for LIF (LIF-binding subunit, LIF receptor, and nonbinding signal transducer, gp130), is present on the PGC surface, thus strongly suggesting a direct action of LIF on PGCs in culture. It has still not been determined, however, whether LIF or other related cytokines (e.g., oncostatin M, ciliary neurotrophic factor) have a role in the normal development of PGCs. In this regard, it has been reported that mice deficient in LIF are fertile (Stewart et al. 1992), and that a targeted mutation of the LIF receptor does not result in a reduced number of PGCs (Ware et al. 1995).

A second growth factor which exert a very important action directly on PGCs is the already mentioned SCF. Using feeder layers culture for PGCs, we and other groups have confirmed that SCF is essential for PGC growth in vitro, and that the PGC life-supporting effect of feeder cells is partly attributable to the production of such growth factor (Dolci

Table 1. Growth factors and compounds reported to regulate positively or negatively the survival and/or proliferation of mouse PGCs in culture

Growth factor/compound	Effect	Reference
Survival factors		
Stem cell factor	+	Dolci et al. 1991;
		Pesce et al. 1993
Leukemia inhibitory factor	+	De Felici and Dolci 1991
Oncostatin M	+	Cheng et al. 1994
Ciliary neurotrophic factor	+	Cheng et al. 1994
GAS-1	+	Matsubara et al. 1996
Proliferation factors		
cAMP	+	Dolci et a. 1993;
		De Felici et al. 1993
Retinoic acid	+	Koshimizu et al. 1995,
		Pesce et al. 1996b
Tumor necrosis factor-α	+	Kawase et al. 1994
Stem cell factor	+	Matsui et al. 1991
Basic fibroblast growth factor	+	Resnick et al. 1992
Interleukin-3	+	Rich 1995
Interleukin-4	+	Cooke et al. 1996
Pituitary adenylate cyclase activating peptides	+	Pesce et al. 1996a
Transforming growth factor-β	–	Godin and Wylie 1991
GAS-1	+	Mastubara et al. 1996

et al. 1991 and 1993; Matsui et al. 1991; Godin et al. 1991). In particular, experiments performed in our laboratory have shown that: (a) a soluble form of recombinant mouse SCF added to PGCs grown on their own embryonic somatic cells significantly increases the number of PGCs without directly stimulating their proliferation (Dolci et al. 1993), and (b) the addition of anti-c-kit antibody (ACK-2) inhibits PGC survival on STO cell feeder layers (our unpublished observations). Moreover, our data about the temporary antiapoptotic effect of soluble SCF on isolated PGCs reported above and several other sources of experimental evidence widely discussed in Donovan (1994) indicate that the soluble form of SCF is less efficient than membrane-bound SCF at supporting PGC survival. The membrane forms of SCF is probably also involved in promoting PGC adhesion to somatic cells, as recently reported by Pesce et al. (1997).

Another important observation from PGC feeder layer culture is that dbcAMP or cAMP agonists such as forskolin and cholera toxin stimulate markedly PGC proliferation (De Felici et al. 1993). More recently we have found that, among many peptides known to increase intracellular cAMP via specific receptors, pituitary adenylate cyclase activating peptides (PACAPs) are able to stimulate PGC proliferation by activating adenylate cyclase. In addition, evidence about the presence of these peptides in the fetal gonads has also been found (Pesce et al. 1996a).

Finally, we have discovered that retinoic acid promotes proliferation of PGCs both on feeder layers of their own embryonic somatic cells and of TM4 or STO cells (Pesce et al. 1996b), a result reported simultaneously by Koshimizu et al. (1995). Whether PGCs come into contact with retinoic acid in vivo, and whether they have RA receptors are not known yet.

An important question about the feeder-dependent PGC culture systems is whether they allow the normal differentiation of PGCs in oocytes and prospermatogonia. As we have previously reported, PGCs in culture, identifiable as AP-positive cells or for some surface antigens, progressively disappear after 6–7 days of culture. This suggests that PGCs die after ending proliferation. However, these markers are also lost when PGCs differentiate in vivo. Therefore, given the impossibility to follow differentiating PGCs in culture and the absence of markers for fetal oocytes and prospermatogonia, no definitive conclusion can be reached about this.

Although we do not know about normal differentiation of PGCs in long-term culture, an intriguing transformation occurs in such cells when certain combinations of growth factors are employed. Two groups (Matsui et al. 1992; Resnick et al. 1992), reported that in the presence of a combination of LIF and basic fibroblast growth factor (bFGF) or the two of these with SCF some PGCs continue to proliferate beyond the time at which they would normally stop dividing. Eventually they form colonies of densely packed cells that continue to growth and proliferate. The resultant cell lines, which have been termed embryonic germ (EG) cells, closely resemble embryonic stem (ES) cells. EG cells can give rise to multiple differentiated cell phenotypes in culture and to teratocarcinomas when injected into nude mice and contribute to chimeras and populate the germ line (Matsui et al. 1992; Stewart et al. 1994). Recently it has been reported that EG cells can also be derived with a combination of LIF and either forskolin or retinoic acid (Koshimizu et al. 1995).

Taken together, the results of these in vitro studies suggest that the maintenance and proliferation of germ cell populations depends on a combination of several polypeptides, some of which probably have yet to be defined. Moreover, PGCs in culture seem responsive to a variety of compounds whose physiological relevance in vivo remain to be confirmed. In vitro, under the influence of a mixture of some growth factors and compounds, PGCs can certainly be reprogrammed in undifferentiated, pluripotent, and potentially tumorigenic cells. It will be important to verify whether such event can occur in vivo under normal or pathological conditions and its relevance for teratocarcinogenesis.

2.5 Reaggregation of Gonadal Tissues and Formation of Chimeric Gonad in Culture

What determines the phenotypic sex of germ cells, i.e., whether they undergo oogenesis or spermatogenesis?

Until the time that mouse germ cells enter the gonadal ridges their appearance and behavior seems identical regardless of whether they are in a female or a male embryo. However, around 13.5 dpc in the female, germ cells enter the prophase of meiosis; in the male they undergo mitotic arrest and differentiate as prospermatogonia in the G_1 stage of the cell cycle. Since many studies show that PGCs can differentiate into oocytes or prospermatogonia in organ culture, we devised a method to make and culture chimeric gonads in vitro in order to study the effect of the somatic environment on this process (Dolci and De Felici 1990). In particular, three-dimensional reaggregates of gonad tissues of different ages and sex was made to investigate whether entering into meiosis in oocytes and the arrest in G_1 in prospermatogonia are under the control of positive and/or negative signals from the gonadal somatic cells, as suggested by some authors (i.e., Byskov and Saxen 1976). The results showed that 12.5-dpc germ cells from female embryos enter and progress through meiotic prophase in reaggregates made with somatic cells from ovaries but not those made from testis. Male germ cells of the same age were unable to enter into meiosis in either types of reaggregates. These results strongly support the existence of a meiosis-preventing substance in the fetal testis, but not of a meiosis inducing substance in the fetal ovary. Using an approach similar to ours, McLaren and Southee

(1997) recently reached the same conclusions. In addition, they showed that PGCs isolated from early stages (10.5 and 11.5 dpc) can enter meiosis in vitro irrespective of sex when reaggregated with somatic cell from ovaries, and even when reaggregated with somatic cells from lung.

2.6 Conclusions and Future Prospects

The availability of methods to isolate, purify, and culture mouse PGCs has yielded valuable information about mechanisms and factors controlling many aspects of their biology. However, it should be pointed out that the importance of some of these factors in the intact embryo must yet be confirmed. Because PGCs cannot be cultured successfully in the absence of feeder layers, is sometimes impossible to distinguish the direct effects of experimental treatments on them from the indirect effect on feeder cells. Other, undefined factors produced by the feeders or present in the serum added to the culture medium make the interpretation of some results difficult.

The derivation of EG cells from PGCs may represent a way to study some aspects of PGC development and offer the possibility of obtaining ES cells in other species. However, since it is likely that EG cells are PGCs that have dedifferentiated to become ES cells, they are of little use in studying processes proper of the PGC development, such as their migration or differentiation.

An important contribution to elucidating many aspects of the PGC biology would be the establishment of immortalized PGC lines. Somatic cell lines of gonadal origin may also be an important source of PGC growth factors. Further information about growth factors and other molecules involved in PGC development is also likely to come in the future from newly derived "knockout" and transgenic mice.

References

Buehr M (1997) The primordial germ cells of mammals: some current perspectives. Exp Cell Res 232:194–207

Byskov AG, Saxen L (1976) Induction of meiosis in fetal mouse testis in vitro. Dev Biol 52:193–200

Cheng L, Gearing DP, White LS, Compton DL, Schooley K, Donovan P (1994) Role of leukemia inhibitory factor and its receptor in mouse primordial germ cell growth. Development 120:3145–3153

Cooke JE, Heasman J, Wylie CC (1996) The role of interleukin-4 in the regulation of mouse primordial germ cell numbers. Dev Biol 174:14–21

De Felici M, Dolci S (1989) In vitro adhesion of mouse fetal germ cells to extracellular matrix components. Cell Differ Dev 26:87–96

De Felici M, Dolci S (1991) Leukemia inhibitory factor sustains the survival of mouse primordial germ cells cultured on TM$_4$ feeder layers. Dev Biol 147:281–284

De Felici M, McLaren A (1982) Isolation of mouse primordial germ cells. Exp Cell Res 142:476–482

De Felici M, McLaren A (1983) In vitro culture of mouse primordial germ cells. Exp Cell Res 144:417–427

De Felici M, Pesce M (1994) Growth factors in mouse primordial germ cell migration and proliferation. Progr Growth Factor Res 5:135–145

De Felici M, Pesce M (1995) Immunoaffinity purification of migratory mouse primordial germ cells. Exp Cell Res 216:277–279

De Felici M, Dolci S, Pesce M (1992) Cellular and molecular aspects of mouse primordial germ cell migration and proliferation in culture. Int J Dev Biol 36:205–213

De Felici M, Dolci S, Pesce M (1993) Proliferation of mouse primordial germ cells in vitro: a key role for cAMP. Dev Biol 157:227–280

De Felici M (1997) Isolation and culture of germ cells from mouse embryo. In: Celis JC (ed) Cell biology: a laboratory handbook. Academic, New York, pp 68–80

Dolci S, De Felici M (1990) A study of meiosis in chimeric mouse fetal gonads. Development 109:37–40

Dolci S, Williams DE, Ernst MK, Resnick JL, Braman CI, Fock LF, Lyman SD, Boswell SH, Donovan PJ (1991) Requirements for mast cell growth factor for primordial germ cell survival in culture. Nature 352:809–811

Dolci S, Pesce M, De Felici M (1993) Combined action of stem cell factor, leukemia inhibitory factor, and cAMP on in vitro proliferation of mouse primordial germ cells. Mol Repr Dev 35:134–139

Donovan PJ (1994) Growth factor regulation of mouse primordial germ cell development. In: Pedersen RA (ed) Current topics in developmental biology. Academic, New York, pp 189–225

ffrench-Constant C, Hollingsworth A, Heasman J, Wylie CC (1991) Response to fibronectin of mouse primordial germ cells before, during and after migration. Development 113:1365–1373

Garcia-Castro M, Anderson R, Heasman J, Wylie CC (1997) Interactions between germ cells and extracellular matrix glycoproteins during migration and gonad assembly in the mouse embryo. J Cell Biol 138:471–480

Godin I, Wylie CC (1991) TGFβ$_1$ inhibits proliferation and has a chemotropic effect on mouse primordial germ cells in culture. Development 113:1451–1457

Godin I, Deed R, Cooke J, Zsebo K, Dexter M, Wylie CC (1991) Effect of the *Steel* gene product on mouse primordial germ cells in culture. Nature 352:807–809

Kawase E, Yamamoto HKH, Nakatsui N (1994) Tumor necrosis factor α (TNF-α) stimulates proliferation of mouse primordial germ cells in culture. Dev Biol 162:91–95

Koshimizu U, Watanabe M, Nakatsuji N (1995) Retinoic acid is potent growth activator of mouse primordial germ cell in vitro. Dev Biol 168:683–685

Koshimizu U, Taga T, Watanabe M, Saito M, Shirayoshi Y, Kishimoto T, Nakatsuji N (1996) Functional requirement of gp130-mediated signaling for growth and survival of mouse germ cells in vitro and derivation of embryonic germ (EG) cells. Development 122:1235–1242

Mastubara N, Takahashi Y, Nishina Y, Mukouyama Y, Yanagisawa M, Watanabe T, Nakano T, Nomura K, Arita H, Nishimune Y, Obinata Y, Matsui Y (1996) A receptor proteinchinasy, Sky, and its ligand Gas 6 are expressed in gonads and support primordial germ cell growth or survival in culture. Dev Biol 180:499–510

Matsui Y, Zsebo K, Hogan BLM (1990) Embryonic expression of a haemotopoietic growth factor encoded by the Steel locus and the ligand of c-kit. Nature 347:666–669

Matsui Y, Toksoz D, Nishikawa S, Nishikawa S-I, Williams D, Zsebo K, Hogan BLM (1991) Effect of Steel factor and leukemia inhibitory factor on murine primordial germ cells in culture. Nature 353:750–752

Matsui Y, Zsebo K, Hogan BLM (1992) Derivation of pluripotential embryonic stem cells from murine primordial germ cells in culture. Cell 70:841–847

McLaren A (1994) Germline and soma: interactions during early mouse development. Semin Dev Biol 5:43–49

McLaren A, Southee D (1997) Entry of mouse embryonic germ cells into meiosis. Dev Biol 187:107–113

Pesce M, Farace MG, Piacentini M, Dolci S, De Felici M (1993) Stem cell factor and leukemia inhibitory factor promote primordial germ cell survival by suppressing programmed cell death (apoptosis). Development 118:1089–1094

Pesce M, De Felici M (1994) Apoptosis in mouse primordial germ cells: a study by transmission and scanning electron microscope. Anat Embryol 189:435–440

Pesce M, De Felici M (1995) Purification of mouse primordial germ cells by MiniMACS magnetic separation system. Dev Biol 170:722–72

Pesce, M, Canipari R, Ferri GL, Siracusa G, De Felici M (1996a) Pituitary adenylate cyclase activating-polypeptide (PACAP) stimulates adenylate cyclase and promotes proliferation of mouse primordial germ cells. Development 122:215–221

Pesce M, Di Carlo A, Cerrito MG, De Felici M (1996b) All-trans retinoic acid effects on mouse primordial germ cells in culture. Biol Repr 54:414

Pesce M, Di Carlo A, De Felici M (1997) The c-kit receptor is involved in the adhesion of mouse primordial germ cells to somatic cells in culture. Mech Dev (in press)

Rich IV (1995) Primordial germ cells are capable of producing cells of the hematopoietic system in vitro. Blood 86:463–472

Resnick JL, Bixler LS, Cheng L, Donovan PJ (1992) Long term proliferation of mouse primordial germ cells in culture. Nature 359:550–551

Stewart CL, Kaspar P, Brunet LJ, Bhatt H, Gadi I, Kontgen F, Abbondanzo SJ (1992) Blastocyst implantation depends on maternal expression of leukemia inhibitory factor. Nature 359:76–79

Stewart CL, Gadi I, Bhatt H (1994) Stem cell from primordial germ cells reenter the germ line. Dev Biol 161:626–628

Tam PPL, Snow MHL (1981) Proliferation and migration of primordial germ cells during compensatory growth in mouse embryo. J Embryol Exp Morphol 64:133–147

Ware C, Horowitz MC, Renshaw BR, Hunt JS, Liggitt D, Koblar SA, Gliniak BC, McKenna HJ, Papayannopoulos T, Thoma B, Cheng L, Donovan PJ, Peschon J, Bartlett PF, Willis CR, Wright BD, Carpenter MK, Davison BL, Gearing DP (1995) Targeted disruption of the low-affinity leukemia inhibitory factor receptor gene causes placental, skeletal, neural and metabolic defects and results in perinatal death. Development 121:1283–1299

Wylie CC, Heasman J (1993) Migration, proliferation and potency of primordial germ cells. Seminars in Dev Biol 4:161–170

Wylie CC, Stott D, Donovan PJ (1986) Primordial germ cell emigration. In: Browder L (ed) The cellular basis of morphogenesis. Plenum, New York, pp 433–450

3 Spermatogonial Transplantation

L.D. Russell, M. Nagano, and R.L. Brinster

3.1 Introduction

Germ cells are unique in that they are the only cell line able to transmit heritable characteristics. The germ cells and certain cells of the early developing embryo are pluripotent and thus are targeted as the only plausible sites to modify the genome to produce heritable transgenesis. Male and female germ cell lines are developmentally very different. The male continues to produce gametes after puberty while the female germ cells arrest in meiosis prior to birth and complete meiosis only at fertilization. Thus any approach to genetically manipulate germ cells must be quite different in the male and female.

Transgenesis may be defined as the introduction of foreign DNA into the germ cell population. Usually transgenic technology has allowed only one or a few genes to be introduced into the heritable, germ cell population. More recently Brinster and colleagues have substituted the entire heritable male genome from one animal into another through the technique of germ cell transplantation (Brinster and Avarbock 1994; Brinster and Zimmerman 1994; Clouthier et al. 1996). This technique shows great promise for future basic and applied research. This review describes briefly the technique of spermatogonial transplantation and emphasizes some of the directions for basic research important to the future of this technology.

3.2 Spermatogonial Transplantation Technique

The technique of spermatogonial transplantation is described in detail by Ogawa et al. (1997). To summarize, procedural details are separated into (a) preparation of donor cells, (b) preparation of the recipient testis, and (c) transplantation of cells.

3.2.1 Preparation of Donor Cells

Briefly, donor germ cells can be isolated in animals ranging in development from the late neonatal period through adulthood. Enzymatic dispersion of donor cells is accomplished by first removing the tunica albuginea and subsequently incubating the parenchyma in calcium-free Hanks' balanced salt solution containing collagenase. Tubules are freed of Leydig cells by mechanical dissection and the Leydig cell strands removed. Subsequently cells are dispersed after incubation with EDTA, DNase, and trypsin while gently pipetting and agitating the isolated tubules. Fetal bovine serum is added to terminate trypsin activity. Large tissue aggregates are removed by filtration through a nylon mesh screen. The filtrate is gently centrifuged and the supernatant discarded. Germ cells are resuspended in sperm media (Brinster and Avarbock 1994; Brinster and Zimmerman 1994) or Eagle's medium containing fetal bovine serum. The concentration is adjusted to about $100–200\times10^6$ cells and cooled to 5°C where the temperature is held constant until injection (1–4 h later). The range of injection volume required for a mouse recipient is 50–100 µl, of which about 10 µl enter the tubules.

The initial reports of spermatogonial transplantation utilized freshly harvested (Brinster and Avarbock 1994; Brinster and Zimmerman 1994; Clouthier et al. 1996) or frozen (Avarbock et al. 1996) donor cells. More recently mouse donor cells have been cultured for a period of almost 4 months prior to their introduction into a recipient animal (Nagano and Brinster 1998). The culture medium used was a modified Eagle's medium with and without pyruvate and lactate. In some experiments STO feeder layers similar to those employed for embryonic stem cell culture were used with the donor germ cells. Cultures were maintained for up to 132 days and cells transplanted thereafter.

3.2.2 Preparation of the Recipient Testis

Recipient mice that produce spermatogenesis from donor animals must first be largely deprived of endogenous spermatogenesis so that introduced stem cells do not compete with endogenous cells. Although there are a number of chemical and physical means to deplete spermatogenesis, most have not been tested and compared. Brinster and colleagues used the alkylating agent busulfan. In high concentration busulfan is known to kill all but the most resistant type A spermatogonial cells (Bucci and Meistrich 1987). At least 1 month is necessary to realize the full extent of germ cell depletion produced by busulfan. Testes of busulfan-treated mice are small due to massive germ cell death and depletion. The seminiferous tubules contain Sertoli cells and occasional spermatogonia. Depending on the dose, mice treated with busulfan may demonstrate reinitiation of spermatogenesis several months after busulfan treatment.

One way in which mouse-to-mouse transplants can be shown to be unequivocally successful is if a donor cell marker is used for histological identification of cells. Brinster's laboratory has utilized donor cells from a transgenic strain in which most of the germ cells express the LacZ gene. The histochemical demonstration of the gene product, β-galactosidase, is evidence of the presence of donor cells in a recipient testis. Using the substrate X-gal, the histochemical procedure stains any cells expressing LacZ a deep blue color.

In addition, animals possessing a genetically related block to spermatogenesis have been used as recipients. This animal model, used by Brinster and colleagues, takes advantage of the sterility produced by mutations at the W-locus. The sterility in W-locus mice is due to a mutation affecting the c-kit receptor on spematogonia. The few spermatogonia that are present do not develop to advanced spermatogonial types but undergo apoptosis early and are eliminated. Most seminiferous tubules of the W-locus mice appear to be Sertoli cell-only although some tubules possess a few spermatogonia.

If there are indications that histocompatibility may be a factor in transplantation success, "nude" (lacking B cells) or "SCID" (lacking B and T cells) mice treated with busulfan may be utilized as recipients. These mice are fragile, given their defective immune system, and must receive special care to ensure their survival.

3.2.3 Transplantation of Cells

The original reports of spermatogonial transplantation utilized a microinjection technique whereby cells were introduced directly into seminiferous tubules (Brinster and Avarbock 1994; Brinster and Zimmerman 1994; Clouthier et al. 1996). Subsequently other techniques have been shown effective. Filling of seminiferous tubules may also be obtained by microinjection of germ cells into the rete or the efferent ductules (Ogawa et al. 1997; Fig. 1). A knowledge of the anatomy of the male duct system in the testis is essential to understanding fluid flow in the testis. Whether injected into seminiferous tubules, the rete, or the efferent ducts, the flow of the injection fluid is retrograde to fill the majority of seminiferous tubules. Since liquid is virtually incompressible, there must be a temporary expansion of the duct system and seminiferous tubules to accommodate both the endogenous secreted fluid and the injected material. Injection volumes or injection pressures in excess of a certain critical limit cause rupture of the rete or seminiferous tubules, and the cell suspension leaks into the interstitial space. A small amount of leakage of germ cell suspensions is apparently not detrimental to filling of seminiferous tubules and establishment of donor spermatogenesis.

A micromanipulator with a movable platform to adjust the position of the animal is used to visualize and position a micropipette for microinjection. An abdominal incision is made and the testes exteriorized. Micropipettes, made with a pipette puller with a diameter of about 50 µm and angled tips, are used to inject cell suspensions. For seminiferous tubule injections the tunica albuginea is cut and the micropipette

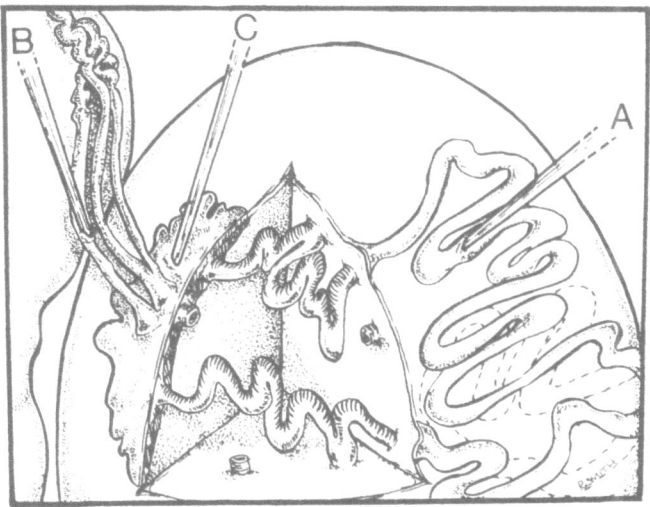

Fig. 1. Sites of introduction of donor cells into the testis of recipient mice. Germ cells may be introduced into seminiferous tubules by microinjection directly into the seminiferous tubule lumen (*A*), the efferent ductules (*B*), or the rete (*C*). (With permission of the publisher from Ogawa et al. 1997)

needle aligned in parallel with one of the protruding seminiferous tubules. To inject efferent ductules the investigator must carefully dissect them in the fat-filled space between the head of the epididymis and the testis. Rete testis injections first require that the vein draining the testis be located as it leaves the testis. The rete lies under this region, and the rete may be entered by puncturing the tunica albuginea just cephalad to the site where the vein enters the testis. After the micropipette is inserted into a seminiferous tubule, ductuli efferentes, or the rete, the fluid pressure is gradually increased with a pressure injector to start the flow of the cell suspension. Adding a small amount of trypan blue to the injection medium allows monitoring of the filling of tubules. Generally, 5–30 min is required to fill from 70%–100% of surface seminiferous tubules. After injection the testes are restored to their abdominal position and the abdominal wall sutured.

Active donor spermatogenesis in a recipient mouse testis has been observed over 18 months posttransplantation and is presumed to remain active during the life of the animal. A variety of techniques may be utilized to demonstrate the presence of donor spermatogenesis. Donor cells with the LacZ gene may be demonstrated histochemically by staining for enzymatic activity of the gene product β-galactosidase. This enzyme is present in donor germ cells from whole or sectioned tubules as well as sperm found within the lumen of the epididymis. Donor spermatogenesis in W-locus animals has been demonstrated by light and electron microscopy (Russell and Brinster 1996; Russell et al. 1996). Microscopy can also be used to determine species-related characteristics of germ cells in xenogenic transplants (Russell and Brinster 1996). Finally, donor spermatogenesis can be demonstrated in breeding studies when the LacZ gene is propagated to and identified in cells of the progeny (Brinster and Brinster 1994).

3.3 Significant Findings Utilizing the Transplantation Technique

Donor spermatogenesis can be initiated and maintained in mammals by microinjection of donor germ cell suspensions into recipient seminiferous tubules. Transplantation between histocompatible mice (Brinster and Avarbock 1994; Brinster and Zimmerman 1994) as well as nonhis-

---

Fig. 2A–D. Example of mouse testes before transplantation (**A, B**) and after ▶ transplantation (**C, D**) with donor cells from a histocompatible mouse. **A,B** the testis of a sterile adult mouse recipient. The mouse (Wᵛ/Wᵛ) used as a recipient is from the line carrying the W-locus mutation (Wᵛ/Wᵛ). **A** Numerous tubules are shown that prominently display vacuolations within the epithelium. **B** The tubules are shown at higher magnification to contain only Sertoli cells (*isolated arrow*) and occasional spermatogonia (*isolated arrowhead*). What have been termed "balls" (*b*) of Sertoli cells are frequently central within tubules (Russell and Brinster 1996; Russell et al. 1996). **C** Some tubules that are spermatogenically active and some that are inactive after approximately 3 months of transplantation. Tubules with spermatogenesis are considerably larger than those that lack spermatogenesis. **D** At higher magnification a small number of seminiferous tubules are shown with active spermatogenesis. All major classes of germ cells can be seen in tubules that appear slightly disorganized. In addition, several degenerating germ cells including elongated spermatids are noted (*isolated arrowheads*)

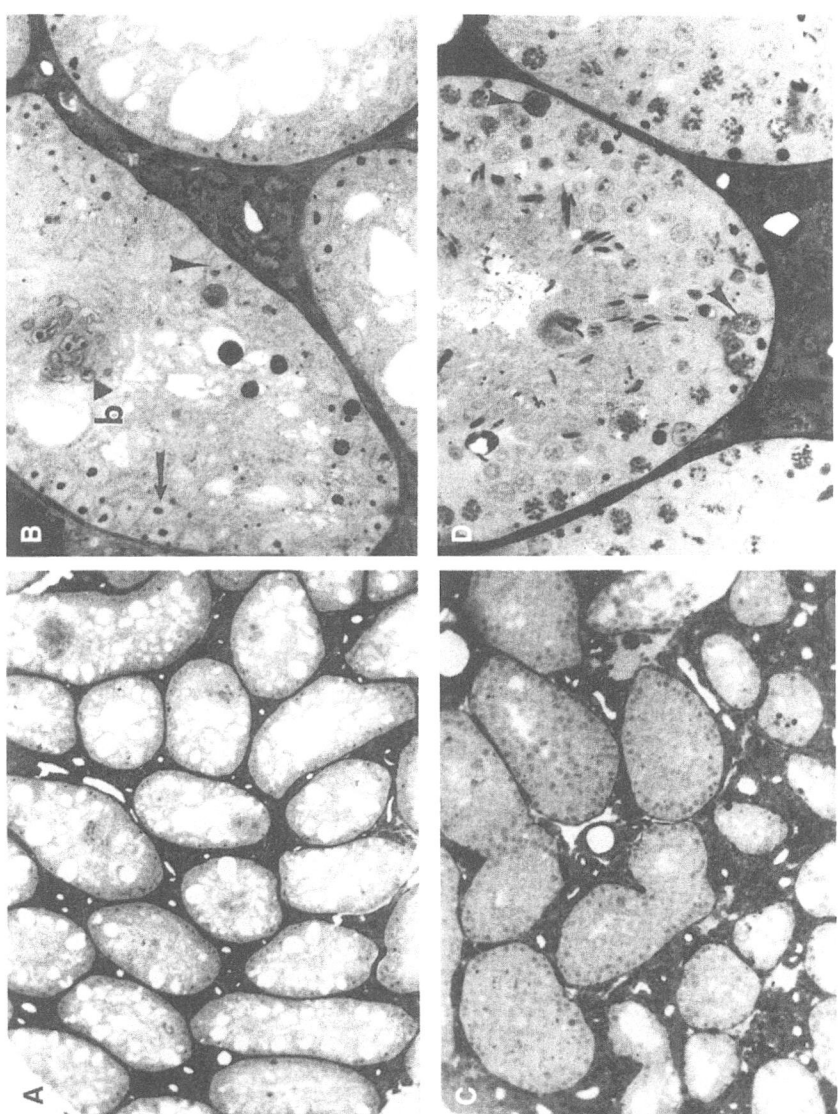

Fig. 2A–D

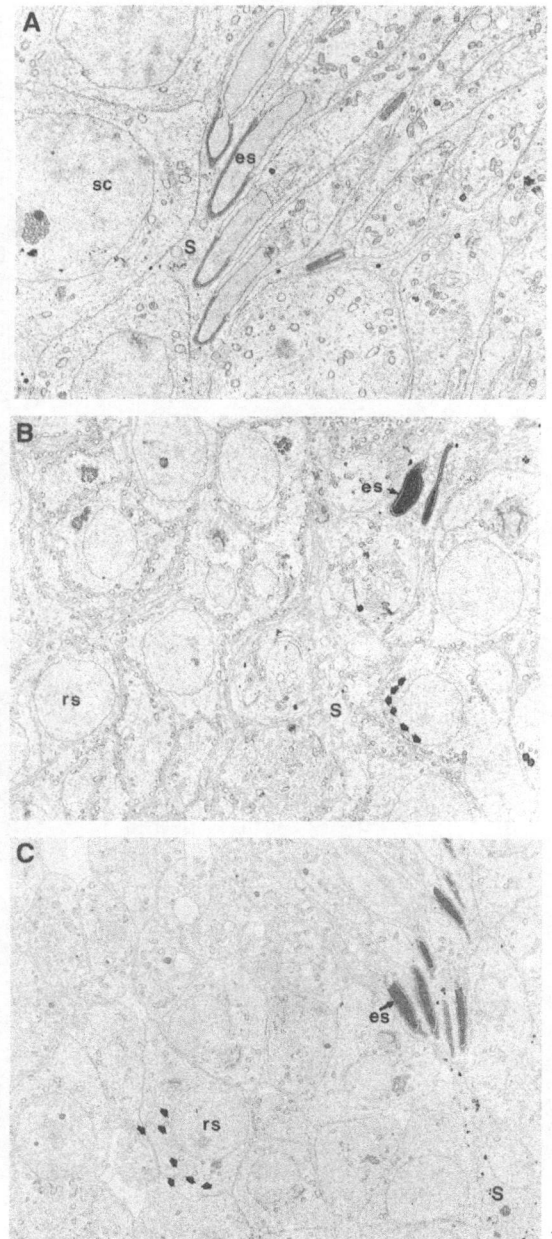

Fig. 3A–C

tocompatible species (xenogenic transplantation; Clouthier et al. 1996) from rat donors into immunodeficient mice has been successful in establishing spermatogenesis. This is the first demonstration of transplantation of isolated germ cells from one mammalian species to a recipient followed by complete and continuing spermatogenesis (Figs. 2, 3).

In mouse-to-mouse transplants, breeding studies show that up to 80% of progeny are from donor cells (Brinster and Brinster 1994), demonstrating heritable transmission of the donor germ cell line. In xenogenic transplants (rat to mouse) up to one in 50 sperm in the mouse epididymis is morphologically characteristic of the rat (Clouthier et al. 1996).

Subsequent to the reports of the initial transplantations success from Brinster's laboratory, Jiang and Short (1995) reported intraluminal spermatogenesis in busulfan-treated rats after intraluminal injection of isolated (90% pure) rat primordial germ cells. Since intraluminal spermatogenesis occurred only in busulfan-treated animals receiving germ cell injections and not in sham-injected rats, the authors concluded that the presence of intraluminal spermatogenesis was due solely to the transplanted tissue. Tissue markers to identify transplanted cells were not utilized.

Germ cells can be frozen for extended periods prior to transplantation. Donor germ cells that have been frozen for periods of up to 5

◄ **Fig. 3A–C.** Electron micrographs of the seminiferous epithelium of germ cell transplants. **A** The transplanted cells were from a mouse into a histocompatible W-locus sterile recipient. **B,C** The transplant was from a Sprague-Dawley rat into a immunodeficient "nude" mouse rendered sterile with busulfan. After approximately 3–4 months the testes were examined, with the result that active spermatogenesis was found in both groups. The germ cell types shown are spermatocytes (*sc*), round spermatids (*rs*), elongate spermatids (*es*), and all appear normal and present in recognized cell associations (stages). The Sertoli cell (*S*) processes are seen extending between germ cells in a relationship typical of that seen in normal animals. **B,C** Both rat and mouse spermatogenesis are present, respectively, in the same testis. The rat cells are from the transplant and the mouse cells are from recovery of endogenous spermatogenesis after busulfan treatment. Mouse spermatids and rat spermatids can be distinguished by the location of the mitochondria in round cells. In the mouse mitochondria are randomly scattered along within the cytoplasm (*short arrows* in **C**) whereas in the rat they become aligned along the plasma membrane (*short arrows* in **B**)

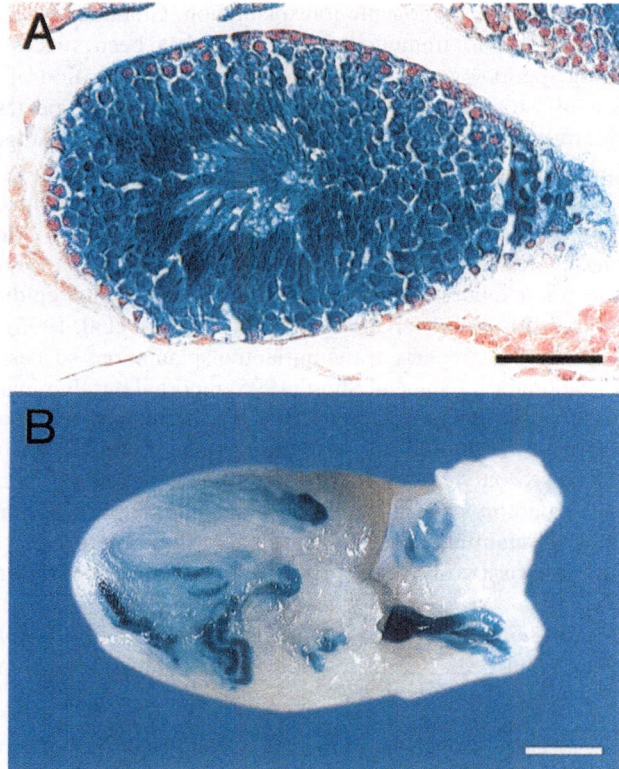

Fig. 4. A Seminiferous tubule showing donor spermatogenesis in a mouse recipient in which adult donor cells were cultured for 19 days prior to transplantation. *Deep blue color*, histochemical demonstration of β-galactosidase activity (using X-gal as substrate), the product of the LacZ gene which is expressed
only in germ cells from the donor. **B** Establishment of donor spermatogenesis
from 10-day-old neonate cells cultured 111 days prior to transplantation. Donor spermatogenesis is evidenced in this testis 108 days after transplantation
by the deep blue colored portions of tubules, indicating the presence of β-
galactosidase activity expressed by donor cells. (Figures used with permission
of Nagano and Brinster1998)

months are capable of establishing successful spermatogenesis after transplantation (Avarbock et al. 1996). Freezing of donor cells demonstrates our ability to stabilize a germ cell line indefinitely such that it can be utilized at a later time. Freezing can preserve the germ line of rare or endangered species as well as preserve the genome of males considered valuable for agricultural purposes.

Cultured donor cells produce spermatogenesis in a recipient male. Mouse cells cultured for periods up to about 4 months produce spermatogenesis in mouse recipients (Fig. 4). Our ability to culture stem cells represents an important step toward the goal of transfecting stem cells. Stable transfection of stem cell spermatogonia occurs when DNA is incorporated into the cell genome during cell division.

Spermatogenesis must be initiated from stem cell spermatogonia. Since spermatogenesis resulting from germ cell transplantation is a continuous process lasting many months postinjection (Russell and Brinster 1996; Russell et al. 1996; Brinster and Avarbock 1994; Brinster and Zimmerman 1994), the process must be generated anew by stem cells. Stem cells are the only cell type capable of continually producing spermatogenesis and, at the same time, capable of self-renewal. Given that spermatogenesis was active for at least 18 months in recipient testis, it is assumed to be a continuous process and to result from the cell division in stem cell line. If spermatogenesis were initiated by non-stem cell elements, the germ cell population would be depleted from the seminiferous epithelium after about 1 month due to failure of self-renewal of germ cell elements.

Stem cells relocate from the tubule lumen to the basal compartment of the seminiferous tubule after injection. The normal position for spermatogonia is at the periphery of the seminiferous tubule, lying along the basal lamina (Russell and Brinster 1996; Russell et al. 1996). Although spermatogonia are injected with a variety of other cell types, they relocate to their normal position along the basal lamina. Relocation involves selective movement of stem cell spermatogonia between adjoining Sertoli cells through Sertoli-Sertoli junctions. Specific recognition factors must be operative in the recipient Sertoli cells to recognize stem cell spermatogonia injected into the lumen of seminiferous tubules and to transport them radially through the Sertoli cell barrier to reside on the basal lamina of the seminiferous tubule. These recognition factors must be operative in mouse Sertoli cells such that they can identify and reposition stem cells of both mouse and rat.

Although donor Sertoli cells are injected with germ cells, spermatogenesis takes place in an environment in which recipient Sertoli cells are in association with donor germ cells. Both LacZ markers and electron microscopy confirm that donor Sertoli cells rarely take up residence in the testis of the recipient animal (Brinster and Avarbock 1994; Brinster and Zimmerman 1994; Russell et al. 1996). Electron microscopy has never revealed rat Sertoli cells among rat germ cells within a mouse seminiferous tubule. This observation becomes especially significant in xenogenic transplants where rat spermatogenesis is occurring within the mouse testis. The mouse Sertoli cell is thus capable of supporting rat spermatogenesis, indicating that although 10–11 million years of evolution have transpired since rat and mouse diverged on the evolutionary scale, there is considerable capability in the Sertoli cells of one species to support germ cells of another species.

Spermatogenesis with morphological characteristics of two species can take place simultaneously within the testis of a mouse. Both rat and mouse spermatogenesis occur simultaneously in the mouse testis after rat cells are transplanted into the busulfan-treated mouse testes. Establishment of rat spermatogenesis occurs simultaneously with the recovery of endogenous mouse spermatogenesis; however, there appears to be no admixture of rat and mouse cells in the same cross-sectioned tubule.

The *testis can support spermatogenesis of differing cycle lengths.* Although the rat and mouse are closely related species, their spermatogenic cycle lengths differ by approximately 50%. The cycle length difference is not prohibitory to the development of rat spermatogenesis in a mouse. It is also possible that the cycle length of rat germ cells in the mouse testis is altered by the milieu of the recipient Sertoli cells.

Spermatogenesis is not as efficient in the recipient animals as in the normal, untransplanted animal. Germ cell degeneration, phagocytosis of released sperm, and malformed sperm are seen more frequently in transplanted spermatogenesis than in the untransplanted, normal, control animal (Russell and Brinster 1996; Russell et al. 1996). The reason for these abnormalities found in apparently histocompatible donors and recipients is not known but may be related to damage to Sertoli cells resulting from chemical treatment or prolonged inactivity. One might suggest that the environment provided by the Sertoli cell in xenogenic transplants into immunodeficient recipients is less than optimal to support qualitatively normal spermatogenesis. Macrophages are present in the tubular lumen of all recipients and may be a reflection of the increased need to scavenge and eliminate abnormal germ cells. Sertoli cell-only areas of seminiferous tubules phagocytose released sperm from another part of a tubule.

Spermatogenesis resulting from germ cell transplantation demonstrates normal cell associations. Moreover, these cell associations are characteristic of the donor species. In mouse-to-mouse transplants the cell associations, or stages, are those characteristic of the mouse (Russell et al. 1990). In rat-to-mouse transplants the cell associations in which rat cells are seen are characteristic of the rat (Leblond and Clermont 1952; Russell et al. 1990). The ability to form cell associations characteristic of the donor species therefore is an endogenous property of germ cells.

3.4 Applications of Transplant Technology to Basic Research

Shortly after the initial publication of the technique of spermatogonial transplantation the popular media focused on potential clinical and "futuristic" applications of spermatogonial transplant technology. Here we put forward some of the questions related primarily to basic application of spermatogonial technology that can be answered.

There is great need to study and improve the transplantation technology itself to increase the efficiency of seminiferous tubule germ cell colonization. Five months after injection of the germ cell suspension the transplanted testes showed less than half of the seminiferous tubules colonized by transplanted cells. It is important to determine the factors that would improve transplantation success. Currently a variety of cell types are injected. Would procedures for isolation and purification of stem cells or even isolation and purification of type A spermatogonia enhance transplantation colonization? Is it necessary to microinject cell types other than type A spermatogonia to achieve transplantation success? Are there growth factors that can be supplied to the testis that would enhance the spreading and development of stem cells? What is the developmental progression of transplanted cells? Does spermatogenesis in the transplanted animal result from a few or many seeding sites? Assuming more than one seeding site, how are seeding sites distributed throughout the testis? Do stem cells colonize the testis and can studying transplants after injection give us insights into the kinetics of spermatogenesis? Do injected germ cells more advanced than type A spermatogonia seed the testis and develop into sperm? Does the timing of spermatogenesis reflect which cell is the stem cell (A_0, A_4, or A_s), suggesting which model of spermatogonial renewal is the best (Clermont and Bustos-Obregon 1968; Huckins and Oakberg 1978a,b)? When does spermatogenesis first reach completion in transplanted testes? Does a wave of spermatogenesis form in transplanted testes? Is the profile of hormones (testosterone and gonadotropins) similar in transplanted and nontransplanted testes? How do xenogenic transplants affect the hormonal status and secretory products of the testis compared with a normal animal? Can stem cell spermatogonia be stably transfected in culture prior to transplantation? Can cryopreservation techniques be utilized in conjunction with in vitro methods to stably transfect the germ cell line?

Transplantation protocols are especially useful in discriminating the role of the Sertoli cell from that of the germ cell in the spermatogenic process. As an example, assume that a transgenic animal is produced that shows some abnormality of spermatogenesis. The question might be asked: "Is the abnormality a direct consequence of a germ cell defect or a Sertoli cell defect?" The latter can often be suspected in some situations on the grounds that the Sertoli cell is well known to support spermatogenesis (Russell and Griswold 1993), and that defective Sertoli cells often lead to a secondary loss in germ cells (Russell et al. 1990). Transplantation of stem cell spermatogonia from the transgenic animal to a histocompatible recipient should discriminate which cell, the Sertoli cell or the germ cell, is the primary target of the transgene. Normal growth and development of the transplanted transgenic cells in a wild type highly suggest that the somatic cell population (most likely the Sertoli cell) is in some way defective in the mutant animal.

The transplant model should prove useful in understanding the duration and timing of spermatogenesis. Xenogenic transplants in which rat germ cells are transplanted into mice testes show spermatogenesis morphologically characteristic of both species. The duration of the cycle of the seminiferous epithelium in the rat and mouse differ by about 50%. The question may be asked: "Do rat cells developing within a seminiferous tubule speed up their development when transplanted into a mouse to a rate characteristic of mouse cells, or does the mouse testes maintain two separate cycle lengths, one for mouse and one for rat?" The answer to this question has implications for determining which cells – the germ cells or the surrounding somatic cells – control germ cell cell-cycle length.

Xenogenic transplants may also prove useful in determining how cell-to-cell junctions work in the testis. There is an abundance of junctional types in the testis that physically connect the germ cells and Sertoli cells and serve functions that support spermatogenesis (Russell 1993). Our observations (unpublished) suggest some of these junctions do not form normally in mouse testes transplanted with rat cells. The consequence of abnormal junctions might provide useful information about the role of specific junctional types. Given that donor spermatogenesis is not completely normal in transplanted animals, junctional formation may be responsible for a quantitative deficit in normal sperm. Thus further study along these lines is needed.

Little is known about the immunology of the testis. The testis is thought to be an immunoprivileged site due to the locally high steroid levels, the secretion of immunosuppressant substances (Bellgrau et al. 1995) by Sertoli cells and by the presence of a Sertoli cell barrier. Transplantation from one mouse strain to another (allogenic transplants) or from one species to another (xenogenic transplants) makes it possible to study the immune system. Can the immune system in the testis can be suppressed to improve transplantation success as well as improve the quality of spermatogenesis without the necessity of having to use genetically immunodeficient mice?

Acknowledgements. We thank Carl Hausler for reading and improving the manuscript. Financial support was provided from the National Institutes of Health (NICHD 23657), USDA/NRI Competitive Grants Program (95-37205-2353), Commonwealth and General Assembly of Pennsylvania, and the Robert J. Kleberg, Jr. and Helen C. Kleberg Foundation.

References

Avarbock MR, Brinster CJ, Brinster R (1996) Reconstitution of spermatogenesis from frozen spermatogonial stem cells. Nat Med 2:693–696

Bellgrau D, Gold D, Selawry H, Moore J, Franzusoff A, Duke RC (1995) A role for CD95 ligand in preventing graft rejection. Nature 377:630–632

Brinster RL, Avarbock MR (1994) Germline transmission of donor haplotype following spermatogonial transplantation. Proc Natl Acad Sci USA 91:11303–11307

Brinster RL, Zimmerman JW (1994) Spermatogenesis following male germ-cell transplantation. Proc Natl Acad Sci USA 91:11298–11302

Bucci LR, Meistrich M (1987) Effects of busulfan on murine spermatogenesis: cyto-toxicity, sterility, sperm abnormalities and dominant lethal mutations. Mutat Res 176:159–268

Clermont Y, Bustos-Obregon E (1968) Re-examination of spermatogonial renewal in the rat by means of seminiferous tubules mounted "in toto." Am J Anat 122:237–248

Clouthier DE, Avarbock MR, Maika SD, Hammer RE, Brinster RL (1996) Rat spermatogenesis in mouse testes following spermatogonial stem cell transplantation. Nature 381:418–421

Huckins C, Oakberg EF (1978a) Morphological and quantitative analysis of spermatogonia in mouse testis using whole mounted seminferous tubules. I. The normal testis. Anat Rec 192:519–528

Huckins C, Oakberg EF (1978b) Morphological and quantitative analysis of spermatogonia in mouse testis using whole mounted seminferous tubules. II. The irradiated testis. Anat Rec. 192:529–54

Jiang F-X, Short RV (1995) Male germ cell transplantation in rats: apparent synchronization of spermatogenesis between host and donor seminferous epithelia. Int J Androl 18:326–330

Leblond CP, Clermont Y (1952) Spermiogenesis of rat, mouse, hamster, and guinea pig as revealed by the periodic acid-fuchsin sulfurous acid technique. Am J Anat 90:167–210

Nagano M, Brinster R (1998) Spermatogonial transplantation and reconstitution of donor cell spermatogenesis in recipient males. Acta Pathol Microsc Immunol Scand 106 (in press)

Ogawa T, Arechanga JM, Avarbock MR, Brinster RL (1997) Transplantation of testis germinal cells into mouse seminiferous tubules. Int J Dev Biol 41:111–122

Russell LD (1993) Morphological and functional evidence for Sertoli-germ cell relationships. In: Russell LD, Griswold MD (eds) The Sertoli cell. Cache River. Clearwater, pp 365–390

Russell LD, Brinster RL (1996) Transplants of rat spermatogonia into mice seminiferous tubules: preliminary ultrastructural observations. J Androl 17:615–627

Russell LD, Griswold MD (1993) The Sertoli cell. Cache River, Clearwater

Russell LD, Ettlin RA, Sinha Hikim AP, Clegg ED (1990) Histological and histopathological evaluation of the testis. Cache River, Clearwater

Russell LD, Franca LR, Brinster RL (1996) Syngeneic spermatogonial transplants in mice: Ultrastructural observations. J Androl 117:603–614

4 Genetic Control of Meiosis and the Onset of Spermiogenesis in Drosophila

M.T. Fuller and H. White-Cooper

4.1 Introduction

Male gametogenesis constitutes one of the most dramatic examples of cellular differentiation in the body. During spermiogenesis male germ cells change from round to long and streamlined and almost every subcellular organelle is remodeled. In addition, male germ cells undergo three different types of cell division program in the course of spermatogenesis: stem cell divisions, mitotic amplification divisions, and meiosis. During the specialized cell division of meiosis, regulation of cell cycle progression is drastically altered by the differentiation program. Work in our laboratory seeks to discover the genes and genetic circuitry that drive the dramatic cellular differentiation of spermatogenesis and coordinate it with the meiotic cell cycle program. To facilitate this genetic approach we study spermatogenesis in *Drosophila* as a model system.

4.2 Overview of Spermatogenesis in *Drosophila*

The overall program of spermatogenesis in *Drosophila* greatly resembles spermatogenesis in mammals (Fig. 1; for an extensive review of spermatogenesis in *Drosophila*, see Fuller 1993; Lindsley and Tokuyasu 1980). Sperm are produced continuously throughout reproductive life from a relatively small number of dedicated male germ line stem cells. In *Drosophila* the male germ line stem cells are located at the apical tip of the testes, where they lie clustered around a specialized set of somatic cells termed the apical hub (Hardy et al. 1979). The germ line stem cells are each flanked by a pair of somatic stem cells, the cyst progenitor cells (Gonczy and DiNardo 1996; Hardy et al. 1979). When a germ line stem cell divides, one daughter remains in contact with the apical hub and retains stem cell identity, while the other daughter is displaced away from the hub and initiates differentiation as a founder gonial cell. Similarly, when the cyst progenitor cells divide, the daughters that remain in contact with the hub retain stem cell identity, while the daughters displaced away from the hub differentiate as cyst cells. Two cyst cells enclose each founder gonial cell to form a cyst, the major differentiation unit of spermatogenesis in *Drosophila*. The two cyst cells never divide again, but enclose the descendants of the founder gonial cell throughout the entire differentiation process. Although little is known about the somatic cyst cells, they may be the functional equivalent of Sertoli cells in mammals.

The founder gonial cell initiates four rounds of mitotic amplification division, resulting in a cluster of 16 cells. Cytokinesis is incomplete during the gonial amplification divisions, and therefore the germ cells descended from a founder gonial cell remain connected by cytoplasmic bridges (Hardy et al. 1979; Hime et al. 1996) and divide in synchrony. After the fourth gonial division the 16 germ cells in the developing cyst initiate the meiotic program and together enter premeiotic DNA synthesis. Premeiotic S phase is followed by an extended, specialized G_2 phase of the cell cycle, meiotic prophase. *Drosophila* males differ from male mammals in that homologous chromosomes do not undergo recombination. There is no synaptonemal complex, and the landmark cytological stages of meiotic prophase, which are based on chromosome morphology, are not visible.

4.2.1 The Primary Spermatocyte Period of Growth and Gene Expression

The primary spermatocyte period in *Drosophila*, as in mammals, is characterized by extensive cell growth and new transcription. A large number of different mRNAs are expressed in male germ cells during the primary spermatocyte stage, including transcripts from novel genes expressed only in the testis, for example the CGP repeat family of male-specific transcripts thought to encode sperm tail components (Kuhn et al. 1991; Schafer et al. 1993), or genes encoding testis-specific isoforms of proteins involved in general cellular function, for example β-tubulin (Kemphues et al. 1979). In many cases genes expressed in other tissues utilize testis-specific promoters to produce novel transcripts in primary spermatocytes; for example, the *dhod* gene utilizes a different transcription start site for expression of a male-specific transcript in primary spermatocytes (Yang et al. 1995) and the *gonadal* gene is transcribed as a novel bicistronic message in the male germ line (Schulz et al. 1990). As in mammals (Geremia et al. 1977; Monesi 1964), many genes required for subsequent spermatid differentiation are transcribed in primary spermatocytes, and bulk transcription decreases sharply at around the onset of the first meiotic division. Unlike in mammals, however, in *Drosophila* no transcription has been detected in haploid spermatids by bulk autoradiographic studies (Olivieri and Olivieri 1965), and few genes transcribed in the haploid stages have been identified to date (Bendena et al. 1991)

4.2.2 Spermatid Differentiation

Following meiosis the haploid round spermatids undergo the extensive cellular and subcellular differentiation of spermiogenesis. The mitochondria in each spermatid fuse into two giant mitochondria, which wrap around each other to form a specialized mitochondrial derivative called the Nebenkern (Tates 1971; Tokuyasu 1975). The centriole inserts into the base of the nucleus and is converted into a basal body (Tates 1971). A microtubule-based axoneme grows out from the basal body and, along with the mitochondrial derivative, elongates to extend the full length of the spermatid flagellum (a distance of 1.8 mm in *Drosophila melanogaster*; Lindsley and Tokuyasu 1980). Nuclear DNA condenses, and the spermatid nucleus is converted from round to a long, thin, hooked shape (Tokuyasu 1974). The dramatic cellular and subcellular morphogenesis of spermatid differentiation in *Drosophila* is mediated by transcripts expressed prior to the meiotic divisions, probably most if not all during the primary spermatocyte growth and gene expression phase. As in mammals, translational control plays a prominent role in regulating the timing of gene product expression during male germ cell differentiation in *Drosophila* (Schafer et al. 1995).

4.2.3 Genetic Analysis of Spermatogenesis in *Drosophila*

Drosophila offers a superb model system in which to investigate the genetic mechanisms that regulate and mediate the differentiation program of male gametogenesis. The landmark stages of spermatogenesis (Fig. 1) in *Drosophila* are easily visible by phase-contrast light microscopy in unfixed, squashed preparations that take only a few minutes to make and examine. The ability to rapidly gain an overview of the process of spermatogenesis greatly facilitates genetic screens for male sterile mutations that cause defects at specific stages. The dramatic changes in cellular and subcellular morphology throughout spermato-genesis provide a wealth of cytological markers for analysis of mutant phenotypes, allowing identification of defects in many different specific morphogenetic events (for an overview of mutations affecting spermato-genesis in *Drosophila* see Fuller 1993). Several large-scale screens for male sterile mutations in *Drosophila* have been or are currently being carried out (Hackstein 1991; Castrillon et al. 1993; references cited in Fuller 1993; P.G. Wilson and M.T. Fuller, unpublished; B.T. Wakimoto, D. Lindsley, and C. Zucker, work in progress), providing raw material for identification of genes of interest by examination of mutant pheno-types.

4.3 Coordinate Control of Meiosis and Spermatid Differentiation

The central goal of our work is to understand the genetic circuitry that regulates and coordinates the meiotic divisions with onset of the sper-matid differentiation program. In this review we summarize our work on a set of key regulatory genes required for both meiotic cell cycle pro-gression and onset of spermatid differentiation in *Drosophila*. We have identified a set of three genes, *cannonball (can)*, *meiosis I arrest (mia)*, and *spermatocyte arrest (sa)*, that act together or in a pathway to activate tissue and stage-specific transcription in primary spermatocytes of a suite of target genes that act during postmeiotic spermatid differentia-tion. Wild type function of these three regulatory genes is also required for meiotic cell cycle progression, suggesting a cross-regulatory control to ensure that spermatocytes arrest at the G_2/M transition of meiosis I until genes required for postmeiotic differentiation have been tran-scribed. Finally, we have identified a gene, *always early (aly)*, as a candidate to act earlier in the pathway to regulate both meiotic cell cycle progression and the transcription program for spermatid differentiation.

4.3.1 Spermatid Differentiation Is Independent of Completion of Meiosis

During normal spermatogenesis in wild type, meiotic division always precedes onset of spermatid differentiation. The simplest way to specify this order of events would be to make the onset of spermatid differentiation dependent on completion of the meiotic cell cycle. Genetic analysis of spermatogenesis in *Drosophila*, however, indicates that spermatid differentiation can proceed independently of completion of meiosis. The G_2/M transition of mitosis in eukaryotes is regulated by the function of cell cycle phosphatase *cdc25* which removes inhibitory phosphate groups from the cell cycle kinase *cdc2*, allowing activation of the cdc2/Cyclin B complex (Dunphy and Kumagai 1991; Gautier et al. 1991). There are two *Drosophila* homologs of the *S. pombe cdc25* gene, *string* and *twine*. Wild type function of *string* is required for mitosis (Edgar and O'Farrell 1989), while wild type function of *twine* is required for meiosis (Alphey et al. 1992; Courtot et al. 1992).

In the testis *string* is expressed in the mitotically dividing spermatogonial cells, while transcription of *twine* initiates in early primary spermatocytes in preparation for meiotic division. In males mutant for *twine* the mitotic spermatogonial divisions proceed, and mature primary spermatocytes are produced. However, the male germ cells skip the major events of meiosis (Alphey et al. 1992; Courtot et al. 1992). The chromosomes initiate but do not complete condensation, no spindle is assembled, and there is no chromosome segregation or cytokinesis. Nevertheless, extensive spermatid differentiation proceeds, and the sixteen 4×N spermatids resulting from the failure in meiotic division form mitochondrial derivatives and undergo flagellar elongation and nuclear shaping (White-Cooper et al. 1993; Lin et al. 1996). Similar results were observed in mutant males carrying a temperature sensitive allele of the cell cycle kinase *cdc2*. When *cdc2^{ts}* males were raised at permissive temperature and then shifted to nonpermissive temperature, spermatocytes failed to undergo the meiotic divisions, but spermatid differentiation proceeded (Sigrist et al. 1995).

4.3.2 Genes Required for Both Meiotic Cell Cycle Progression and Onset of Spermatid Differentiation

Spermiogenesis in the absence of meiotic division as observed in *twine* and $cdc2^{ts}$ mutant males indicates that the pathway that regulates spermatid differentiation is independent of the pathway controlling meiotic cell cycle progression. However, the phenotype of certain other male sterile mutations in *Drosophila* indicates that spermatogenesis proceeds by a branched pathway rather than by two independent pathways. We have identified at least eight genes, the meiotic arrest class, that are required for both completion of the meiotic cell cycle and onset of spermatid differentiation (Lin et al. 1996; White-Cooper et al. 1998; A. MacQueen, B.T, Wakimoto, and H. White-Cooper, unpublished data). Our detailed analysis of the cytological and molecular phenotype of four of these genes, described below, indicates that spermatid differentiation and meiotic cell cycle progression are coordinated at least two points. First, the *aly* gene acts in primary spermatocytes to directly or indirectly allow transcription of genes in both the meiotic cell cycle program and the spermatid differentiation program. Second, the *can*, *mia*, and *sa* genes act in primary spermatocytes both to turn on transcription of spermatid differentiation genes and to activate the G_2/M transition of meiosis I through post-transcriptional control of *twine* protein accumulation.

Wild type function of the *aly*, *can*, *mia*, and *sa* genes of *Drosophila* is required for male germ cells to complete meiosis and initiate spermatid differentiation. The requirement for function of these genes appears to be specific to male gametogenesis, as mutant flies are viable and female fertile (Lin et al. 1996). Males mutant for any one of the four loci are sterile. The early stages of spermatogenesis appear normal and primary spermatocytes form and grow to mature size. However, cells in meiotic division and spermatid differentiation stages are completely absent, and mature primary spermatocytes with partially condensed chromosomes accumulate to fill the testis (Figs. 1, 2; Lin et al. 1996). Primary spermatocytes appear to arrest at or within the G_2/M transition of meiosis I in the mutant testes. In wild type young adult males, a cyst of 16 cells entering the first meiotic division is seen on average roughly once in every two testes squashes examined. However, in testes from flies mutant for *aly*, *can*, *mia*, or *sa* each testis contains many mature

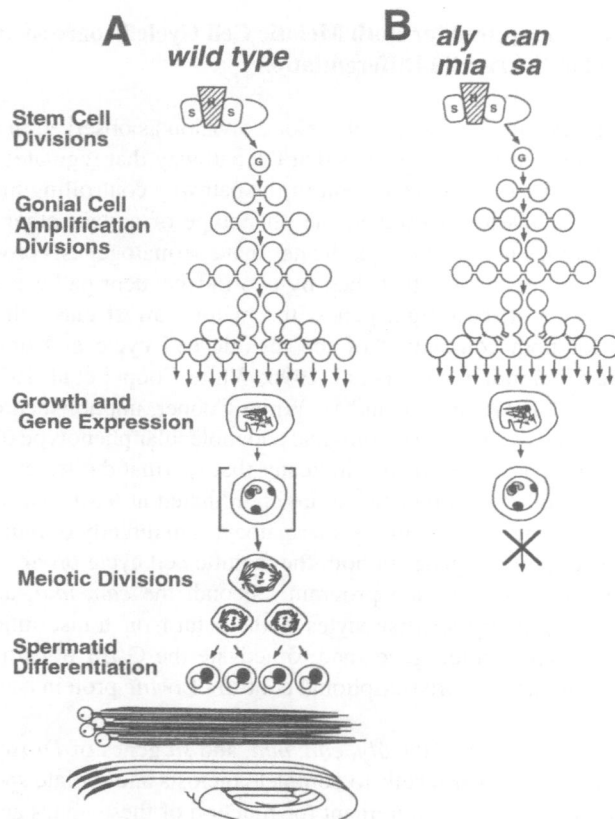

Fig. 1A,B. Diagram of male germ cell differentiation in wild type and meiotic arrest mutant *Drosophila*. **A** Spermatogenesis in wild type. For simplicity, only one of the 16 primary spermatocytes in a cyst is shown. In actuality, all 16 primary spermatocytes grow and undergo meiosis, resulting in a bundle of 64 interconnected haploid spermatids that proceed through spermiogenesis in synchrony. *Brackets*, the G_2/M transition of meiosis I. In wild type this stage proceeds so rapidly that there is an average of only one cyst of 16 spermatocytes undergoing the G_2/MI transition per two young adult testes examined by phase contrast light microscopy (Lin et al. 1996). **B** Spermatogenesis in males mutant for any one of the meiotic arrest mutants *aly, can, mia,* or *sa*. Male germ cell differentiation proceeds through the spermatocyte growth phase, but cells arrest at the G_2/M transition of meiosis I and cells with partially condensed chromosomes accumulate to fill the testis (Lin et al. 1996). Cells also fail to undergo spermatid differentiation. Diagram adapted from (Lin et al. 1996)

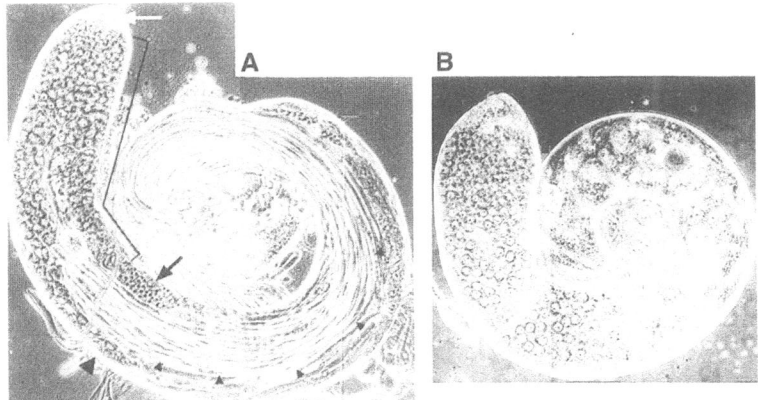

Fig. 2A,B. Whole wild type and meiotic arrest mutant *Drosophila* testes.
A Whole wild type testis viewed by phase-contrast microscopy. Male germ line stem cells reside in the germinal proliferation center at the apical tip of the testis (*white arrow*). After four rounds of mitotic amplification divisions at the testis apical tip, germ cells enter the primary spermatocyte phase of growth and gene expression (*brackets*). Spermatocyte cysts are displaced away from the apical tip as they grow, and cells thus enter meiotic divisions near the start of the coiled part of the testis (*large arrowhead*). Cysts of haploid early round spermatids at the "onion stage" are easily identified by their regular array of phase light spherical nuclei paired with phase dark mitochondrial derivatives (*black arrow*). Ropelike bundles each containing 64 elongating spermatids stretch up the testis lumen (*small arrowheads*). (From Fuller 1998). **B** Whole testis from *aly* mutant male. Early stages of germ cell differentiation at the apical tip of the testis are present and appear normal. Mature primary spermatocytes fill the testis, and no cells in meiotic division or the spermatid differentiation stages are visible. The arrested spermatocytes eventually degenerate in the basal part of the testis. Note that the mutant testis is shorter than wild type, probably due to lack of the elongating spermatid stages

primary spermatocytes with partially condensed chromosomes, indicating arrest at onset of the G2/M transition (Lin et al. 1996).

The phenotype of *Drosophila* males mutant for *aly*, *can*, *mia*, or *sa* bears uncanny resemblance to the clinical description of meiosis I maturation arrest azoospermia in humans. Meiosis I maturation arrest is one of the more common forms of azoospermia (Colgan et al. 1980; Meyer et al. 1992; Wong et al. 1973) and is characterized by lack of cells in meiotic division or the spermatid differentiation stages, and accumulation of what appear to be mature primary spermatocytes with partially condensed chromosomes (Soderstrom and Suominen 1980). The similarities between the meiotic arrest phenotype of the *Drosophila* mutants and the clinical description of meiosis I maturation arrest in humans raises the intriguing possibility that the genetic circuitry that regulates and coordinates meiosis and spermatid differentiation in *Drosophila* might be conserved to mammals.

To elucidate the molecular mechanisms by which the *aly*, *can*, *mia*, and *sa* genes of *Drosophila* act to regulate spermatogenesis, we have investigated the effect of mutations in each of the four genes on the expression of two sets of potential targets. To explore the mechanism of action of the genes in controlling cell cycle progression, we have examined the expression of mRNA and protein for the core cell cycle regulators *cyclin A*, *cyclin B*, and *twine* during male meiosis. To understand the role of the meiotic arrest genes in controlling onset of spermatid differentiation, we have examined the expression in primary spermatocytes of a suite of genes involved in spermatid differentiation.

4.4   Expression of Cell Cycle Control Genes in Male Meiosis

The G_2/M transition of meiosis I in wild type *Drosophila* males is regulated by many of the same core cell cycle genes that regulate the G_2/M transition of mitosis. As discussed above, when adult males carrying a *ts* allele of *cdc2* are shifted to non-permissive temperature, spermatocytes failed to undergo the meiotic divisions (Sigrist et al. 1995). The *cyclin A* and *cyclin B* genes are also expressed in primary spermatocytes and are likely to play similar roles in regulating the G_2/M transition of meiosis I as in the G_2/M transition of mitosis. Both *cyclin A* and *cyclin B* mRNAs are present at the tip of the testis, where the gonial cells are undergoing mitotic proliferation. *cyclin A* but not *cyclin B* message remains present during premeiotic S phase (White-Cooper et al. 1998). Both *cyclin A* and *cyclin B* mRNAs are expressed at high levels in primary spermatocytes, starting early in the primary spermatocyte growth period (Table 1, Fig. 3).

The mRNA for *twine*, the *cdc25* homolog required for the G_2/M transition of male meiosis, is first expressed in the testis early in the

Table 1. Expression of cell cycle control genes in wild type meiosis

	Growing primary spermatocytes	Late primary spermatocytes	Meiotic division	Postmeiotic spermatids
cyclin A mRNA	+	+	+ Degraded during divisions	–
cyclin B mRNA	+	+	+ Degraded during divisions	–
twine mRNA	+	+	+ Degraded during divisions	–
Cyclin A protein	+ (Cytoplasmic)	+ (Cytoplasmic)	Enters nucleus at G$_2$/MI Degraded by metaphase I	–
Cyclin B protein	–	+ (Cytoplasmic)	Enters nucleus after cyclin A Degraded at metaphase I Reappears for meiosis II	+/– (low Lewels)
twine-LacZ fusion protein	–	+	+	N/A

primary spermatocyte growth period (Alphey et al. 1992; Courtot et al. 1992). In wild type the *cyclin A*, *cyclin B*, and *twine* mRNAs remain present in late primary spermatocytes, but decrease greatly or disappear by the early haploid spermatid stage (Table 1, Fig. 3; White-Cooper et al. 1998). Message for the *Drosophila* gene *boule*, which is required for progression of meiosis through the G$_2$/MI transition (Eberhart et al. 1996), also first accumulates in early primary spermatocytes, but persists into the early elongation stages of spermiogenesis (Fig. 3). *boule* encodes a predicted RNA binding protein homolog of the mammalian gene *Dazla*, which has been shown to be required for spermatogenesis (Ruggiu et al. 1997).

The expression and subcellular location of cell cycle control proteins in primary spermatocytes (Table 1) suggests a mechanism for regulation of the timing of the G$_2$/M transition of meiosis I. Cyclin A protein is expressed throughout the early stages of spermatogenesis. It is nuclear in cells near the apical tip of the testes, in the region where early germ cells are undergoing mitosis and or premeiotic DNA replication. Cyclin A protein is cytoplasmic in early primary spermatocytes and remains there until the onset of the G$_2$/M transition, when it enters the nucleus (Gonczy et al. 1994; Lin et al. 1996). In wild type testes, Cyclin A protein is degraded by metaphase I. This degradation is dependent on the activity of *twine* (Lin et al. 1996) and thus, by inference, active *cdc2* kinase. Although expression of *cyclin B* message begins early in the primary spermatocyte growth phase, the level of cyclin B protein in

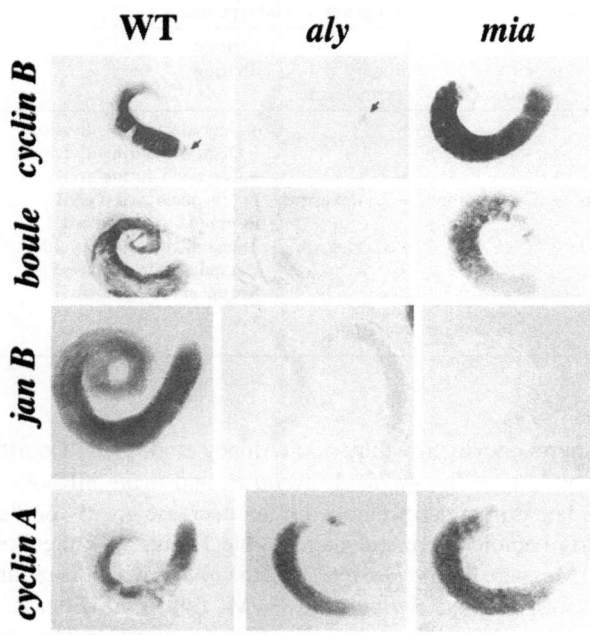

Fig. 3. Transcription of cell cycle control and spermatid differentiation genes in wild type (*WT*) and meiotic arrest mutant testes. Whole-mount *Drosophila* testes probed by in situ hybridization for expression of specific transcripts. Wild type function of *aly* is required for transcription in primary spermatocytes of the meiotic cell cycle control genes *cyclin B* (shown) and *twine* (White-Cooper et al. 1998) and many spermatid differentiation genes (White-Cooper et al. 1998; *janB* is shown). Wild type function of *aly* is also required for transcription of *boule* (shown) a gene required for both meiotic cell cycle progression and certain aspects of spermatid differentiation (Eberhart et al. 1996). *cyclin A* (shown) and many other mRNAs are expressed in *aly* mutant spermatocytes (White-Cooper et al. 1998), indicating that wild type function of *aly* is not required for all transcription at this stage. Note that expression of *cyclin B* mRNA in the mitotic cells at the apical tip of the testis does not require wild type *aly* function (*arrow*). mRNAs for the cell cycle genes *cyclin B*, *boule*, *cyclin A* (shown), and *twine* (White-Cooper et al. 1998) are expressed in spermatocytes from *mia* (shown), *can*, and *sa* mutant testes (White-Cooper et al. 1998). However, wild type function of *can*, *mia*, and *sa* is required for transcription of many spermatid differentiation genes (White-Cooper et al. 1998) including *janB* (shown for *mia*). In wild type, transcription of these spermatid differentiation genes begins early in the primary spermatocyte growth period, days before the arrest point of the mutants

primary spermatocytes remains low until just before cells enter the G2/MI transition. Cyclin B protein begins to accumulate in the cytoplasm of primary spermatocytes as chromatin condensation initiates, is present at high levels at prometaphase, then enters the nucleus and is almost immediately degraded at metaphase (White-Cooper et al. 1998).

Analysis of the expression of a *twine-lacZ* reporter fusion protein suggests that expression of *twine* protein, like cyclin B, is delayed for days after the first appearance of the message in primary spermatocytes. Although mRNA for the *twine-lacZ* fusion, as with the endogenous *twine* message, is expressed starting early in the primary spermatocyte stage, the β-galactosidase activity of the reporter construct is not detected until just before the onset of the first meiotic division (White-Cooper et al. 1998). The delay in accumulation of cyclin B protein and the *twine-lacZ* reporter fusion protein suggests that timing of the G2/M transition of meiosis I in wild type males is regulated by post-transcriptional control mechanisms, possibly developmentally regulated translational control or changes in protein stability of cyclin B and the *twine* cdc25 cell cycle phosphatase.

Accumulation of the *twine* protein cannot be the sole rate limiting step regulating timing of the G2/MI cell cycle transition, as expression of the *twine* homolog *string* under a heterologous promoter is able to partially rescue meiotic cell cycle progression in a *twine* mutant background but does not cause primary spermatocytes to enter the first meiotic division prematurely (Sigrist et al. 1995). Requirement for accumulation of cyclin B protein or another unidentified cell cycle control factor might limit the capacity of younger spermatocytes to enter the G2/MI transition under these conditions.

4.4.1 *aly* Regulates Transcription of Meiotic Cell Cycle Genes

Wild type function of *aly* is required for transcription in primary spermatocytes of at least three genes required for the G2/M transition of meiosis I: *cyclin B*, *twine*, and *boule* (Table 2; White-Cooper et al. 1998). *twine* and *boule* are not required for mitosis and are first expressed in the testis in primary spermatocytes, where their expression requires *aly* (White-Cooper et al. 1998). Regulation of *cyclin B* mRNA expression appears to be more complex. *cyclin B* mRNA is present in

Table 2. Expression of cell cycle control genes in meiotic arrest (*aly, can, mia, sa*) and meiotic control (*twine*) mutants

	Wildtype	*aly*	*can, mia, sa*	*twine*
cyclin A mRNA	+	+ Persists	+ Persists	+ Gone after meiosis
Cyclin A protein	+	+ Persists	+ Persists	+ Nuclear in early spermatids Gradually turns over
cyclin B mRNA	+	–	+ Persists	+ Gone after meiosis
Cyclin B protein	+	–	+ Persists	+ Does not enter nucleus Gone after meiosis
twine mRNA	+	–	+	+
twine-lacZ fusion protein	+	–	–	N/A

gonial cells undergoing mitotic division in *aly* mutant males (Fig. 3, arrow). However expression of *cyclin B* mRNA in primary spermatocytes is *aly* dependent (Fig. 3, Table 2). Wild type function of *aly* is not required for expression of all cell cycle control genes utilized during meiosis. Transcripts for *cyclin A*, *pelota*, *roughex*, and *polo* are all expressed in *aly* mutant testes (White-Cooper et al. 1998).

The *aly* gene appears to sit at the head of a pathway regulating meiotic cell cycle progression in primary spermatocytes. However, *aly* is not likely to encode a global regulator of the primary spermatocyte growth and gene expression program, as mature primary spermatocytes with relatively normal size and morphology are present in *aly* mutant testes (Lin et al. 1996).

4.5 Expression of Spermatid Differentiation Genes in Primary Spermatocytes

Many genes required for spermatid differentiation are first transcribed during the primary spermatocyte growth and gene expression period. A number of genes identified by male specific transcripts have been studied as model systems for translational control. *Mst87F*, *Mst84D*, and *Mst98C* are members of the CGP family of related genes thought to encode sperm tail components (Schafer et al. 1993). Members of this family are transcribed in primary spermatocytes, but the mRNAs are not translated until days after completion of the meiotic divisions (Kuhn et al. 1988, 1991; Schafer et al. 1993, 1995). The *dhod*, *janB*, and *don juan (dj)* genes are also transcribed in primary spermatocytes but the mRNAs are not translated until after meiosis (Santel et al. 1997; Yang et al. 1995; Yanicostas and Lepesant 1990). The *fuzzy onions (fzo)* gene of *Drosophila* encodes a mitofusin protein required for the developmentally regulated fusion of mitochondria that takes place in early haploid spermatids (Hales and Fuller 1997). Although the *fzo* gene is transcribed starting in early spermatocytes, the protein product is not detected on mitochondria until late anaphase II. These are no doubt only a few of the many genes required for spermatid differentiation that are expressed during the primary spermatocyte stage, as in *Drosophila* there is little new transcription during the haploid stages of spermatogenesis (Olivieri and Olivieri 1965).

4.5.1 *can*, *mia*, and *sa* Regulate Transcription of Spermatid Differentiation Genes

Wild type function of *can*, *mia*, and *sa* is required for transcription in primary spermatocytes of several genes that act during spermatid differentiation. Transcripts for *Mst87F*, *Mst84D*, *Mst98C*, *janB*, *dj*, and *fzo* are greatly reduced compared to wild type in primary spermatocytes from *can*, *mia*, or *sa* mutant testes (Fig. 3; White-Cooper et al. 1998). To date we have tested 18 different genes normally transcribed in wild type spermatocytes for expression in *can*, *mia*, and *sa* mutant testes. Eight required wild type function of *can*, *mia*, and *sa* for normal expression. For the six of these where the stage of action of the gene product is known, the genes function during postmeiotic spermatid differentiation. The ten genes transcribed at normal levels in *can*, *mia*, and *sa* spermatocytes are all known to function either in meiotic or premeiotic stages. The striking correlation between stage of action and requirement for *can*, *mia*, and *sa* suggests that the *can*, *mia*, and *sa* genes may activate a transcription program specific for spermiogenesis.

The same set of spermatid differentiation genes that require *can*, *mia*, and *sa* for expression are also not transcribed in testes from males mutant for *aly* (White-Cooper et al. 1998). Failure to activate the spermiogenesis transcription program may explain the lack of spermatid differentiation seen in *aly* as well as in *can*, *mia*, and *sa* mutant testes.

4.6 *can*, *mia*, and *sa* May Regulate the G2/MI Cell Cycle Transition by a Post-Transcriptional Control Mechanism

Transcripts encoding *cyclin B*, *twine* and the *twine-lacZ* reporter fusion are all expressed in early primary spermatocytes and persist through the arrested spermatocyte stage in *can*, *mia*, or *sa* males (White-Cooper et al. 1998). Cyclin B protein is expressed in *can*, *mia*, and *sa* spermatocytes as the cells approach the G_2/MI transition. However, the *twine-lacZ* reporter fusion protein is not expressed in *can*, *mia*, or *sa* mutant testes (Table 2; White-Cooper et al. 1998).

Spermatocytes from males mutant for either *aly*, *can*, *mia*, or *sa* all arrest at the same point in spermatogenesis – the G2/M transition of meiosis I (Lin et al. 1996). We hypothesize that the mutants cause arrest at the G2/MI transition due to failure to produce active *cdc2*/cyclin B complex. However, the meiotic arrest mutants appear to affect formation of an active *cdc2*/cyclin B complex by different biochemical mechanisms (Fig. 4). Wild type function of *aly* is required for transcription in primary spermatocytes of key cell cycle control genes, including *cyclin B*, *twine*, and *boule* (White-Cooper et al. 1998). In contrast, wild type function of *can*, *mia*, and *sa* appear to be required for expression of *twine* protein (White-Cooper et al. 1998), the critical cell cycle phosphatase required to activate the *cdc2/cyclin B* complex (Sigrist et al. 1995).

Accumulation of twine and Cyclin B protein at the end of the primary spermatocyte growth period appears to be under different genetic control. The former requires wild type function of *can*, *mia*, and *sa* while the latter does not. It may be that accumulation of twine protein in primary spermatocytes is the cell cycle readout of the *can mia*, and *sa* pathway, while accumulation of Cyclin B protein just before onset of the meiotic divisions is the cell cycle readout of a different genetic pathway. Progression through the G2/MI cell cycle transition at the end of the primary spermatocyte extended G2 phase would thus require activation of both pathways.

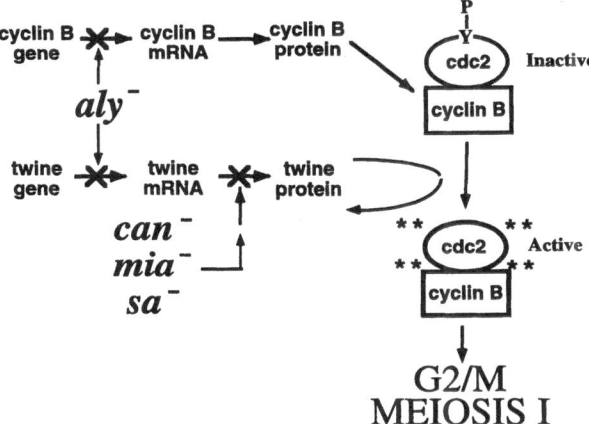

Fig. 4. Mutations in *aly*, *can*, *mia*, and *sa* block meiotic cell cycle progression at the same point, but by different molecular mechanisms. Model for the mechanism of cell cycle arrest in the meiotic arrest mutants *aly*, *can*, *mia*, and *sa*. All four mutants cause arrest at the G_2/M transition of meiosis I, presumably due to failure to produce active *cdc2*/Cyclin B complex (** **) required for this cell cycle transition. Mutations in *aly* cause arrest due to failure to express transcripts for certain cell cycle control genes, for example *cyclin B* and the activating cell cycle phosphatase *twine*. Mutations in *can*, *mia*, and *sa* appear to cause failure to accumulate twine protein (White-Cooper et al. 1998), thus affecting cell cycle progression via a post-transcriptional mechanism. The effect of *can*, *mia*, and *sa* on twine protein expression may be indirect, through action of another gene or genes

4.7 Model for Coordinate Control of Spermiogenesis and Meiotic Cell Cycle Progression

We propose that the wild type products of *can*, *mia*, and *sa* act together or in a pathway in primary spermatocytes to turn on transcription of a number of genes required for spermatid differentiation (Fig. 5; White-Cooper et al. 1998). Failure to turn on this stage- and tissue-specific transcription program in *can*, *mia*, or *sa* mutant males results in the global lack of spermatid differentiation observed in the mutant testes. We hypothesize that the arrest of meiosis at the G_2/MI transition in *can*,

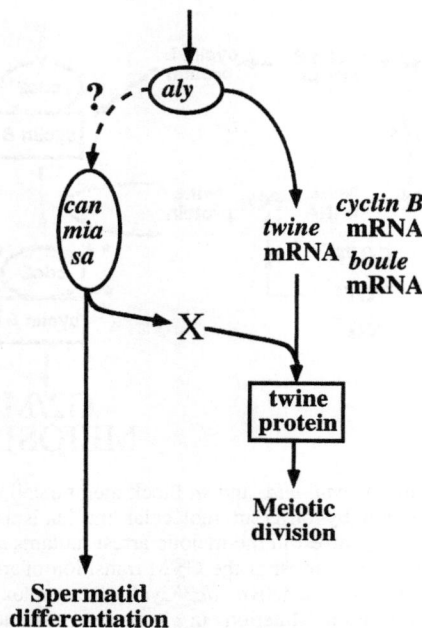

Fig. 5. Model for the genetic circuitry that coordinately regulates meiotic cell cycle progression and spermatid differentiation in *Drosophila*. The wild type *aly* gene product directly or indirectly activates transcription of *cyclin B*, *twine*, and *boule* in primary spermatocytes to regulate the specialized cell cycle of meiosis. Wild type *aly* also controls onset of spermatid differentiation, possibly by activating *can*, *mia*, and/or *sa*. The wild type products of the *can*, *mia*, and *sa* genes act together or in a pathway to turn on tissue and stage specific transcription in primary spermatocytes of a suite of genes required for post-meiotic spermatid differentiation. Mutations in *can*, *mia*, and *sa* cause meiotic cell cycle arrest because a hypothetical gene or genes (*X*) expressed as part of the *can*, *mia*, and *sa* dependent spermatid differentiation program is required to allow accumulation of twine protein, either by alleviating translational repression on the *twine* mRNA or by stabilizing the twine protein in mature primary spermatocytes. (Adapted from White-Cooper et al. 1998)

mia, and *sa* mutant testes stems from a cross-regulatory control mechanism where a gene or genes (X in Fig. 5) expressed as part of the spermatid differentiation program act(s) to allow expression of twine protein in mature primary spermatocytes, either by relieving translational repression or by inhibiting protein turnover. In wild type spermatocytes this cross-regulatory mechanism ensures that the cells do not begin meiotic division until genes required for spermatid differentiation have been transcribed.

We also propose that *aly* acts upstream of *can*, *mia*, and *sa* to regulate onset of the transcription program for spermatid differentiation (White-Cooper et al. 1998). We place *aly* in the *can*, *mia*, and *sa* pathway because testes from *aly* mutant males have the same phenotype and lack the same spermatid differentiation transcripts as testes from *can*, *mia*, and *sa* mutant males. We suggest that *aly* acts upstream in the pathway because *aly* mutants affect expression of other transcripts not dependent on *can*, *mia*, or *sa*.

4.8 Future Directions

Our work to date has identified the outlines of the genetic circuitry that regulates the onset of spermiogenesis and coordinates meiotic cell cycle progression with the differentiation program in *Drosophila*. We now stand in an excellent position to elucidate the molecular mechanisms that underlie this genetic control. To determine how *can*, *mia*, and *sa* act to turn on the stage- and tissue-specific expression of spermatid differentiation genes during the primary spermatocyte period, we are cloning the genes to learn the molecular nature of their products. We are also using reporter constructs to identify the *cis*-acting sequences that bring transcription of several target genes under control of *can*, *mia*, and *sa*. To learn how the *can*, *mia*, and *sa* transcription program is activated we are cloning *aly* and investigating its mode of action and regulation. To uncover the mechanism of the cross-regulatory control that makes the G_2/M transition of meiosis I dependent on the transcription program governed by *can*, *mia*, and *sa*, we are identifying the *cis*-acting sequences that delay accumulation of twine protein and searching for the *trans*-acting factor(s) that allow twine protein accumulation at the end of meiotic prophase. Finally, we are screening a new, large-scale collection of male sterile mutations (B.T. Wakimoto and C. Zucker) to identify additional genes required for both meiotic cell cycle progression and onset of spermiogenesis. This screen has already yielded four new genes of the meiotic arrest class.

One intriguing long range goal of our studies is to test whether the genetic regulatory circuitry that we have identified in *Drosophila* is conserved and functions similarly during spermatogenesis in mammals. To do so, we plan to identify mouse homologs of *aly*, *can*, *mia*, and *sa* expressed in the testis and determine whether mutations in these genes cause defects in spermatogenesis. The demonstration that the *Drosophila* gene *boule* and its mouse homolog *Daz-like (Dazla)* are both required for normal spermatogenesis (Eberhart et al. 1996; Ruggiu et al. 1997) supports the possibility that the genetic regulatory circuitry of spermatogenesis might be conserved from flies to mammals. If so, it will be interesting to test whether mammalian homologs of *aly*, *can*, *mia*, and *sa* are mutated in cases of meiosis I maturation arrest in humans.

Acknowledgements. We thank Ting-Yi Lin, Mark Hiller, and all the other members of the Fuller laboratory for many discussions and helpful comments. H.W.-C. was supported by a Stanford Medical School Dean's Postdoctoral Fellowship and the Walter and Idun Berry Fellowship Fund. This work was supported by NIH grant no. HD32936 to M.T.F.

References

Alphey L, Jimenez J, White-Cooper H, Dawson I, Nurse P, Glover DM (1992) *twine*, a *cdc25* homologue that functions in the male and female germlines of *Drosophila*. Cell 69:977–988

Bendena WG, Ayme SA, Garbe JC, Pardue ML (1991) Expression of heat-shock locus hsr-omega in nonstressed cells during development in *Drosophila melanogaster*. Dev Biol 144:65–77

Castrillon DH, Gonczy P, Alexander S, Rawson R, Eberhart CG, Viswanathan S, DiNardo S, Wasserman SA (1993) Toward a molecular genetic analysis of spermatogenesis in *Drosophila melanogaster*: characterization of male-sterile mutants generated by single P element mutagenesis. Genetics 135:489–505

Colgan TJ, Bedard YC, Strawbridge TG, Buckspan MB, Klotz PG (1980) Reappraisal of the value of testicular biopsy in the investigation of infertility. Fertil Steril 33:56–60

Courtot C, Frankhauser C, Simanis V, Lehner C (1992) The *Drosophila cdc25* homolog *twine* is required for meiosis. Development 116:405–416

Dunphy WG, Kumagai A (1991) The cdc25 protein contains an intrinsic phosphatase activity. Cell 67:189–196

Eberhart CG, Maines JZ, Wasserman SA (1996) Meiotic cell cycle requirement for a fly homologue of human deleted in azoospermia. Nature 381:783–785

Edgar BA, O'Farrell PH (1989) Genetic control of cell division patterns in the *Drosophila* embryo. Cell 57:177–187

Fuller MT (1993) Spermatogenesis. In: Bate M, Martinez-Arias A (eds) The development of *Drosophila*, vol 1. Cold Spring Harbor, Cold Spring Harbor, pp 71–147

Fuller MT (1998) Genetic control of cell proliferation and differentiation in *Drosophila* spermatogenesis. In: Bellve A (ed) The male germ cell: migration to fertilization. Academic, London (in press)

Gautier J, Solomon MJ, Booher RN, Bazan JF, Kirschner MW (1991) *cdc25* is a specific tyrosine phosphatase that directly activates p34cdc2. Cell 67:197–211

Geremia R, Boitani C, Conti M, Monesi V (1977) RNA synthesis in spermatocytes and spermatids and preservation of meiotic RNA during spermatogenesis in the mouse. Cell Differentiation 5:343–355

Gonczy P, DiNardo S (1996) The germ line regulates somatic cyst cell proliferation and fate during *Drosophila* spermatogenesis. Development 122:2437–2447

Gonczy P, Thomas BJ, DiNardo S (1994) *roughex* is a dose-dependent regulator of the second meiotic division during *Drosophila* spermatogenesis. Cell 77:1015–1025

Hackstein JHP (1991) Spermatogenesis in *Drosophila*. A genetic approach to cellular and subcellular differentiation. Eur J Cell Biol 56:151–169

Hales KG, Fuller MT (1997) Developmentally regulated mitochondrial fusion mediated by a conserved novel predicted GTPase. Cell 90:121–129

Hardy RW, Tokuyasu KT, Lindsley DL, Garavito M (1979) The germinal proliferation center in the testis of *Drosophila melanogaster*. J Ultrastruct Res 69:180–190

Hime GR, Brill JA, Fuller MT (1996) Assembly of ring canals in the male germ line from structural components of the contractile ring. J Cell Sci 109:2779–2788

Kemphues KJ, Raff RA, Kaufman TC, Raff EC (1979) Mutation in a structural gene for a β-tubulin specific to testis in *Drosophila melanogaster*. Proc Natl Acad Sci USA 76:3991–3995

Kuhn R, Schafer U, Schafer M (1988) Cis-acting regions sufficient for spermatocyte-specific transcriptional and spermatid-specific translational control of the *Drosophila melanogaster* gene *mst(3)gl-9*. EMBO J 7:447–454

Kuhn R, Kuhn C, Borsch D, Glatzer KH, Schafer U, Schafer M (1991) A cluster of four genes selectively expressed in the male germ line of *Drosophila melanogaster*. Mech Dev 35:143–151

Lin T-Y, Viswanathan S, Wood C, Wilson PG, Wolf N, Fuller MT (1996) Coordinate developmental control of the meiotic cell cycle and spermatid differentiation in *Drosophila* males. Development 122:1331–1341

Lindsley D, Tokuyasu KT (1980) Spermatogenesis. In: Ashburner M, Wright TRF (eds) Genetics and biology of *Drosophila*, vol 2d. Academic Press, New York, pp 225–294

Meyer JM, Maetz JL, Rumpler Y (1992) Cellular relationship impairment in maturation arrest of human spermatogenesis: an ultrastructural study. Histopathology 21:25–33

Monesi V (1964) Ribonucleic acid synthesis during mitosis and meiosis in the mouse testis. J Cell Biol 22:521–532

Olivieri G, Olivieri A (1965) Autoradiographic study of nucleic acid synthesis during spermatogenesis in *Drosophila melanogaster*. Mutat Res 2:366–380

Ruggiu M, Speed R, Taggart M, McKay SJ, Kilanowski F, Saunders P, Cooke HJ (1997) The mouse *Dazla* gene encodes a cytoplasmic protein essential for gametogenesis. Nature 389:73–77

Santel A, Winhauer T, Blümer N, Renkawitz-Pohl R (1997) The *Drosophila don juan* (*dj*) gene encodes a novel sperm specific protein component characterised by an unusual domain for repetitive amino acid motif. Mech Dev 64:19–30

Schafer M, Borsch D, Hulster A, Schafer U (1993) Expression of a gene duplication encoding conserved sperm tail proteins is translationally regulated in *Drosophila melanogaster*. Mol Cell Biol 13:1708–1718

Schafer M, Nayernia K, Engel W, Schafer U (1995) Translational control in spermatogenesis. Dev Biol 172:344–352

Schulz RA, Miksch JL, Xie XL, Cornish JA, Galewsky S (1990) Expression of the *Drosophila gonadal* gene: alternative promoters control the germ-line expression of monocistronic and bicistronic gene transcripts. Development 108:613–622

Sigrist S, Ried G, Lehner CF (1995) Dmcdc2 kinase is required for both meiotic divisions during *Drosophila* spermatogenesis and is activated by the Twine/cdc25 phosphatase. Mech Dev 53:247–260

Soderstrom K-O, Suominen M (1980) Histopathology and ultrastructure of meiotic arrest in human spermatogenesis. Arch Pathol Lab Med 104:476–482

Tates AD (1971) Cytodifferentiation during spermatogenesis in *Drosophila melanogaster:* an electron microscope study. Rijksuniversiteit, Leiden

Tokuyasu KT (1974) Dynamics of spermiogenesis in *Drosophila melanogaster*. IV. Nuclear transformation. J Ultrastruct Res 48:284–303

Tokuyasu KT (1975) Dynamics of spermiogenesis in *Drosophila melanogaster*. VI. Significance of "onion" nebenkern formation. J Ultrastruct Res 53:93–112

White-Cooper H, Alphey L, Glover DM (1993) The *cdc25* homologue *twine* is required for only some aspects of the entry into meiosis in Drosophila. J Cell Sci 106:1035–1044

White-Cooper H, Schafer MA, Alphey LS, Fuller MT (1998) Transcriptional and post-transcriptional control mechanisms coordinate the onset of spermatid differentiation with meiosis I in *Drosophila*. Development 125:125–134

Wong TW, Straus FH, Warner NE (1973) Testicular biopsy in the study of male infertility. Arch Pathol 95:151–159

Yang J, Porter L, Rawls J (1995) Expression of the dihydroorotate dehydrogenase gene, *dhod,* during spermatogenesis in *Drosophila melanogaster*. Mol Gen Genet 246:334–341

Yanicostas C, Lepesant JA (1990) Transcriptional and translational cis-regulatory sequences of the spermatocyte-specific *Drosophila janusB* gene are located in the 3' exonic region of the overlapping *janusA* gene. Mol Gen Genet 224:450–458

5 Chromatin Structure and Gene Expression During Spermatogenesis

W.M. Baarends, H.P. Roest, J.W. Hoogerbrugge,
P.J.M. Hendriksen, J.H.J. Hoeijmakers, and J.A. Grootegoed

5.1 Introduction

The developmental series of events during spermatogenesis that leads to the enclosure of a haploid genome in the head of the highly specialized spermatozoon requires strict control of gene expression (Grootegoed 1996). This control of gene expression shows different properties during the mitotic, meiotic, and postmeiotic phases of spermatogenesis. However, these phases form a continuum. This is most evident for the transition of meiotic spermatocytes into postmeiotic spermatids, since spermatocytes already express a number of genes which encode proteins that are essential for sperm function rather than for meiotic events. Spermatogonia may have a similar foresight. The mitotic step from B spermatogonia to preleptotene primary spermatocytes is often considered as the point of entry into meiosis, but it should be noted that A1 spermatogonia already have embarked on a one-way pathway leading to the meiotic prophase.

The meiotic prophase in spermatocytes and in oocytes shows many common features, including sex-specific gene expression. Consequently the end products of male and female meiosis are remarkably different: one primary spermatocyte gives rise to four haploid spermatids that can develop into spermatozoa capable of specific binding to the zona pellucida and fusion with the oocyte, whereas the oocyte which is arrested in the late prophasic dictyate stage first grows and forms a zona pellucida, and then is able to generate one haploid ovum and two polar bodies at ovulation and at the first steps of fertilization.

The description presented in this chapter of chromatin structure and gene expression during spermatogenesis is not comprehensive but rather provides a number of examples to illustrate some of the principles involved. Focused is principally upon the mouse. Many important and classical articles cannot be acknowledged within the limits of the present chapter. The list of references gives selected key articles and recent reviews, and the reader is also referred to references therein.

5.2 The Route to Meiosis

Embryonic primordial germ cells reach the undifferentiated anlagen of the gonads through a migration process which depends on interaction of stem cell factor (SCF) with the Kit receptor. The germ cells encounter soluble and membrane-bound SCF along their migration route, and interaction of this factor with the Kit receptor at the surface of the germ cells stimulates their proliferation and survival (Fleischman 1993). After arrival of the germ cells in the undifferentiated gonads, the first differences between spermatogenesis and oogenesis are determined by the absence or presence of embryonic expression of *Sry* (the sex determining region of the Y-chromosome gene). The product of this gene, a DNA-binding factor that regulates the expression of other genes, stands at the basis of the differentiation of the indifferent gonad into a testis (Koopman et al. 1991). Upon formation of a testis the primordial germ cells are enclosed in testicular tubules together with the precursor Sertoli cells.

The onset of meiosis is still far away, awaiting gonadotropic stimulation of the testis around puberty. This gonadotropic stimulation induces maturation of Sertoli cells and the onset of spermatogenesis, starting with differentiation of undifferentiated A spermatogonia into differentiating A spermatogonia, followed by mitotic divisions leading from A1–A4 spermatogonia to intermediate and B spermatogonia, and then into the meiotic prophase. We are still far from understanding the control of this long route to meiosis, which is very different from the relatively short and rapid embryonic pathway leading oogonia into the meiotic prophase. It is clear, however, that the surrounding precursor Sertoli cells play an active role. This is indicated by the fact that XY germ cells which go astray during embryonic migration and arrive in an ectopic location such as the adrenal gland, start meiosis following a female schedule (for review, see Handel and Hunt 1992).

5.3 X and Y Chromosomes During Spermatogenesis

In oocytes the two X chromosomes are transcriptionally active during the meiotic prophase. In marked contrast, the X and Y chromosomes in primary spermatocytes are heterochromatic, forming the so-called sex body, which is first visible at the early pachytene stage of the meiotic prophase. Autoradiographic incorporation studies using radiolabeled uridine have indicated the very low, if any, transcriptional activity of the sex body chromatin (Monesi et al. 1978). Very little is known about the molecular mechanism of sex chromosome inactivation during spermatogenesis, although recent data suggest the presence of the XY-associated proteins XY40 and XY77 (Alsheimer et al. 1997; Kralewski and Benavente 1997; Kralewski et al. 1997). Our own recent data (Baarends et al. 1998) show marked ubiquitination of histone H2A in the sex body (see Sect. 5.8), although it is not yet clear whether this ubiquitination plays an active role in XY inactivation.

Interestingly, extratesticular spermatocytes that enter meiosis during fetal development do not form a sex body, and this suggests a testicular cell-to-cell signal for sex chromatin inactivation in spermatocytes (Handel and Hunt 1992). When spermatocytes do not contain a Y chromosome but yet go through spermatogenesis, such as can occur in XO female mice, the single X chromosome shows an inactive chromatin

configuration (Handel and Hunt 1992), which indicates that the inactivation signal is not generated by the Y chromosome. This is supported
by the observation that there is no stable pairing between the X and Y
chromosomes in oocytes in ovaries of XY female mice, where the two
sex chromosomes segregate at random (Lovell-Badge and Robertson
1990). Hence there is indeed a testicular signal acting on spermatocytes
to induce sex body formation, or, alternatively, it is the specific series of
mitotic spermatogonial divisions which leads to expression of cellular
factors resulting in XY inactivation in the ensuing meiotic prophase.

A known participant in X chromosome inactivation in female somatic cells is RNA transcribed from the *Xist* gene. This RNA does not
encode a protein but rather exerts a direct inhibitory effect on gene
transcription of the X chromosome from which it is transcribed (Kay et
al. 1993; Kuroda and Meller 1997). When *Xist* RNA expression was
found in spermatocytes, this led to the suggestion that the female somatic mechanism of X-chromosome inactivation might also be involved
in X inactivation in spermatocytes (McCarrey and Dilworth 1992).
However, *Xist* RNA is present in spermatogenic cells from type A
spermatogonia up to and including spermatids (McCarrey and Dilworth
1992), whereas X-chromosome inactivation is probably confined to
primary spermatocytes. In spite of the presence of *Xist* RNA in spermatids, we have observed postmeiotic transcriptional activity of the X
chromosome (Hendriksen et al. 1995; see Sect. 5.4). Moreover, the level
of *Xist* RNA in testis is far lower than in female somatic tissues (Kay et
al. 1993). Finally, it has now been shown that *Xist*-deficient mice are
defective in female X-chromosomal dosage compensation, but not in
spermatogenesis (Marahrens et al. 1997). Taken together, it is clear that
Xist RNA expression in the testis does not play a crucial role in sex body
formation. It is possible that *Xist* RNA expression in spermatogenic
cells is related to changes in methylation of the *Xist* gene, in relation to
paternal imprinting of the X chromosome (Norris et al. 1994).

5.4   Postmeiotic Expression of the X and Y Chromosomes

Postmeiotic expression of the X and Y chromosomes, or for that matter
all haploid gene expression, might lead to inequality between spermatozoa. However, it is now well established that the haploid spermatids are

functionally diploid, by sharing mRNAs and proteins through the cytoplasmic bridges which interconnect the spermatogenic cells also after completion of the meiotic divisions (Braun et al. 1989). It is not certain that all gene products are being shared, as indicated by observations on transmission of t-complex mutations (Lyon 1986), but there seems to be no decisive biological reason against transcription of the X and Y chromosomes in spermatids. Indeed, several years ago postmeiotic transcription was reported for two Y-chromosomal genes; *Zfy* (Nagamine et al. 1990) and *Sry* (Capel et al. 1993; Rossi et al. 1993). We have also obtained evidence for postmeiotic transcription of Y-chromosomal genes, *Sry* and *Ube1y*, and in addition transcription of the X chromosome in spermatids was discovered for the genes *Ube1x* and *mHR6A* (Hendriksen et al. 1995).

From the available data it seems that most if not all genes on the Y chromosome are expressed in spermatids. Some of this expression is probably nonfunctional. This is clearest for *Sry* expression because the main transcript in the testis is circular, prohibiting its translation (Capel et al. 1993; Dolci et al. 1997), although it remains to be shown that this circular RNA does not have a function by itself.

Postmeiotic transcription of the X chromosome certainly is much more selective than that of the Y chromosome. Several X-chromosomal genes that are silenced in spermatocytes (*Pgk-1, Pdha-1, G6pd*) are not reactivated in spermatids (Eddy 1995; Hendriksen et al. 1995, 1997).

Intriguingly, the products of the X- and Y-chromosomal genes *Ube1x, Ube1y,* and *mHR6A*, which are expressed in spermatids, are all involved in the ubiquitin system. This system seems to play a prominent role in spermatogenesis (see below).

5.5 The Ubiquitin System in Spermatogenesis

Ubiquitin is a ubiquitous, highly conserved protein of 76 amino acid residues that can be covalently attached to cellular acceptor proteins through a multistep enzymatic process that involves activities of ubiquitin-activating E1 enzymes (such as Ube1x and Ube1y), ubiquitin-conjugating E2 enzymes (such as mHR6A), and ligating E3 enzymes (Fig. 1). Polyubiquitination often marks proteins for selective destruction by the 26-S proteasome, a large multisubunit ATP-dependent pro-

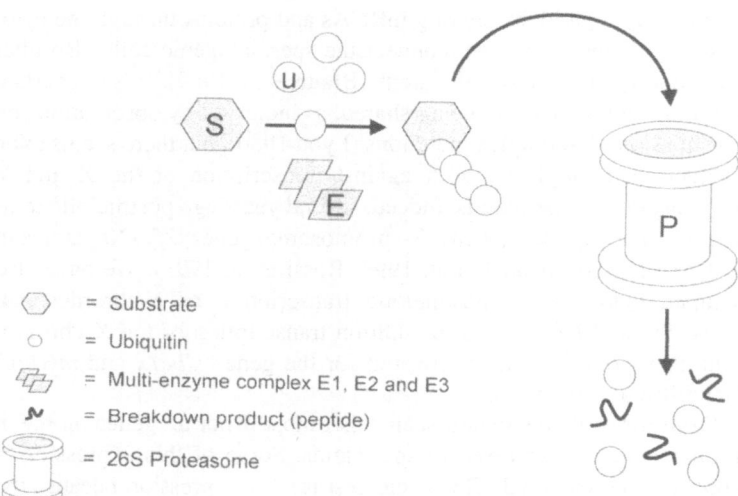

◇   = Substrate

○   = Ubiquitin

▱▱   = Multi-enzyme complex E1, E2 and E3

∿   = Breakdown product (peptide)

⬚   = 26S Proteasome

Fig. 1. Ubiquitin-dependent protein degradation. Ubiquitination of protein substrates generally requires the successive actions of three different enzymes, E1, E2, and E3 (see Sect. 5.5). The enzymes are depicted as a single complex, but this is hypothetical. These activities join the C-terminal carboxyl group of ubiquitin via isopeptide linkage to a lysine ε-amino group of the substrate. Polyubiquitinated proteins are recognized by the 26-S proteasome and de-graded, and intact ubiquitin is released from the peptide fragments. Note: mono- and polyubiquitination may have consequences other than proteolysis, such as functional alteration of the substrate and ligand-mediated endocytosis of integral membrane proteins (for review, see Hochstrasser 1996a,b; Var-shavsky 1997)

tease. In addition, the ubiquitin system has other functions, such as a role in endocytosis of integral membrane proteins and a chaperone function in protein (re)folding (for review, see Varshavsky 1997).

The observation that enzymes from the ubiquitin system are present in spermatogenic cells is not at all surprising in view of the fact that the entire pathway is highly ubiquitous indeed. However, the ubiquitin system in spermatogenic cells seems to have become specialized to meet particular requirements of spermatogenesis.

Whereas *Ube1x* is expressed in many tissues in the mouse, *Ube1y* is expressed only in the testis, and it has been designated a candidate spermatogenesis gene (Kay et al. 1991; Mitchell et al. 1991). Other and recent observations on peculiar aspects of the ubiquitin system in testis from different species, include the following. The level of a ubiquitin-like protein (UBL1) is elevated in human testis (Shen et al. 1996). Expression of ubiquitin itself is high in chicken (Agell and Mezquita 1988) and mammalian (Lanneau and Loir 1982) testis, and testis-specific mRNAs are produced through alternative splicing of a heat shock inducible polyubiquitin gene in chicken (Mezquita et al. 1997). Several ubiquitin-conjugating enzymes show increased or exclusive expression in testis of rat [HR6A and HR6B (Koken et al. 1996), E217 kb (Wing and Jain 1995) and the isoform 8A (Wing et al. 1996)] and human [hUBC9 (Kovalenko et al. 1996; Yasugi et al. 1996), and UbcH-ben (Yamaguchi et al. 1996)]. The same has been reported for a ubiquitin protease in rat (Kajimoto et al. 1992); these proteases release ubiquitin from proteins or peptides.

The findings in this list may be related to the fact that a high turnover of proteins occurs during spermatogenesis, such as the turnover of nuclear proteins during the postmeiotic histone-to-protamine transition (Agell and Mezquita 1988; Oliva and Dixon 1991). This requirement for rapid and massive downregulation of the cellular concentration of proteins could pose a high demand on ubiquitin-dependent proteolysis, carried out by the 26-S proteasome. In *Drosophila* and *Xenopus* the proteasome contains testis-specific subunits that are highly expressed (Fuji et al. 1993; Yuan et al. 1996). An additional possible function of the ubiquitin system in spermatogenesis is related to several recent findings that show involvement of RAD6 (see Sect. 5.7) and the ubiquitin system in aspects of gene silencing (Henchoz et al. 1996; Moazed and Johnson 1996; Huang et al. 1997). Thus ubiquitination of nuclear proteins during spermatogenesis could also play an important role in the regulation of chromatin structure and gene expression.

Recently we have reported that homozygous inactivation of the gene encoding the ubiquitin-conjugating enzyme *mHR6B* (an autosomally encoded isoenzyme of mHR6A) results in male infertility in mice (Roest et al. 1996). To try to explain these observations we first introduce chromatin reorganization during spermatogenesis (see Sect. 5.6) and mHR6A and *mHR6B* (see Sect. 5.7) in more detail.

5.6 Changes in Chromatin Structure
During Spermatogenesis

Extensive activities related to germ cell specific changes in chromatin structure occur during spermatogenesis. First, genomic imprints are erased, and a paternal mode of genomic imprinting is imposed, most likely during the premeiotic phase (Kafri et al. 1992). Second, during the meiotic prophase, homology search of the autosomes, synapsis, and homologous recombination take place (Heyting 1996). In this context, an exciting new area of research in mammals concerns the functions of several proteins of the DNA repair machanisms in meiotic homologous recombination, as revealed by specific infertility phenotypes of knock-out mouse models of the DNA mismatch repair genes *Pms2* and *Mlh1* (Baker et al. 1995, 1996). Also, complex protein-protein interactions detected by immunocytochemistry have visualized meiosis-specific functions of certain proteins involved in DNA repair (Baker et al. 1996; Plug et al. 1996; Barlow et al. 1997; Moens et al. 1997; Scully et al. 1997).

Third, the composition of chromatin in germ cells changes dramatically while they develop from mitotic spermatogonia into meiotic spermatocytes and subsequently into postmeiotic haploid spermatids. In general there are two waves of histone synthesis during the meiotic prophase of male mouse germ cells, first during preleptotene and then during pachytene (Bhatnagar et al. 1985). A number of histone genes are expressed exclusively in male germ cells, and the encoded proteins partially replace their somatic isotypes (Fig. 2). In rat testis, a testis-specific H3 protein is expressed already in spermatogonia. Subsequently, testis-specific tH2A and tH2B start to accumulate in preleptotene spermatocytes, and testis-specific H1t is synthesized in pachytene spermatocytes (Meistrich et al. 1985; Unni et al. 1995a; Drabent et al. 1996). In mouse and rat a second testis-specific H2B gene (ssH2B) is expressed exclusively in postmeiotic spermatids (Moss and Orth 1993; Unni et al. 1995b). Finally, during spermatid development the nucleus elongates and subsequently condenses. This process requires the replacement of nucleosomal histones by transition proteins and subsequently by protamines (Oliva and Dixon 1991; Kistler et al. 1996).

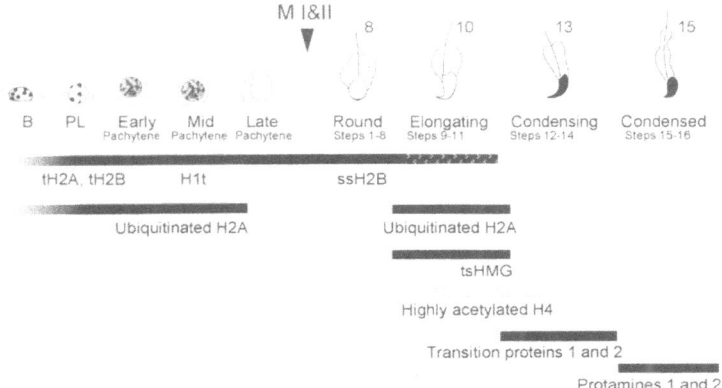

Fig. 2. Histone-to-protamine transition during mouse spermatogenesis. *From left to right*, subsequent stages of germ cell development schematically represent the last step of entry into meiosis and the subsequent meiotic and postmeiotic development. *Bars*, the presence or absence of specific proteins involved in chromatin structure; *upper bar*, the presence of histones, packaged in nucleosomes during spermatogenesis. The onset of expression of various testis-specific histones is shown. Histones remain present until spermatid nuclei have elongated. Then they are efficiently removed (in the mouse; see Sect. 5.9) and replaced by transition proteins and subsequently by protamines (*bars*). The removal of histones is preceded by a marked increase in the immunohisto-chemical detection of tH2B (*patterned region of the histone bar*). The testis-specific tsHMG DNA-binding protein may contribute to changes in chromatin structure through modulation of topoisomerase I activity. *Open bar*, histone H4 hyperacetylation during nuclear elongation indicating that this has been reported for rat germ cells; this has not been studied in the mouse. Ubiquitinated H2A was detected in pachytene spermatocytes, associated with the sex body and the autosomes, and in steps 8–12 spermatids (see Sect. 5.8). *B*, spermatogonium B; *PL*, preleptotene spermatocyte; *MI, MII*, meiotic divisions I and II

In the mouse and the human there are two transition proteins, TP1 and TP2, and two protamines, P1 and P2 (Fig. 2). This drastic histone removal is preceded by a number of posttranslational modifications of histones, such as H4 acetylation, most thoroughly investigated in rat testis (Meistrich et al. 1992). Also, tH2B immunoexpression is enhanced in elongating spermatids of rat and mouse (Unni et al. 1995a; Roest et al. 1996). Furthermore, a testis-specific member of the high mobility group (tsHMG) family of proteins is expressed exclusively during nuclear elongation (Boissonneault and Lau 1993; Alami-Ouahabi et al. 1996). This DNA-binding protein may contribute to changes in chromatin structure through modulation of topoisomerase I activity (Alami-Ouahabi et al. 1996).

The association of protamines with DNA forms linear side-by-side arrays of chromatin. This results in the formation of a nucleus containing tightly compacted DNA, at least six times as compacted as the DNA in mitotic chromosomes (Balhorn 1982; Ward and Coffey 1991). The condensation, and thereby transcriptional inactivation, of the genome in spermatids precedes the shutoff of protein synthesis, and many mRNAs in spermatids are stored and subjected to translational regulation (Hecht 1995; Kleene 1996; Schmidt and Schibler 1997).

5.7   From Yeast to Mouse and Human

The mouse gene *mHR6A* is a highly conserved homologue, structural and functional, of the *Saccharomyces cerevisiae RAD6* gene. In addition to the X-chromosomal *mHR6A* gene, the mouse genome contains an autosomal homologue, the *mHR6B* gene. The mHR6A and mHR6B proteins are almost identical (96% identical amino acid residues). The human genome also contains two genes, X-chromosomal *hHR6A* and autosomal *hHR6B*, and the encoded proteins are 100% identical with the mouse proteins (Koken et al. 1991). In the yeast *Saccharomyces cerevisiae*, RAD6 is required for a variety of cellular functions, including postreplication DNA repair, DNA damage-induced mutagenesis, and sporulation (for review, see Lawrence 1994). Both human genes can complement part of the DNA repair and mutagenesis defect in a yeast *rad6* mutant (Koken et al. 1991). In view of the very strong evolutionary conservation of RAD6/HR6B from yeast to mouse and human it is to be expected that the mammalian homologues are involved in cellular processes that require similar molecular mechanisms.

The *mHR6B* knockout mouse obtained by gene targeting (Roest et al. 1996) is the first mouse model for inactivation of a gene that takes part in the ubiquitin system (Ciechanover 1996). In these mice the impairment of spermatogenesis becomes overt during the postmeiotic condensation of chromatin in spermatids, which involves histone-to-protamine transition (see Sect. 5.6). Also other signs of impairment of the normal function of the spermatogenic epithelium are apparent, such as formation of vacuoles in Sertoli cells, increased apoptosis of spermatocytes, and premature release of immature round germ cells from the epithelium (Roest et al. 1996). It cannot be excluded that these are secondary effects following derailment of nuclear condensation in spermatids. Surprisingly, the effect on spermatogenesis was the only observed phenotypic expression of the gene knockout. Growth and development of male and female knockout mice was found to be normal, and the females show normal ovarian function and fertility.

A role of the mammalian RAD6 homologues in postreplication DNA repair has not yet been found, most likely because mHR6A can compensate for lack of mHR6B in virtually all cell types of the *mHR6B* knockout mice, assuming that the two enzymes have similar specificity. However, spermatogenic cells form an exception in view of the impairment of spermatogenesis in the *mHR6B* knockout mice. This may be explained by the fact that, although the mRNA expression levels of *mHR6A* and *mHR6B* are elevated in testis, the amount of mHR6B protein in spermatids is relatively high compared to the amount of mHR6A protein (Koken et al. 1996). The relative abundance of the B protein occurs in spite of the postmeiotic expression of the X-chromosomal *mHR6A* gene (see Sect. 5.4).

An obvious question at this point is whether the molecular mechanism for impairment of spermatogenesis in *mHR6B* knockout mice is in some way related to the activities of RAD6 in yeast. The *RAD6* epistasis group is involved in what has been called the "pathway for restoration of replication competence" (Lawrence 1994). This system arose early in evolution to overcome the problems associated with replicating a damaged DNA template. Within the process of postreplication repair two subpathways can be discerned. First, an error-prone translesion synthesis mechanism has been described in which replication continues over the damage, taking the risk of making a mistake. This subpathway is responsible for most of the damage-induced mutagenesis. Second, an error-free daughter-strand repair system has been postulated, involving reinitiation of DNA replication downstream of the lesion, followed by filling of the resulting gap by recombination with the duplicated, intact complementary DNA strand. Both subpathways are in fact damage-tolerance mechanisms because the original lesion is not removed, and the RAD6 protein appears to be implicated in both mechanisms.

Since RAD6 can mono- and polyubiquitinate histones in vitro (see Sect. 5.8), one option is that the ubiquitin-conjugating activity of the protein is required for inducing local changes in chromatin structure, in the context of the events described above. Another possibility is that RAD6 functions in assembly and/or disassembly of the replication or recombination machineries at the site of the lesion. The pleiotropic phenotype of *rad6* mutants indicates that the protein is engaged in other processes as well. In particular, the sporulation defect in yeast provides an intriguing parallel with the spermatogenesis abnormalities registered in the *mHR6B* knockout mice.

In view of the high functional conservation the RAD6 homologues mHR6A and mHR6B are probably also involved in postreplication DNA repair. Hence the primary cause of the derailment of spermatogenesis, as is observed in the *mHR6B* knockout mice, may be found in mitotic spermatogonia and/or in the preleptotene spermatocytes in which the last DNA replication of spermatogenesis takes place. However, it is also possible that the role of the mammalian RAD6 homologues in the ubiquitin system in spermatogenesis concerns some other aspect(s) of chromatin restructuring.

As a working hypothesis we have postulated that mHR6B plays an important role in particular in postmeiotic chromatin reorganization in condensing spermatids. As a first step in trying to provide evidence for this hypothesis we have studied histone ubiquitination during mouse spermatogenesis.

5.8 Histone Ubiquitination in Spermatocytes and Spermatids

It has been shown that the yeast and rabbit RAD6 proteins can ubiquitinate histone H2A and, to a lesser extent, H2B in vitro (Haas et al. 1991). Two prominent types of histone modifications have been documented during spermatogenesis. In rat spermatids the occurrence of highly acetylated H4 is associated with histone displacement (Meistrich et al. 1992). Furthermore, during chicken and trout spermatogenesis the presence of ubiquitinated histones has been detected at late stages when nucleosomes are disassembled (Agell et al. 1983; Oliva and Dixon

1991). To investigate the role of histone ubiquitination during mouse spermatogenesis and the possible function of mHR6A and/or mHR6B therein we have started a study on histone ubiquitination in mouse testis.

It was observed that ubiquitinated histone H2A (uH2A) represents the major ubiquitinated histone species in mouse testis (Baarends et al. 1998). This conclusion is based on sodium dodecyl sulfate polyacrylamide gel electrophoresis/western blot analysis of basic nuclear proteins isolated from total testis of 30-day-old mice using a polyclonal antibody directed against ubiquitin and a monoclonal antibody that specifically recognizes uH2A.

The cellular localization of testicular uH2A was studied by immunohistochemistry, using the monoclonal anti-uH2A on formaldehyde-fixed testis tissue sections. A marked and distinct staining pattern was observed during the meiotic prophase. In early pachytene spermatocytes uH2A was first observed in a specific subregion located at the nuclear periphery. This region most likely represents the sex body, containing the heterochromatic X and Y chromosomes (see Sect. 5.3), which was confirmed using cytological preparations of the spermatocytes. In addition, during midpachytene, a granular pattern of anti-uH2A staining covering the autosomes became visible. Late pachytene spermatocytes lost most of the signal, and finally also the sex body became uH2A negative. No staining was apparent during diplotene and the subsequent meiotic divisions. Postmeiotically uH2A was observed only in nuclei of steps 8–12 elongating spermatids (Baarends et al. 1998; Fig. 2).

In somatic cells of many species approximately 10% of histone H2A and not more than 2% of H2B are ubiquitinated (West and Bonner 1980). The function of histone ubiquitination in somatic cells is not clear. There are some indications that histone ubiquitination results in destabilization of the H2A-H2B dimer, which may facilitate replacement by newly synthesized histones and/or potentiate DNA transcription (Li et al. 1993). Similarly, histone ubiquitination in steps 8–12 spermatids may be involved in replacement of histones by transition proteins (Fig. 2). As yet it is unknown whether there is a major defect in histone ubiquitination in spermatogenic cells in the testis of the *mHR6B* knockout mice. In view of the severe impairment of spermatogenesis, in particular spermiogenesis, in the *mHR6B* knockout mice, this is difficult to study. Moreover, it is important to note that mHR6A and mHR6B may not be the only ubiquitin-conjugating E2 enzymes involved in histone ubiquitination during spermatogenesis (see Sect. 5.5). Eventually the ubiquitin system will prove to be involved in many different aspects of posttranslational regulation of protein function during spermatogenesis.

5.9 Concluding Remarks

Readers may ask: what is the relevance of data on the mouse for our understanding of human male fertility and infertility? There is no short answer to that question, but we can indicate the following. As discussed above, many of the genes involved in the spermatogenic machinery are highly conserved in evolution. The mouse and human *HR6A* and *HR6B* genes are a special example, by encoding proteins showing 100% mouse/human identity. The *mHR6B* knockout mice still produce a small number of spermatozoa which show a wide range of morphological abnormalities (Roest et al. 1996), resembling oligo-astheno-teratozoospermia as is often observed in infertile human males. Furthermore, male fertility is not compromised in *mHR6B* heterozygote –/+ male mice, and also not in female –/– mice, which implies that an inactivating mutation of the *mHR6B* gene can be easily transmitted. Taken together, it is worthwhile to evaluate whether some male infertility patients carry homozygous mutations in the hHR6B gene.

Another point related to chromatin reorganization during spermatogenesis in human is that chromatin packaging in human spermatozoa shows marked intersperm and interindividual variation, with persistence of variable amounts of histones in the protamine/DNA complex (Gatewood et al. 1987, 1990; Manicardi et al. 1995; Bianchi et al. 1996; Roijen et al. 1998). It seems that overall the histone-to-protamine replacement process in human spermatids is less complete than what is observed in experimental animals such as rat and mouse. The partial persistence of histones in human spermatozoa might play a functional role, for example, in reactivation of the male haploid genome in the male pronucleus upon fertilization of the ovum. However, it can also be suggested that persistence of histones in spermatozoa is a negative hallmark of sperm quality because it may result in poor chromatin packaging and enhanced genome instability. For mouse and human spermatozoa a correlation has been reported between chromatin packaging and the occurrence of DNA nicks (Manicardi et al. 1995; Sakkas et al. 1995).

Hence gene expression and chromatin structure during spermatogenesis offer an exciting area for basic research, and the outcome of this research is relevant in the context of our understanding of human male fertility and infertility.

References

Agell N, Mezquita C (1988) Cellular content of ubiquitin and formation of ubiquitin conjugates during chicken spermatogenesis. Biochem J 250:883–889

Agell N, Chiva M, Mezquita C (1983) Changes in nuclear content of protein conjugate histone H2A-ubiquitin during rooster spermatogenesis. FEBS Lett 155:209–212

Alami-Ouahabi N, Veilleux S, Meistrich ML, Boissonneault G (1996) The testis-specific high-mobility-group protein, a phosphorylation-dependent DNA-packaging factor of elongating and condensing spermatids. Mol Cell Biol 16:3720–3729

Alsheimer M, Imamichi Y, Heid H, Benavente R (1997) Molecular characterization and expression pattern of XY body-associated protein XY40 of the rat. Chromosoma 106:308–314

Baarends WM, Roest HP, Hoogerbrugge JW, Vreeburg JTM, Hoeijmakers JHJ, Grootegoed JA (1998) Chromatin remodeling during spermatogenesis is reflected by changes in the nuclear deposition of ubiquitinated H2A in mice. Miniposter, 10th European Workshop on Molecular and Cellular Endocrinology of the Testis, Capri, Italy

Baker SM, Bronner CE, Zhang L, Plug AW, Robatzek M, Warren G, Elliott EA, Yu J, Ashley T, Arnheim N, Flavell RA, Liskay RM (1995) Male mice defective in the DNA mismatch repair gene PMS2 exhibit abnormal chromosome synapsis in meiosis. Cell 82:309–319

Baker SM, Plug AW, Prolla TA, Bronner CE, Harris AC, Yao X, Christie DM, Monell C, Arnheim N, Bradley A, Ashley T, Liskay RM (1996) Involvement of mouse Mlh1 in DNA mismatch repair and meiotic crossing over. Nat Genet 13:336–342

Balhorn R (1982) A model for the structure of chromatin in mammalian sperm. J Cell Biol 93:298–305

Barlow AL, Benson FE, West SC, Hulten MA (1997) Distribution of the Rad51 recombinase in human and mouse spermatocytes. EMBO J 16:5207–5215

Bhatnagar YM, Romrell LJ, Bellvé AR (1985) Biosynthesis of specific histones during meiotic prophase of mouse spermatogenesis. Biol Reprod 32:599–609

Bianchi PG, Manicardi GC, Umer F, Campana A, Sakkas D (1996) Chromatin packaging and morphology in ejaculated human spermatozoa: evidence of hidden anomalies in normal spermatozoa. Mol Hum Reprod 2:139–144

Boissonneault G, Lau Y-FC (1993) A testis-specific gene encoding a nuclear high-mobility-group box protein located in elongating spermatids. Mol Cell Biol 13:4323–4330

Braun RE, Behringer RR, Peschon JJ, Brinster RL, Palmiter RD (1989) Genetically haploid spermatids are phenotypically diploid. Nature 337:373–376

Capel B, Swain A, Nicolis S, Hacker A, Walter M, Koopman P, Goodfellow P, Longfellow P, Lovell-Badge R (1993) Circular transcripts of the testis-determining gene Sry in adult mouse testis. Cell 73:1019–1030

Ciechanover A (1996) Ubiquitin-mediated proteolysis and male sterility. Nat Med 2:1188–1190

Drabent B, Bode C, Bramlage B, Doenecke D (1996) Expression of the mouse testicular histone H1t during spermatogenesis. Histochem Cell Biol 106:247–251

Dolci S, Grimaldi P, Geremia R, Pesce M, Rossi P (1997) Identification of a promoter region generating Sry circular transcripts both in germ cells from male adult mice and in male mouse embryonal gonads. Biol Reprod 57:1128–1135

Eddy EM (1995) 'Chauvinist genes' of male germ cells: gene expression during mouse spermatogenesis. Reprod Fertil Dev 7:695–704

Fleischman RA (1993) From white spots to stem cells: the role of the Kit receptor in mammalian development. Trends Genet 9:285–290

Fuji G, Tashiro K, Emori Y, Saiko K, Shiokawa K (1993) Molecular cloning of cDNAs for two Xenopus proteasome subunits and their expression in adult tissues. Biochim Biophys Acta 1216:65–72

Gatewood JM, Cook GR, Balhorn R, Bradbury EM, Schmid CW (1987) Sequence specific packaging of DNA in human sperm chromatin. Science 236:962–964

Gatewood JM, Cook GR, Balhorn R, Schmid CW, Bradbury EM (1990) Isolation of four core histones from human sperm chromatin representing a minor subset of somatic histones. J Biol Chem 265:20662–20666

Grootegoed JA (1996) The testis: spermatogenesis. In: Hillier SG, Kitchener HC, Neilson JP (eds) Scientific essentials of reproductive medicine. Saunders, Philadelphia, pp 172–184

Haas AL, Reback PB, Chau V (1991) Ubiquitin conjugation by the yeast RAD6 and CDC34 gene products. Comparison to their putative rabbit homologs, E2 (20 K) and E2 (32 K). J Biol Chem 15:5104–5112

Handel MA, Hunt PA (1992) Sex-chromosome pairing and activity during mammalian meiosis. BioEssays 14:817–822

Hecht NB (1995) The making of a spermatozoon: a molecular perspective. Dev Gen 16:95–103

Henchoz S, Rubertis D, Pauli D, Spierer P (1996) The dose of a putative ubiquitin-specific protease affects position-effect variegation in Drosophila melanogaster. Mol Cell Biol 16:5717–5725

Hendriksen PJM, Hoogerbrugge JW, Themmen APN, Koken MHM, Hoeijmakers JHJ, Oostra BA, Lende T van der, Grootegoed JA (1995) Post-meiotic transcription of X and Y chromosomal genes during spermatogenesis in the mouse. Dev Biol 170:730–733

Hendriksen PJM, Hoogerbrugge JW, Baarends WM, Boer P de, Vreeburg JTM, Vos EA, Lende T van der, Grootegoed JA (1997) Testis-specific expression of a functional retroposon encoding glucose-6-phosphate dehydrogenase in the mouse. Genomics 41:350–359

Heyting C (1996) Synaptonemal complexes: structure and function. Curr Opin Cell Biol 8:389–396

Hochstrasser M (1996a) Protein degradation or regulation: Ub the judge. Cell 84:813–815

Hochstrasser M (1996b) Ubiquitin-dependent protein degradation. Annu Rev Genet 30:405–439

Huang H, Kahana A, Gottschling DE, Prakash L, Liebman SW (1997) The ubiquitin-conjugating enzyme Rad6 (Ubc2) is required for silencing in Saccharomyces cerevisiae. Mol Cell Biol 17:6693–6699

Kafri T, Ariel M, Brandeis M, Shemer R, Urven L, McCarrey J, Cedar H, Razin A (1992) Developmental pattern of gene-specific DNA methylation in the mouse embryo and germ line. Genes Dev 6:705–714

Kajimoto Y, Hashimoto T, Shirai Y, Nishino N, Kuno T, Tanaka C (1992) cDNA cloning and tissue distribution of a rat ubiquitin carboxyl-terminal hydrolase PGP9.5. J Biochem 112:28–32

Kay GF, Ashworth A, Penny GD, Dunlop M, Swift S, Brockdorff N, Rastan S (1991) A candidate spermatogenesis gene on the mouse Y chromosome is homologous to ubiquitin-activating enzyme E1. Nature 354:486–489

Kay GF, Penny GD, Patel D, Ashworth A, Brockdorff N, Rastan S (1993) Expression of Xist during mouse development suggest a role in the initiation of X chromosome inactivation. Cell 72:171–182

Kistler WS, Henriksen K, Mali P, Parvinen M (1996) Sequential expression of nucleoproteins during rat spermiogenesis. Exp Cell Res 225:374–381

Kleene KC (1996) Patterns of translational regulation in the mammalian testis. Mol Reprod Dev 43:268–281

Koken MHM, Reynolds P, Jaspers-Dekker I, Prakash L, Prakash S, Bootsma D, Hoeijmakers JHJ (1991) Structural and functional conservation of two human homologs of the yeast DNA repair gene RAD6. Proc Natl Acad Sci USA 88:8865–8869

Koken MHM, Hoogerbrugge JW, Jaspers-Dekker I, Wit J de, Willemsen R, Roest HP, Grootegoed JA, Hoeijmakers JHJ (1996) Expression of the ubiquitin-conjugating DNA repair enzymes HHR6A and B suggests a role in spermatogenesis and chromatin modification. Dev Biol 173:119–132

Koopman P, Gubbay J, Vivian N, Goodfellow P, Lovell-Badge R (1991) Male development of chromosomally female mice transgenic for Sry. Nature 351:117–121

Kovalenko OV, Plug AW, Haaf T, Gonda DK, Ashley T, Ward DC, Radding CM, Golub EI (1996) Mammalian ubiquitin-conjugating enzyme Ubc9 interacts with Rad51 recombination protein and localizes in synaptonemal complexes. Proc Natl Acad Sci USA 93:2958–2963

Kralewski M, Benavente R (1997) XY body formation during rat spermatogenesis: an immunocytochemical study using antibodies against XY body-associated proteins. Chromosoma 106:304–307

Kralewski M, Novello A, Benavente R (1997) A novel Mr 77,000 protein of the XY body of mammalian spermatocytes: its localization in normal animals and in Searle's translocation carriers. Chromosoma 106:160–167

Kuroda MI, Meller VH (1997) Transient Xist-ence. Cell 91:9–11

Lanneau M, Loir M (1982) An electrophoretic investigation of mammalian spermatid-specific nuclear proteins. J Reprod Fertil 65:163–170

Lawrence C (1994) The RAD6 DNA repair pathway in Saccharomyces cerevisiae: what does it do, and how does it do it? Bioessays 16:253–258

Li W, Nagaraja S, Delcuve GP, Hendzel J, Davie JR (1993) Effects of histone acetylation, ubiquitination and variants on nucleosome stability. Biochem J 296:737–744

Lovell-Badge R, Robertson E (1990) XY female mice resulting from a heritable mutation in the primary testis-determining gene Tdy. Development 109:635–646

Lyon MF (1986) Male sterility of the mouse t-complex is due to homozygosity of the distorter genes. Cell 44:357–363

Manicardi GC, Bianchi PG, Pantano S, Azzoni P, Bizzaro D, Bianchi U, Sakkas D (1995) Presence of endogenous nicks in DNA of ejaculated human spermatozoa and its relationship to chromomycin A3 accessibility. Biol Reprod 52:864–867

Marahrens Y, Panning B, Dausmán J, Strauss W, Jaenisch R (1997) Xist-deficient mice are defective in dosage compensation but not spermatogenesis. Gen Dev 11:156–166

McCarrey JR, Dilworth DD (1992) Expression of Xist in mouse germ cells correlates with X-chromosome inactivation. Nat Genet 2:200–203

Meistrich ML, Bucci LR, Trostle-Weige PK, Brock WA (1985) Histone variants in rat spermatogonia and primary spermatocytes. Dev Biol
112:230–240

Meistrich ML, Trostle-Weige PK, Lin R, Bhatnagar YM, Allis CD (1992)
Highly acetylated H4 is associated with histone displacement in rat spermatids. Mol Reprod Dev 31:170–181

Mezquita J, Pau M, Mezquita C (1997) Heat-shock inducible polyubiquitin
gene UBI undergoes alternative initiation and alternative splicing in mature
chicken testes. Mol Reprod Dev 46:471–475

Mitchell MJ, Woods DR, Tucker PK, Opp JS, Bishop CE (1991) Homology of
a candidate spermatogenic gene from the mouse Y chromosome to the
ubiquitin-activating enzyme E1. Nature 354:484–486

Moazed D, Johnson AD (1996) A deubiquitinating enzyme interacts with SIR4
and regulates silencing in S. cerevisiae. Cell 86:667–677

Moens PB, Chen DJ, Shen Z, Kolas N, Tarsounas M, Heng HHQ, Spyropoulos
B (1997) Rad51 immunocytology in rat and mouse spermatocytes and oocytes. Chromosoma 106:207–215

Monesi V, Geremia R, D'Agostino, Boitani C (1978) Biochemistry of male
germ cell differentiation in mammals: RNA synthesis in meiotic and postmeiotic cells. Current Topics Developm Biol 12:11–36

Moss SB, Orth JM (1993) Localization of a spermatid-specific histone 2B protein in mouse spermiogenic cells. Biol Reprod 48:1047–1056

Nagamine CM, Chan K, Hake LE, Lau Y-FC (1990) The two candidate testis-
determining Y genes (Zfy-1 and Zfy-2) are differentially expressed in fetal
and adult mouse tissues. Genes Dev 4:63–74

Norris DP, Patel D, Kay GF, Penny GD, Brockdorff N, Sheardown SA, Rastan
S (1994) Evidence that random and imprinted Xist expression is controlled
by preemptive methylation. Cell 77:41–51

Oliva R, Dixon GH (1991) Vertebrate protamine genes and the histone-to-protamine replacement reaction. Progr Nucl Acid Res Mol Biol 40:25–94

Plug AW, Xu J, Reddy G, Golub EI, Ashley T (1996) Presynaptic association
of Rad51 protein with selected sites in meiotic chromatin. Proc Natl Acad
Sci USA 11:5920–5924

Roest HP, Klaveren J van, Wit J de, Gurp CG van, Koken MHM, Vermey M,
Roijen JH van, Vreeburg JTM, Baarends WM, Bootsma D, Grootegoed JA,
Hoeijmakers JHJ (1996) Inactivation of the HR6B ubiquitin-conjugating
DNA repair enzyme in mice causes a defect in spermatogenesis associated
with chromatin modification. Cell 86:799–810

Roijen JH van, Ooms MP, Spaargaren M, Baarends WM, Weber RFA, Grootegoed JA, Vreeburg JTM (1998) Immunoexpression of testis-specific histone
2B (TH2B) in human spermatozoa and testis tissue. Human Reprod (in the
press)

Rossi P, Dolci S, Albanesi C, Grimaldi P, Geremia R (1993) Direct evidence that the mouse sex-determining gene Sry is expressed in the somatic cells of male fetal gonads and in the germ cell line in the adult testis. Mol Reprod Dev 34:369–373

Sakkas D, Manicardi G, Bianchi PG, Bizzaro D, Bianchi U (1995) Relationship between the presence of endogenous nicks and sperm chromatin packaging in maturing and fertilizing mouse spermatozoa. Biol Reprod 52:1149–1155

Schmidt EE, Schibler U (1997) Developmental testis-specific regulation of mRNA levels and mRNA translational efficiencies for TATA-binding protein mRNA isoforms. Dev Biol 184:138–149

Scully R, Chen J, Plug AW, Xiao Y, Weaver D, Feunteun J, Ashley T, Livingston DM (1997) Association of BRCA1 with Rad51 in mitotic and meiotic cells. Cell 88:265–275

Shen Z, Pardington-Purtymun P, Comeaux JC, Moyzis RK, Chen DJ (1996) UBL1, a human ubiquitin-like protein associating with human RAD51/RAD52 proteins. Genomics 36:271–279

Unni E, Mayerhofer A, Zhang Y, Bhatnagar YM, Russell LD, Meistrich ML (1995a) Increased accessibility of the N-terminus of testis-specific histone TH2B to antibodies in elongating spermatids. Mol Reprod Dev 42:210–219

Unni E, Zhang Y, Kangasniemi M, Saperstein W, Moss SB, Meistrich ML (1995b) Stage-specific distribution of the spermatid-specific histone 2B in the rat testis. Biol Reprod 53:820–826

Varshavsky A (1997) The ubiquitin system. Trends Biochem Sci 22:383–387

Ward WS, Coffey DS (1991) DNA packaging and organization in mammalian spermatozoa: comparison with somatic cells. Biol Reprod 44:569–574

West MHP, Bonner WM (1980) Histone 2A, a heteromorphous family of eight protein species. Biochemistry 19:3238–3245

Wing SS, Bédard, Morales C, Hingamp P, Trasler J (1996) A novel rat homolog of the Saccharomyces cerevisiae ubiquitin-conjugating enzymes UBC4 en UBC5 with distinct biochemical features is induced during spermatogenesis. Mol Cell Biol 16:4064–4072

Wing S, Jain P (1995) Molecular cloning, expression, and characterization of a ubiquitin conjugating enzyme (E217kB) highly expressed in rat testis. Biochem J 305:125–132

Yamaguchi T, Kim N-S, Sekine S, Seino H, Osaka F, Yamao F, Kato S (1996) Cloning and expression of cDNA encoding a human ubiquitin-conjugating enzyme similar to the Drosophila bendless gene product. J Biochem 120:494–497

Yasugi T, Howley PM (1996) Identification of the structural and functional human homolog of the yeast ubiquitin-conjugating enzyme UBC9. Nucl Acids Res 24:2005–2010

Yuan X, Miller M, Belote JM (1996) Duplicated proteasome subunit genes in Drosophila melanogaster encoding testes-specific isoforms. Genetics 144:147–157

6 The Control of Testis ACE Expression

K.E. Bernstein and E. Bernstein

6.1 Introduction

The renin-angiotensin system was first discovered by Tigerstedt and Bergman in 1898. These experiments, and the work of Goldblatt et al. in 1934, investigated the role of the renin-angiotensin system in blood pressure control. Since then many laboratories have described the biochemistry by which the protein angiotensinogen is converted into the eight amino acid peptide angiotensin II. The final step in this process, the conversion of the decapeptide precursor angiotensin I into angiotensin II, is catalyzed by angiotensin-converting enzyme (ACE), a dipeptidyl carboxypeptidase (Corvol et al. 1995).

The important role of angiotensin II in blood pressure control led to the development of orally active pharmaceutical inhibitors of ACE. These drugs are now used throughout the world to treat human hypertension, heart failure, and progressive renal disease. Indeed, a variety of data support the idea that the physiological actions of the renin-angiotensin system are more complex than simple blood pressure control. In particular, a unique isozyme of ACE which is made by developing male germ cells appears to play a critical role in male fertility. This isozyme, termed testis ACE, has been studied in ACE-deficient mice; male ACE-deficient animals produce far smaller litters than wild-type mice.

6.2 Somatic ACE

ACE is made by a number of different tissues, including vascular endothelium, renal proximal tubular epithelium, ciliated gut epithelium, and in areas of the brain (Corvol et al. 1995). The ACE isozyme produced by these tissues is identical and is referred to as somatic ACE. ACE is enzymatically promiscuous, and many small peptides in addition to angiotensin I can be cleaved. Other known ACE substrates include bradykinin, enkephalins, neurotensin, substance P, and gonadotropin-releasing hormone.

The cloning of somatic ACE showed that it is a single polypeptide chain containing two homologous domains and two distinct catalytic regions (Soubrier et al. 1988; Bernstein et al. 1989). Both catalytic sites of ACE use zinc, and both catalyze the conversion of angiotensin I to angiotensin II with roughly equal affinities. Other natural substrates, however, are cleaved preferentially by one of the catalytic centers. In the mouse, somatic ACE is synthesized as a 1312 amino acid precursor protein containing a 34 amino acid signal sequence at the amino-terminus. Somatic ACE is an ectoenzyme in which the majority of the protein is extracellular, but ACE remains bound to the cell membrane by a carboxyl-terminal hydrophobic anchor sequence.

6.3 Testis ACE

In 1971 Cushman and Cheung identified a unique form of ACE found within the testis of the rat. While this enzyme is catalytic and able to convert angiotensin I into angiotensin II, it is only about half the size of the somatic ACE protein found in the lung or the kidney. Testis ACE is expressed by postmeiotic male germ cells; high-level expression is found in round and elongating spermatids at step 10 and beyond (Langford et al. 1993). Purification of the enzyme showed it to be approximately 90–110 kDa. cDNA encoding testis ACE was first isolated in 1989 (Ehlers et al. 1989; Kumar et al. 1989; Lattion et al. 1989). These studies showed that testis ACE is identical to the carboxyl domain of somatic ACE with the exception that the amino-terminal 66 amino acids are unique to the testis isozyme. Thus, testis ACE contains only a single catalytic domain and binds a single molecule of zinc.

Southern blot analysis established that both testis ACE and somatic ACE arise from a single genetic locus. In 1990, Howard et al. demonstrated that transcription of testis ACE begins in the 12th intron of the somatic *ACE* gene. The first exon of testis ACE is treated as intronic DNA by somatic tissues. The remainder of the testis ACE protein corresponds to exons 13 through 25 of somatic ACE. Thus it is the unique transcriptional start site that gives rise to a germ cell isozyme containing only the carboxyl-terminal half of the somatic protein. The start of testis ACE 7 kb downstream from the transcription start site of somatic ACE led to the hypothesis that the *ACE* gene contains a testis-specific promoter. To investigate this, Langford et al. (1991) used a transgenic mouse approach in which a 700-bp region of genomic DNA immediately upstream of the start of testis ACE transcription was placed 5' of a *LacZ* reporter construct. Transgenic mice were made with the construct, and the capacity of different tissues to recognize the putative promoter region was tested by measuring β-galactosidase activity. The mice bearing the transgenic construct produced elevated levels of β-galactosidase uniquely in the testis. Histochemical analysis in these animals showed reporter gene expression in the identical cells that express testis ACE, namely round and elongating spermatids. Subsequent work showed that as little as 91 bp genomic DNA taken from the region immediately upstream of the start of testis ACE transcription is sufficient to target reporter gene expression to male germ cells in transgenic mice (Howard et al. 1992). The testis ACE promoter is highly active, and male germ cells produce an abundant amount of testis ACE mRNA and protein. No other tissue has been described as making even small amounts of this gene product. Thus, the testis ACE promoter is a relatively small portion of DNA that directs high-level gene expression in a highly tissue-specific fashion.

A number of in vivo and in vitro studies suggest that the testis ACE promoter contains two important protein-binding DNA motifs (Zhou et al. 1995). One motif is at position −32 relative to the start of testis ACE transcription. This sequence, TCTTAT, while not bearing a great deal of homology to a consensus TATA sequence, appears nevertheless to bind the transcription factor TFIID (Zhou et al. 1996a). A second critical motif is found at position −55. Here the 8-bp motif TGAGGTCA is quite similar to a consensus cAMP response element (CRE) binding site (TGACGTCA). Analysis of these two transcriptional motifs using the technique of in vitro transcription suggested that both DNA motifs are necessary for full testis ACE expression; promoter constructs containing only one of the two motifs were approximately one-third as active as the parent construct in the transcriptional assay (Zhou et al. 1995). Our group has studied mice transgenic for a testis ACE promoter construct in which the endogenous TATA box (TCTTAT) was replaced with a consensus TATA sequence TATAAA (Zhou et al. 1996a). In these animals the pattern of reporter gene expression was identical to that observed in transgenic mice bearing the wild-type testis ACE promoter. Thus the precise sequence of the −32 motif does not appear to specify tissue-specific expression.

We have also used transgenic mice to examine the in vivo role of the −55 motif (Esther et al. 1997a). In vitro analysis had suggested that a single A to G point mutation at position −48, made the element less similar to the consensus CRE-binding site and markedly reduced the transcriptional activity of the testis ACE promoter. When tested in transgenic mice, this same change totally abolished the activity of the testis ACE promoter. Surprisingly, when transgenic mice were prepared with a testis ACE promoter construct in which the testis ACE −55 motif was mutated to the consensus CRE sequence TGACGTCA, we observed a pattern of expression identical to that of the wild-type testis ACE promoter. Thus, at present, the exact biochemical signals specifying germ cell specific utilization of the testis ACE promoter are not fully understood.

In 1993, Delmas et al. described a cAMP response element modifier (CREM) family of transcription factors. One isoform in this family, CREMτ, is expressed at high levels only in developing male germ cells. In contrast to many CREM isoforms, CREMτ is a transcriptional activator, and gel shift studies show that CREMτ is capable of binding to the CRE-like sequence at position −55 of the testis ACE promoter (Zhou et al. 1996b). We have also observed that adding anti-CREM antibody to a testis nuclear extract inhibits the in vitro transcription of the testis ACE promoter in a dose-dependent fashion. Further, transfection experiments using JEG-3 cells have shown that maximal transcriptional efficiency of the testis ACE promoter is achieved when this promoter is cotransfected with the genes encoding CREMτ and protein kinase A. Thus several different approaches suggest an important role of the testis specific transcription factor CREMτ in testis ACE expression.

6.4 Knockout Mice

While progress was made rapidly in understanding the molecular biology of testis ACE transcription, the question remained as to whether the testis specific ACE isozyme plays any physiological role. To investigate this we collaborated with Dr. Mario Capecchi, Howard Hughes Medical Institute at the University of Utah, to create mice with defined changes in the *ACE* gene. These animals were prepared using the technique of targeted homologous recombination in embryonic stem cells. Our group has reported on two separate lines of mice termed ACE.1 and ACE.2. The ACE.1 animals are null for ACE expression; they lack the expression of both somatic and testis ACE (Esther et al. 1996). In contrast, ACE.2 animals have ACE activity circulating in the plasma (Esther et al. 1997b). These animals are unique in that they neither express the tissue bound form of somatic ACE nor do they produce the testis ACE isozyme. Both strains of mice present with the similar phenotype of low blood pressure and an inability to concentrate urine. ACE.1 mice also present with a kidney lesion characterized by marked underdevelopment of the renal medulla and papillae. While the ACE.2 animals have subtle abnormalities in renal structure, they demonstrate a normal development of the renal medulla and papillae.

Both the ACE.1 and ACE.2 strains of mice were created such that they lack the 91-bp testis ACE promoter. This results in the absolute lack of testis ACE expression as measured by both western blot analysis and tissue ACE enzyme activity. Surprisingly, histological study of the testis showed a normal pattern of male germ cell development. Study of sperm motility from ACE knockout mice also showed no differences from wild-type controls. However, male knockout animals from both the ACE.1 and ACE.2 strains have a marked reproductive defect. This was found by mating homozygous mutant male mice with superovulated,

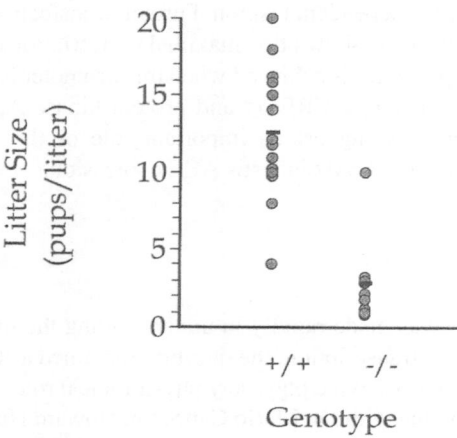

Fig. 1. Decreased fertility of male mice lacking ACE. The fertility of male mice homozygous for the ACE.1 and ACE.2 mutations was tested by mating these animals with wild-type superovulated female mice. The females were killed, and the litter size was determined 18 days after plugging (–/–). As a control we performed the same experiment with littermate wild-type male mice (+/+). While wild-type male mice sire litters in excess of 12 pups, ACE knockout males produce litters that average three pups

wild-type female mice. In this situation a wild-type male mouse sires litters in excess of ten pups. In contrast, the homozygous mutant male animals produce far smaller litters, often containing one or two pups (Fig. 1). In summary, male mice lacking testis ACE can plug females and produce some offspring, but their fertility is markedly lower than wild-type mice. Interestingly, female mice lacking all ACE appear to reproduce in normal fashion when mated to wild-type males.

Several groups have now created and studied angiotensinogen knockout mice (Tanimoto et al. 1994; Kim et al. 1995; Niimura et al. 1996). These animals, which lack all angiotensin II, are similar to the ACE knockout animals in that they present with very low systolic blood pressures and a renal lesion. While the overall health of the angiotensinogen knockout animals appears more compromised than that of the ACE knockout mice, it seems that these animals are capable of reproducing in an uncompromised fashion. This divergence in phenotypes between the angiotensinogen and ACE knockout animals suggests that testis ACE operates on a peptide different from angiotensin I.

In addition to the lack of testis ACE, the knockout mice studied by our group have defects in somatic ACE expression. This phenotype complicates the precise assignment of the fertility defect. We predict that animals lacking only the somatic form of ACE will have normal male reproductive fertility. Tatei et al. (1995) have reported the isolation and characterization of an ACE gene from *Drosophilia* that they call *Race*. The Race protein is 615 amino acids, approximately half the size of somatic ACE, and is thus similar to the mammalian testis ACE isozyme in containing a single catalytic domain. Transheterozygotes for two different lethal alleles of the *Race* gene exhibit male sterility. This finding correlates with results from our studies of knockout mice.

6.5 Conclusion

The study of testis ACE demonstrates that this protein is found only in developing male germ cells. It is the result of a germ cell specific promoter located within the 12th intron of the ACE gene. This promoter is very small; yet in the proper biochemical milieu it is capable of marked transcriptional activity. These features suggest that an understanding of testis ACE expression by phenotypically differentiated cells may yield great insight into the control of gene expression in a tissue-specific fashion.

The study of ACE knockout mice suggests that testis ACE plays a crucial role in male fertility. The lack of the enzyme is associated with a marked reduction in litter size. This does not appear to be the result of a motility deficit. Further investigations are necessary to define the precise physiological role of the testis ACE isoform in reproduction.

112 K.E. Bernstein and E. Bernstein

References

Bernstein KE, Martin BM, Edwards AS, Bernstein EA (1989) Mouse angiotensin I-converting enzyme is a protein composed of two homologous domains. J Biol Chem 264:11945–11951

Corvol P, Williams TA, Soubrier F (1995) Peptidyl dipeptidase A: angiotensin I-converting enzyme. Methods Enzymol 248:283–305

Cushman DW, Cheung HS (1971) Concentrations of angiotensin-converting enzyme in tissues of the rat. Biochim Biophys Acta 250:261–265

Delmas V, van der Hoorn F, Mellstrom B, Jegou B, Sassone-Corsi P (1993) Induction of CREM activator proteins in spermatids: down-stream targets and implications for haploid germ cell differentiation. Mol Endocrinol 7:1502–1514

Ehlers MR, Fox EA, Strydom DJ, Riordan JF (1989) Molecular cloning of human testicular angiotensin-converting enzyme: the testis isozyme is identical to the C-terminal half of endothelial angiotensin-converting enzyme. Proc Natl Acad Sci USA 86:7741–7745

Esther CR Jr, Howard TE, Marino EM, Goddard JM, Capecchi MR, Bernstein KE (1996) Mice lacking angiotensin-converting enzyme have low blood pressure, renal pathology and reduced male fertility. Lab Invest 74:953–965

Esther CR Jr, Marino EM, Howard TE, Corvol P, Capecchi MR, Bernstein KE (1997a) The critical role of tissue angiotensin converting enzyme (ACE) as revealed by gene targeting in mice. J Clin Invest 99:2375–2385

Esther CR Jr, Semeniuk D, Marino EM, Zhou Y, Overbeek PA, Bernstein KE (1997b) Expression of testis angiotensin-converting enzyme is mediated by a cyclic AMP response element. Lab Invest 77:483–488

Goldblatt H, Lynch J, Hanzal RF, Summerville WW (1934) Studies on experimental hypertension. I. The production and persistent elevation of systolic blood pressure by means of renal ischemia. J Exp Med 59:347–380

Howard TE, Shai S-Y, Langford KG, Martin BM, Bernstein KE (1990) Transcription of testicular angiotensin-converting enzyme (ACE) is initiated within the 12th intron of the somatic ACE gene. Mol Cell Biol 10:4294–4302

Howard TE, Balogh R, Overbeek P, Bernstein KE (1992) Sperm specific expression of angiotensin-converting enzyme (ACE) is mediated by a 91 base pair promoter encoding a CRE-like element. Mol Cell Biol 13:18–27

Kim HS, Krege JH, Kluckman KD, Hagaman JR, Hodgin JB, Best CF, Jennette JC, Coffman TM, Maeda N, Smithies O (1995) Genetic control of blood pressure and the angiotensinogen locus. Proc Natl Acad Sci USA 92:2735–2739

Kumar RS, Kusari J, Roy SN, Soffer RL, Sen GC (1989) Structure of testicular angiotensin converting enzyme: a segmental mosaic isozyme. J Biol Chem 264:16754–16758

Langford KG, Shai S-Y, Howard TE, Kovac MJ, Overbeek PA, Bernstein KE (1991) Transgenic mice demonstrate a testis specific promoter for angiotensin converting enzyme (ACE). J Biol Chem 266:15559–15562

Langford KG, Zhou Y, Russell LD, Wilcox JN, Bernstein KE (1993) Regulated expression of testis angiotensin-converting enzyme during spermatogenesis in mice. Biol Reproduct 48:1210–1218

Lattion AL, Soubrier F, Allegrinin J, Hubert C, Corvol P, Alhenc-Gelas F (1989) The testicular transcript of the angiotensin I-converting enzyme encodes for the ancestral, non-duplicated form of the enzyme. FEBS Lett 252:99–104

Niimura F, Labosky PA, Kakuchi J, Okubo S, Yoshida H, Oikawa T, Ichiki T, Naftilan AJ, Fogo A, Inagami T, Hogan BLM, Ichikawa I (1996) Gene targeting in mice reveals a requirement for angiotensin in the development and maintenance of kidney morphology and growth factor regulation. J Clin Invest 96:2947–2954

Soubrier F, Alhenc-Gelas F, Hubert C, Allegrinin J, John M, Tregar G, Corvol P (1988) Two putative active centers in human angiotensin I-converting enzyme revealed by molecular cloning. Proc Natl Acad Sci USA 85:9386–9390

Tanimoto K, Sugiyama F, Goto Y, Ishida J, Takimoto E, Yagami K, Fukamizu A, Murakami K (1994) Angiotensinogen–deficient mice with hypotension. J Biol Chem 269:31334–31337

Tatei K, Cai H, Ip YT, Levine M (1995) Race: a Drosophila homologue of the angiotensin converting enzyme. Mech Dev 51:157–168

Tigerstedt R, Bergman PG (1898) Niere und Kreislauf. Scand Arch Physiol 7–8:223–271

Zhou Y, Delafontaine P, Martin BM, Bernstein KE (1995) Identification of two positive transcriptional elements within the 91-base pair promoter for mouse testis angiotensin converting enzyme (testis ACE). Dev Genet 16:201–209

Zhou Y, Overbeek PA, Bernstein KE (1996a) Tissue specific expression of testis angiotensin converting enzyme is not determined by the −32 nonconsensus TATA motif. Biochem Biophys Res Comm 223:48–53

Zhou Y, Sun Z, Means AR, Sassone-Corsi P, Bernstein KE (1996b) cAMP-response element modulator τ is a positive regulator of testis angiotensin converting enzyme transcription. Proc Natl Acad Sci USA 93:12262–12266

7 Growth Hormone Releasing Hormone and Growth Hormone Releasing Hormone-Related Peptide in the Testis

K.K. Samaddar, T.M. Todoran, and O. Hirsch Pescovitz

7.1   GHRH Overview

Growth hormone releasing hormone (GHRH) is a peptide synthesized in the cell bodies of neurosecretory neurons in the ventromedial and arcuate nuclei of the hypothalamus. When stimulated, GHRH travels down the axons of these neurons and is released into the hypophyseal portal circulation. GHRH binds to receptors on somatotrophs in the anterior pituitary, resulting in growth hormone (GH) gene expression and the secretion of GH. This positive regulation of GH by GHRH is opposed by somatostatin, which is synthesized in neurosecretory cell bodies located in the anterior paraventricular region of the hypothalamus.

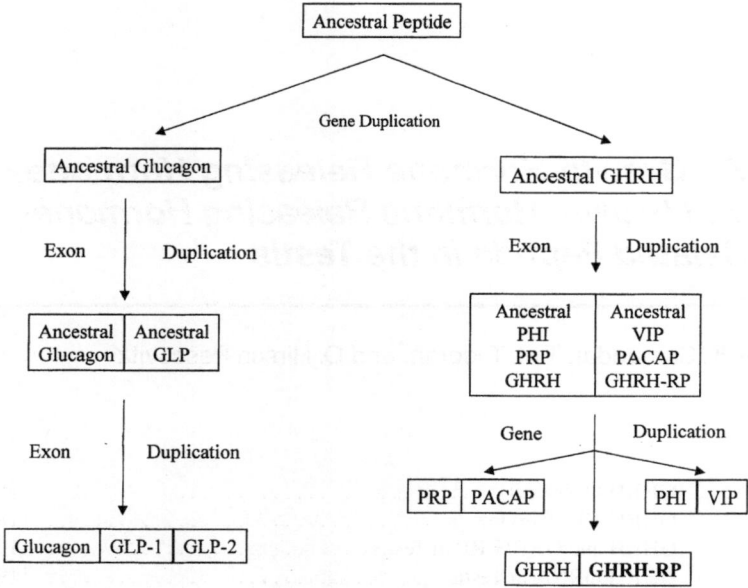

Fig. 1. Evolution of the GHRH peptide family. It is thought that GHRH arose from a single gene 1250 million years ago. *GLP*, Glucagon-like peptide; *PA-CAP*, pituitary adenylate cyclase activating polypeptide; *PRP*, PACAP-related peptide; *PHI*, peptide histidine isoleucine; *VIP*, vasoactive intestinal peptide; *GHRH*, growth hormone-releasing hormone; *GHRH-RP*, growth hormone releasing hormone-related peptide

In 1982, GHRH was isolated from pancreatic tumors obtained from patients who presented with acromegaly (Guillemin et al. 1982; Rivier et al. 1982). Two years later, Ling et al. (1984) isolated GHRH from the hypothalamus. During the past decade the characterization of various peptide hormones led to the recognition that the GHRH gene belongs to a "superfamily" of gut-brain peptides. These peptides include glucagon, glucagon-like peptides 1 and 2 (GLP-1 and GLP-2), secretin, gastric inhibitory protein, vasoactive intestinal polypeptide (VIP), pituitary adenylate cyclase activating polypeptide (PACAP), peptide histidine isoleucine (PHI), and PACAP-related peptide (PRP). The sequence of GHRH shares the greatest homology to other family members with peptide histidine isoleucine (37%–63%) and PRP (35%–55%). To a

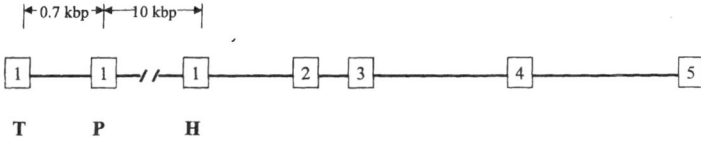

Fig. 2. Schematic representation of the GHRH mRNA. The GHRH mRNA consists of five or six exons. Exons 2–5 are common to testis (*T*), placenta (*P*), and hypothalamus (*H*). Exon 1 is tissue specific. Placenta exon 1 is 10 kbp 5' to hypothalamus exon 1, and testis exon 1 is 0.7 kbp 5' to exon 1 of placenta

lesser degree GHRH is homologous with VIP (25%–43%), glucagon (21%–35%), secretin (22%–37%), PACAP (24%–32%), and GIP (5%–19%) (Campbell and Scanes 1992). It is thought that GHRH arose 1250 million years ago from an ancestral gene that contained a single exon (Fig. 1). This primitive exon, which encoded a 27 amino acid peptide, first underwent gene duplication followed by exon duplication resulting in ancestral GHRH (Campbell and Scanes 1992). A single copy of the GHRH gene has been identified in human, mouse, and rat. The GHRH gene is located on human chromosome 20 (Mayo et al. 1985) and on mouse chromosome 2 (Godfrey et al. 1993).

Since its discovery in 1984, GHRH mRNA transcripts have been identified in many other tissues in addition to the hypothalamus. GHRH mRNA transcripts and GHRH-like peptides have been isolated in human testis (Berry et al. 1992), placenta (Berry et al. 1992; Gonzalez-Crespo and Boronat 1991; Margioris et al. 1990), and leukocytes (Weigent et al. 1990). In rodents GHRH mRNA transcripts and GHRH-like peptides have been identified in several tissues. Similar to humans, transcripts have been isolated in both rat placenta (Baird et al. 1985) and rat testis (Berry et al. 1988). Using reverse transcribed polymerase chain reaction (RT-PCR) and Southern blot analysis, Matsubara et al. (1995), identified GHRH mRNA transcripts in spleen, small intestine, pancreas, kidney, adrenal gland, skeletal muscle, and ovary. These data suggest that GHRH is involved in extrahypothalamic paracrine or autocrine systems.

The GHRH mRNA transcript consists of five or possibly six exons. Hypothalamus, testis, and placenta each share the common exons 2–5 (Fig. 2). Exon 1, however, is probably tissue specific. The GHRH mRNA in hypothalamus and placenta is 750 nucleotides, in contrast to the rat GHRH mRNA in testis which is 1700 nucleotides in length. This difference is most likely due to tissue-specific promoter sequences and alternative splicing of exon 1. The placenta exon 1 is 10 kilobasepairs (kbp) 5' to the exon 1 of hypothalamus (Gonzalez-Crespo and Boronat 1991), and testis exon 1 is 0.7 kbp 5' to exon 1 of placenta (Srivastava et al. 1995).

The GHRH receptor has been cloned from rat, mouse, and human (Mayo et al. 1985) and is similar in all three species. The GHRH receptor has seven hydrophobic domains that span the membrane. The amino-terminus is thought to be extracellular. The GHRH receptor has been localized to chromosome 6 in mouse (Godfrey et al. 1993) and chromosome 7p15 in humans (Wajnrajch et al. 1994). Similar to GHRH, its receptor also belongs to a large distinct family of receptors. When it was first cloned it was thought to include only calcitonin, secretin, and parathyroid hormone receptors. Recently, however, the VIP, GIP, and GLP-1 receptors have been shown to also be included in this family. All the members of this receptor family are coupled to G_s and activate adenylate cyclase resulting in an increase in the second messenger cAMP. In addition to increasing cAMP, each of these receptors is also coupled to pathways that result in an increase in other second messengers (Segre and Goldring 1993).

7.2 GHRH-RP Overview

In addition to the bioactive GHRH peptide produced from the GHRH gene, we hypothesized that a second biologically active peptide is derived from proteolytic processing of the pro-GHRH precursor. We have called this carboxyl-terminal cleavage product of the precursor peptide, growth hormone releasing hormone–related peptide (GHRH-RP; Breyer et al. 1996). Similarly, VIP and PACAP pro-proteins each produce at least two peptides (Fig. 3). The homology that GHRH-RP peptide shares with other members of the GHRH superfamily, especially VIP and PACAP, and its action in Sertoli cells suggest that it may play an important role in autocrine or paracrine signaling.

```
GHRH-RP:   H L D R V W A E D K Q M A L E S I L
PACAP:     H S D . . . . . . . . . . . K Q M A L . . . . .L
VIP:       H S D . . . V . . . . . . D K Q M A L . . S I L
```

Fig. 3. Comparison of GHRH-RP (1–18) amino acid sequence with those of PACAP and VIP

7.3 GHRH and GHRH-RP in Testis

The testis consists of the seminiferous tubules, which contain Sertoli cells, germ cells, peritubular myoid cells, and an interstitium composed of Leydig cells, macrophages, fibroblasts, and blood vessels (Gnessi et al. 1997). Interactions between autocrine and paracrine factors of these cellular compartments are essential for normal spermatogenesis. Numerous hypothalamic neuropeptides were identified in testis prior to the discovery of GHRH in rat and human testis (Berry and Pescovitz 1988; Berry et al. 1992; Ciampani et al. 1992; Gnessi et al. 1997). The exact role of neuropeptides such as pro-opiomelonocortin, corticotropin-releasing hormone, gonadotropin-releasing hormone, and thyrotropin-releasing hormone in the testis is still unknown.

7.4 GHRH mRNA in Testis

Northern blot analysis of testis mRNA indicates that the hypothalamic GHRH mRNA is approximately 750 nucleotides while the testis GHRH mRNA is 1750 nucleotides (Berry and Pescovitz 1988). Variations in GHRH mRNA transcripts explain the differences in GHRH mRNA size. The exon 1 sequence of testis GHRH differs from that of either hypothalamus or placenta (Srivastava et al. 1995). The testicular GHRH mRNA transcript contains a sixth exon in contrast with the five exons present in the placental or hypothalamic transcripts. Moreover, GHRH transcription initiation in testis begins 10.7 kbp 5' to that in the hypothalamus. The tissue-specific expression of GHRH is probably related to distinct promoter and transcription initiation sites (Fig. 4). In contrast with the rodent, the GHRH mRNA in human testis is the same size as that in hypothalamus (Berry et al. 1992). However, since the transcript has not been sequenced, it is unknown whether they are identical.

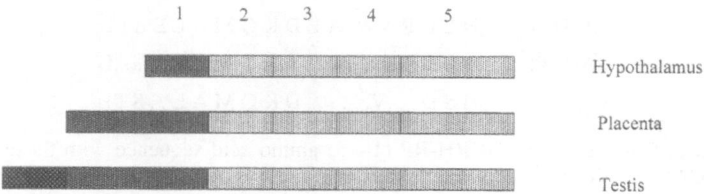

Fig. 4. Comparison of GHRH mRNA transcripts in the hypothalamus, placenta, and testis. The GHRH mRNA from the hypothalamus, placenta, and testis all share exons 2–5. Two different transcripts are found in the testis, with one containing the placental exon 1. Each tissue has a unique first exon

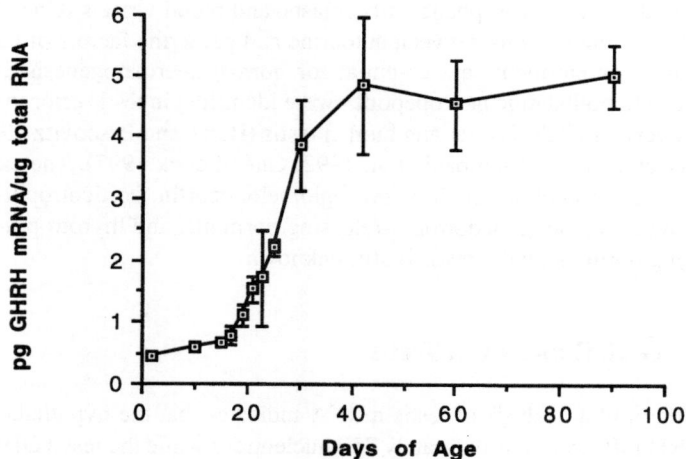

Fig. 5. Ontogeny of testicular GHRH mRNA. Testes from four separate animals were analyzed at each time point, except at 2 days, where 32 individuals were pooled into two individual samples (16/sample). The mean plus or minus SD are shown. (Reproduced with permission from Berry and Pescovitz 1990)

Testicular GHRH mRNA levels increase with age. GHRH mRNA levels are first detectable in testis by 2 days of life in the rat (Berry and Pescovitz 1990). mRNA levels increase at day 21 and reach adult levels by day 30 (Berry and Pescovitz 1990) (Fig. 5). The predominant mRNA species at all ages is approximately 1700 bp by Northern analysis (Berry

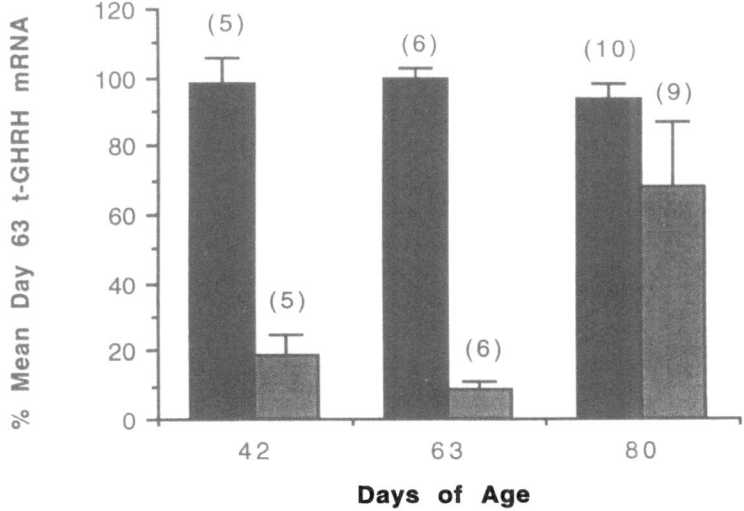

Fig. 6. Effects of hypophysectomy on expression of testicular GHRH mRNA. Total RNA from testes of hypophysectomized or normal rats was analyzed by dot blot. Values were normalized to the mean of day 63 normal values (expressed as a percentage of the day 63 mean). Shown are changes in the testicular levels of hypophysectomized and normal animals for GHRH mRNAs. *Parenthesis above each data bar*, number of animals analyzed in each state. (Reproduced with permission from Berry and Pescovitz 1990)

and Pescovitz 1990). A faint 3350 bp band was also noted in post pubertal animals (Berry and Pescovitz 1990). Testicular GHRH may be regulated by the hypothalamic-pituitary axis (Pescovitz et al. 1990). Hypophysectomy of prepubertal and peripubertal rats results in a large decrease in GHRH mRNA levels while hypophysectomy has little impact on testicular GHRH mRNA levels in postpubertal rats (Berry and Pescovitz 1990) (Fig. 6). When human growth hormone was administered to hypophysectomized prepubertal rats, a small decrease in testicular GHRH mRNA was observed (Berry and Pescovitz 1990). It is still unknown how GH affects testicular GHRH.

A study using ethylene dimethane sulfonate (EDS), a Leydig cell toxin, on prepubertal and postpubertal rats showed a major decrease in testosterone production; however, there was no change in the levels of

GHRH in the testis by northern blot analysis and enzyme-linked immunosorbent assay (ELISA) (Srivastava et al. 1993a). Methoxyacetic acid (MAA), a pachytene spermatocyte toxin, was used to assess whether GHRH is expressed in pachytene spermatocytes (Srivastava et al. 1993a). No effect was observed in the GHRH mRNA levels, probably because of the existence of spermatocytes at various maturation stages in the seminiferous tubules, and because most GHRH mRNA is expressed before the pachytene spermatocyte stage. This explanation is further supported by in situ hybridization analysis (Srivastava et al. 1993a).

In situ hybridization studies and northern gel analysis of mRNA from specific regions of the male reproductive tract and individual testicular cell types have been used to determine the localization of GHRH mRNA. No GHRH mRNA signal was detected in any region of the epididymis or vas deferens (Srivastava et al. 1993a). Even within the testis not all cells produce the GHRH mRNA. Most of the hybridization signal is present at the perimeter of the tubules in early spermatogenic cells and primary spermatocytes (Srivastava et al. 1993a). Some signal is observed in more mature spermatogenic cells; however, no signal is seen in the interstitial cells (Srivastava et al. 1993a). The detection of a GHRH mRNA signal in Leydig cells using RT-PCR may suggest that by using more sensitive techniques, a small amount of message is produced in the interstitium (Srivastava et al. 1994). By isolating specific testicular cell types and extracting the respective RNA, GHRH was detected mostly in spermatocytes and round spermatids with low levels detected in Sertoli cells (Srivastava et al. 1993a). However, no GHRH mRNA signal was detected in elongating spermatids, peritubular myoid cells and Leydig cells (Srivastava et al. 1993a).

7.5   GHRH Immunoactivity in Testis

A GHRH peptide has been localized in testis to mature germ cells and early sperm forms (Pescovitz et al. 1990). However, no GHRH immunoreactivity was detected in Sertoli, interstitial, or endothelial cells by our laboratory (Pescovitz et al. 1990). Others, however, have detected a GHRH-like material in Leydig cells (Ciampani et al. 1992; Moretti et al. 1990). Although these investigators have shown that the peptide possesses similar HPLC elution characteristics as that of hypothalamic rat GHRH release, and that its release is also acutely stimulated by hCG (Ciampani et al. 1992), we do not believe that the GHRH purified from rat testes is identical to synthetic hypothalamic GHRH (Pescovitz et al. 1990). In our studies synthetic GHRH and testicular GHRH have different elution properties on a reverse-phase HPLC column (Pescovitz et al. 1990). However, both synthetic GHRH and GHRH purified from rat testes have comparable biological activity in their ability to stimulate GH release from dispersed anterior pituitary cells in culture (Pescovitz et al. 1990). This indicates that testicular GHRH is bioactive in pituitary cells (Berry and Pescovitz 1990).

7.6   GHRH-RP Immunoactivity in Testis

We hypothesized that the pro-GHRH precursor also produces a second biologically active peptide. To test this hypothesis we synthesized GHRH-RP from the deduced amino acid sequence of the precursor peptide and used this synthetic peptide to generate antisera against it. These antisera were used in immunohistochemical studies to localize GHRH-RP in both hypothalamus and testis (Breyer et al. 1996). In the rat testis GHRH-RP immunoreactivity was seen in the acrosomes of nearly all stages of germ cell development. Specifically, intense staining was evident in stage IV seminiferous tubules in pachytene primary spermatocytes, step 4 secondary spermatocytes, and step 17 elongating spermatids. Incubation of these tissues with an excess of GHRH-RP prior to antisera treatment abolished staining, thus demonstrating the immunospecificity of the findings.

Although a function for GHRH-RP has not yet been found in hypothalamus, results of preliminary studies support a potential role for GHRH-RP in spermatocyte differentiation. In vitro GHRH-RP stimulates stem cell factor (also known as "steel" factor or c-kit ligand; Huang et al. 1990) mRNA expression in primary rat Sertoli cell cultures (Breyer et al. 1996). GHRH also has this effect, but it is less potent by approximately a log factor. Unlike GHRH, however, GHRH-RP does not increase intracellular cAMP (Breyer et al. 1996).

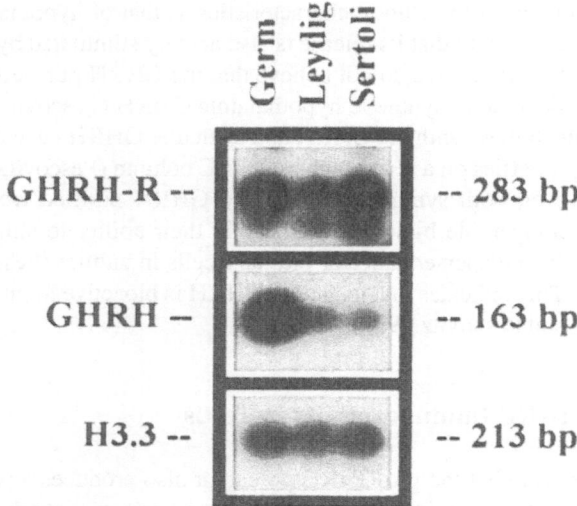

Fig. 7. RT-PCR analysis of testis cell RNAs. RT-PCR products were subjected to electrophoresis on 1.8% agarose gels, transferred to nylon membranes, and hybridized to the indicated probes. *Top*, GHRH receptor mRNA; *center*, GHRH mRNA; *bottom*, histone 3.3 mRNA. (Reproduced with permission from Srivastava et al. 1994)

7.7 GHRH Receptor in Testis

Evidence for GHRH mRNA and peptide expression in testis supports the likelihood of testicular action for the products of pro-GHRH processing. By northern blot analysis, no GHRH receptor could be found in testis (Srivastava et al. 1994). To improve sensitivity RT-PCR was performed on cDNA from whole testis, germ, Sertoli, and Leydig cells (Srivastava et al. 1994). A GHRH receptor mRNA was detected in all cell types with the highest levels of expression in Sertoli and germ cells (Srivastava et al. 1994) (Fig. 7). Sequence analysis demonstrated that the receptor mRNA was identical to pituitary GHRH receptor mRNA (Srivastava et al. 1994). Further, GHRH receptor mRNA expression in Sertoli cells was regulated in a dose-dependent fashion following rat GHRH treatment (Srivastava et al. 1994). Treatment with 10 and 100 nM GHRH for 6 h resulted in 1.4-fold and 2.3-fold increases, respectively, in GHRH receptor mRNA (Srivastava et al. 1994). Interestingly, some studies have reported a downregulation of pituitary GHRH receptors following prolonged treatment with GHRH (Bilezikjian et al. 1986; Wehrenberg et al. 1986). In addition to a GHRH receptor, other investigators have suggested that testicular GHRH functions through a VIP receptor (Ciampani et al. 1992).

7.8   Action of Testicular GHRH and GHRH-RP

GHRH and a GHRH analog stimulated increases in intracellular cAMP, c-fos, and SCF mRNAs in cultured Sertoli cells (Srivastava et al. 1993b). GHRH treatment of Sertoli cells resulted in a twofold increase in cAMP levels (Srivastava et al. 1993b) (Fig. 8). GHRH combined with follicle-stimulating hormone (FSH) increased FSH-induced cAMP production in Sertoli cells (Fabbri et al. 1995). Also, cAMP levels in Leydig cells increase in a dose-dependent fashion with GHRH treatment (Ciampani et al. 1992). This increase is accompanied by an increase in sensitivity to the luteinizing hormone/hCG stimulus for cAMP (Ciampani et al. 1992).

SCF (the product of the *Steel* gene, also called mast cell growth factor, or c-kit ligand) and c-fos are essential for normal spermatogenesis in vivo (Rossi et al. 1991; Tajima et al. 1991; Nakayama et al. 1988) and proliferation of embryonic germ cells in vitro (Matsui et al. 1991; Godin et al. 1991). Therefore we sought to determine whether either GHRH or GHRH-RP regulates SCF expression. A GHRH analog, [His[1], Nle[27]]GHRH(1–32)-NH$_2$, with greater receptor affinity and potency than native GHRH was used to treat cultured Sertoli cells. Stimulation of SCF mRNA was observed at 20 min and 16 h while c-fos mRNA was increased at 20 min (Srivastava et al. 1993b). From 30 min to 4 h of treatment, 100 nM GHRH analog increased SCF mRNA levels at a greater rate than at the 10 nM level (Srivastava et al. 1993b). The same trends were seen with rat GHRH.

Increases in cAMP are abolished when the cells are allowed to preincubate with a GHRH antagonist, (N-Ac-Tyr[1], d-Arg[2])-GRF(1–29)NH$_2$ suggesting that the effect is specific for GHRH (Srivastava et al. 1993b; Fabbri et al. 1995). The increase in SCF mRNA was abolished when the GHRH antagonist was added to the cells 60 min prior to addition of GHRH (Srivastava et al. 1993b).

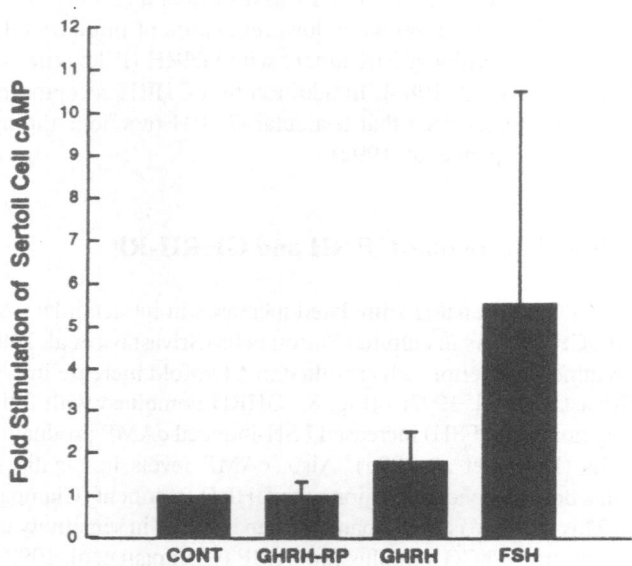

Fig. 8. GHRH and GHRH-RP effects on intracellular cAMP levels. Stimulation of adenylate cyclase in cultured Sertoli cells. Cells were incubated with GHRH-RP, GHRH, FSH or control media and adenylate cyclase stimulation measured (fold stimulation over control). Each bar is representative of five separate experiments. (Reproduced with permission from Breyer et al. 1996)

GHRH-RP treatment resulted in an even greater increase in SCF expression than with GHRH treatment (Breyer et al. 1996) (Fig. 9). At concentrations of 10 nM and 100 nM, GHRH-RP stimulated SCF expression 12-fold and 16-fold, respectively in isolated Sertoli cells (Breyer et al. 1996).

GHRH-RP treatment, however, did not result in an increase in intracellular cAMP (Breyer et al. 1996). Since GHRH-RP does not increase cAMP as GHRH does, GHRH-RP may function via a unique Sertoli cell receptor (Breyer et al. 1996)

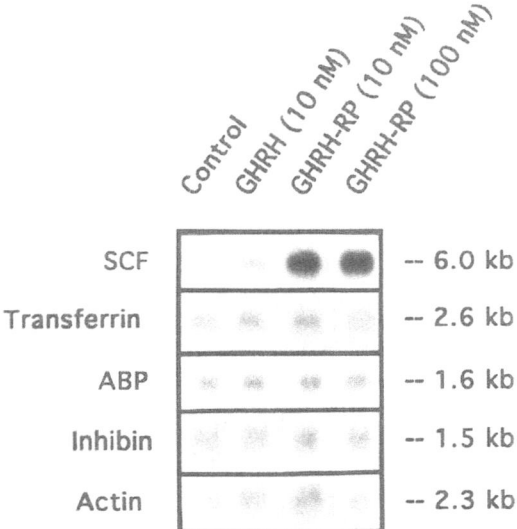

Fig. 9. GHRH-RP action in rat Sertoli cells. Rat Sertoli cells were treated with rat GHRH-RP (10 n*M* and 100 n*M*), rat GHRH (10 n*M*) or control media for 16 h. Northern gel analysis of 10 μg of total Sertoli cell RNA. Blots were probed for SCF, transferrin, ABP, α-inhibin, and γ-actin, as control. (Reproduced with permission from Breyer et al. 1996)

7.9 Conclusion

The functional roles of many neuropeptides isolated in testis have yet to be discovered; however, preliminary data suggest that GHRH and GHRH-RP contribute to the process of spermatogenesis. The GHRH mRNA is expressed in an age-dependent fashion in association with the onset of spermatogenesis. The GHRH mRNA is expressed in spermatocytes and round spermatids but not in elongating spermatids, peritubular myoid cells, interstitial cells, epididymis, or vas deferens. A mature GHRH peptide is present in testicular germ cells and may also be present in Leydig cells. A novel product of the GHRH gene, GHRH-RP, is detected in stage IV seminiferous tubules in pachytene primary spermatocytes, step 4 secondary spermatocytes and step 17 elongating spermatids. A GHRH receptor mRNA identical in sequence to that of the pituitary is detected in Sertoli and germ cells. Both GHRH and GHRH-RP stimulate an increase in stem cell factor expression in Sertoli cells. This effect of GHRH may be mediated by intracellular increases in cAMP and c-fos, but the mechanism by which GHRH-RP acts is still unknown. Further work is intended to further characterize the role of testicular GHRH in autocrine or paracrine actions.

References

Baird A, Wehrenberg WB, Bohlen P, Ling N (1985) Immunoreactive and bio-logically active growth hormone-releasing factor in the rat placenta. Endo-crinology 117:1598–1601

Berry SA, Pescovitz OH (1988) Identification of a rat GHRH-like substance and its messenger RNA in rat testis. Endocrinology 123:661–663

Berry SA, Pescovitz OH (1990) Ontogeny and pituitary regulation of testicular growth hormone-releasing hormone-like messenger ribonucleic acid. Endo-crinology 127:1404–1411

Berry SA, Srivastava CH, Rubin LR, Phipps W, Pescovitz OH (1992) Growth hormone-releasing hormone-like messenger ribonucleic acid and im-munoreactive peptides are present in human testis and placenta. J Clin En-docrinol Metab 75:281–284

Bilezikjian LM, Seifert H, Vale W (1986) Desensitization to growth hormone-releasing factor (GRF) is associated with down-regulation of GRF-binding sites. Endocrinology 118:2045–2052

Breyer PR, Rothrock JK, Beaudry N, Pescovitz OH (1996) A novel peptide from the growth hormone releasing hormone gene stimulates Sertoli cell ac-tivity. Endocrinology 137:2159–2162

Campbell RM, Scanes CG (1992) Evolution of growth hormone-releasing fac-tor (GRF) family of peptides. Growth Regul 2:175–191

Ciampani T, Fabbri A, Isidori A, Dufau ML (1992) Growth hormone-releasing hormone is produced by rat Leydig cell in culture and acts as a positive regulator of Leydig cell function. Endocrinology 131:2785–2792

Fabbri A, Ciocca DR, Ciampani T, Wang J, Dufau ML (1995) Growth hor-mone-releasing hormone in testicular interstitial and germ cells: potential paracrine modulation of follicle stimulating hormone action on Sertoli cell function. Endocrinology 136:2303–2308

Gnessi L, Fabbri A, Spera G (1997) Gonadal peptides as mediators of develop-ment and functional control of the testis: an integrated system with hor-mones and local environment. Endocrinology 8:541–609

Godfrey P, Rahal JO, Beamer WG, Copeland NG, Jenkins NA, Mayo KE (1993) GHRH receptor of little mice contains a missense mutation in the extracellular domain that disrupts receptor function. Nature Genetics 4:227–232

Godin I, Deed R, Cooke J, Zsebo K, Dexter M, Wylie CC (1991) Effects of the steel gene product on mouse primordial germ cells in culture. Nature 352:807–809

Gonzalez-Crespo S, Boronat A (1991) Expression of the rat growth hormone-releasing hormone gene in placenta is directed by an alternative promoter. Proc Natl Acad Sci USA 88:8749–8753

Guillemin R, Brazeau P, Bohlen P, Esch F, Ling N, Wehrenberg WB (1982) Growth hormone-releasing factor from a human pancreatic tumor that caused acromegaly. Science 218:585–587

Huang E, Nocka K, Beier DR, Chu T-Y, Buck J, Lahm H-W, Wellner D, Leder P, Besmer P (1990) The hematopoietic growth factor KL is encoded by the Sl locus and is the ligand of the c-kit receptor, the gene product of the W locus. Cell 63:225–233

Ling N, Esch F, Bohlen P, Brazeau P, Wehrenberg WB, Guillemin R (1984) Isolation, primary structure, and synthesis of human hypothalamic somatocrinin: growth hormone-releasing factor. Proc Natl Acad Sci USA 81:4302–4306

Margioris AN, Brockmann G, Bohler HC, Jr, Grino M, Vamvakopoulos N, Chrousos GP (1990) Expression and localization of growth hormone-releasing hormone messenger ribonucleic acid in rat placenta: in vitro secretion and regulation of its peptide product. Endocrinology 126:151–158

Matsubara S, Sato M, Mizobuchi M, Niimi M, Takahara J (1995) Differential gene expression of growth hormone (GH)-releasing hormone (GHRH) and GRH receptor in various rat tissues. Endocrinology 136:4147–4150

Matsui Y, Toksoz D, Nishikawa S, Nishikawa SI, Williams D, Zsebo K, Hogan BLM (1991) Effect of Steel factor and leukaemia inhibitory factor on murine primordial germ cells in culture. Nature 353:750–752

Mayo KE, Cerelli GM, Lebo RV, Bruce BD, Rosenfeld MG, Evans RM (1985) Gene encoding human growth hormone-releasing factor precursor: structure, sequence, and chromosomal assignment. Proc Natl Acad Sci USA 82:63–67

Monts BS, Breyer PR, Rothrock JK, Pescovitz OH (1996) Peptides of the growth hormone-releasing hormone family. Endocrine 4:73–78

Moretti C, Fabbri A, Gnessi L, Bonifacio V, Bolotti M, Arrizi M, Nassicone Q, Spera G (1990) Immunohistochemical localization of growth hormone-releasing hormone in human gonads. J Endocrinol Invest 13:301–305

Nakayama H, Kuroda H, Hitoshi O, Fujita J, Nishimune Y, Matsumoto K, Nagano T, Suzuki F, Kitamura Y (1988) Studies of Sl/Sld in equilibrium with

+/+ mouse aggregation of chimaeras. Ll. Effect of the steel locus on sper-matogenesis. Development 102:117–126

Pescovitz OH, Berry SA, Laudon M, Ben-Jonathan N, Martin-Meyers A, Hsu S-M, Lambros TJ, Felix AM (1990) Localization and growth hor-mone(GH)-releasing activity of rat testicular GH-releasing hormone-like peptide. Endocrinology 127:2336

Rauch C, Li JY, Croissandeau G, Berthet M, Peillon F, Pagesy P (1995) Char-acterization and localization of an immunoreactive growth hormone-releas-ing hormone precursor form in normal and tumoral and human anterior pi-tuitaries. Endocrinology 136:2594–2601

Rivier J, Spiess J, Thorner M, Vale W (1982) Characterization of growth hor-mone-releasing factor from a human pancreatic islet tumour. Nature 300:276–278

Rossi P, Albanesi C, Grimaldi P, Geremia R (1991) Expression of the mRNA for the ligand of the c-kit in mouse Sertoli cells. Biochem Biophys Res Comm 176:910–914

Segre GV, Goldring SR (1993) Receptors for secretin, calcitonin parathyroid hormone (PTH)/PTH-related peptide, vasoactive intestinal peptide, glu-cagonlike peptide 1, growth hormone-releasing hormone, and glucagon be-long to a newly discovered G-protein-linked receptor family. Trends Endo-crinol Metab 4:309–314

Srivastava CH, Collard MW, Rothrock JK, Peredo MJ, Berry SA, Pescovitz OH (1993a) Germ cell localization of a testicular growth hormone-releasing hormone-like factor. Endocrinology 133:83–89

Srivastava CH, Breyer PR, Rothrock JK, Peredo MJ, Pescovitz OH (1993b) A new target for growth hormone-releasing hormone action in rat: the Sertoli cell. Endocrinology 133:1478–1481

Srivastava CH, Kelley MR, Monts BS, Wilson TM, Breyer PR, Pescovitz OH (1994) Growth hormone-releasing hormone receptor mRNA is present in rat testis. Endocrine 2:607–610

Srivastava CH, Monts BS, Rothrock JK, Peredo MJ, Pescovitz OH (1995) Presence of a spermatogenic-specific promoter in the rat growth hormone-releasing hormone gene. Endocrinology 136:1502–1508

Tajima Y, Onoue H, Kitamura Y, Nishimune Y (1991) Biologically active kit li-gand growth factor is produced by mouse Sertoli cells and is defective in Sld mutant mouse. Development 113:1031–1035

Wajnrajch MP, Chua SC, Green ED, Leibel RL (1994) Human growth hor-mone-releasing hormone receptor (GHRHR) maps to a YAC at chromo-some 7p15. Mammalian Genome 5:595

Wehrenberg WB, Seifert H, Bilezikjian LM, Vale W (1986) Down-regulation of growth hormone-releasing factor receptors following continuous infusion of growth hormone releasing factor in vivo. Neuroendocrinology 43:266–268

Weigent DA, Blalock JE (1990) Immunoreactive growth hormone-releasing hormone in rat leukocytes. J Neuroimmunal 29:1–13

8 Cyclic ADP-Ribose and Calcium Signalling

A. Galione and H.L. Wilson

8.1 Introduction

It is over 100 years since calcium was first implied as an intracellular regulator in heart by Ringer (1882). Since then its universal role as a regulator has become a cornerstone of cell physiology (Campbell 1983), and much progress has been made in our understanding of cellular calcium homeostasis and the way in which cellular stimuli are transduced into transient elevations in intracellular free calcium, here defined as calcium signals.

A major source of calcium for signalling are intracellular stores, predominantly the endoplasmic reticulum. A landmark in calcium signalling research was the finding that inositol 1,4,5-trisphosphate (IP3) coupled receptor-mediated events at the plasma membrane to the opening of calcium release channels present on internal stores (Berridge

1993). Although IP$_3$ appears to operate as a ubiquitous intracellular messenger for calcium mobilization, recent studies indicate that multiple calcium release mechanisms operate in many cells and are regulated by a family of pyridine nucleotide metabolites. The first indication of this concept came from the pioneering work of Lee and his colleagues who showed that β-NAD$^+$ and β-NADP$^+$ can trigger calcium release from sea urchin egg microsomal fractions by a mechanism apparently independent of IP$_3$ (Clapper et al. 1987). Subsequently the structures of the active metabolites have been determined (Lee et al. 1989), and one of them, cyclic adenosine diphosphate ribose (cADPR), has been shown to mobilize calcium in some thirty or so different cell types in a wide range of organisms including plants, invertebrates and mammals (Lee 1997). The enzymes responsible for the synthesis and degradation of cADPR have been shown to be widely distributed, and current work is focusing on the way in which cellular stimuli regulate the production of cADPR.

The mechanism whereby cADPR release and related metabolites stimulate calcium release is of considerable interest, with accumulating evidence suggesting that the major target for cADPR is ryanodine receptors (RyRs; Galione and Summerhill 1996). RyRs are large homotetrameric calcium release channels that were first described as the major calcium release pathways from the sarcoplasmic reticulum during excitation-contraction coupling in skeletal and cardiac muscle (Meissner 1994). However, RyRs have now been shown to be more widespread in cells than originally thought (Sorrentino and Volpe 1993).

Recent research suggests that cADPR is only one of several pyridine nucleotide metabolites regulating calcium signalling, possibly all produced by the same multifunctional enzymes. Other metabolites include 2-phospho-cADPR (cADPRP) which may have a similar action to cADPR, and nicotinic acid adenine dinucleotide phosphate (NAADP) which may regulate a completely new class of calcium release channel.

8.2 Discovery of cADPR and Related Metabolites

In experiments using cuvette-based fluorimetry to measure calcium fluxes across microsomal membranes in sea urchin egg homogenates Lee and colleagues found that in addition to IP$_3$ the pyridine nucleotides

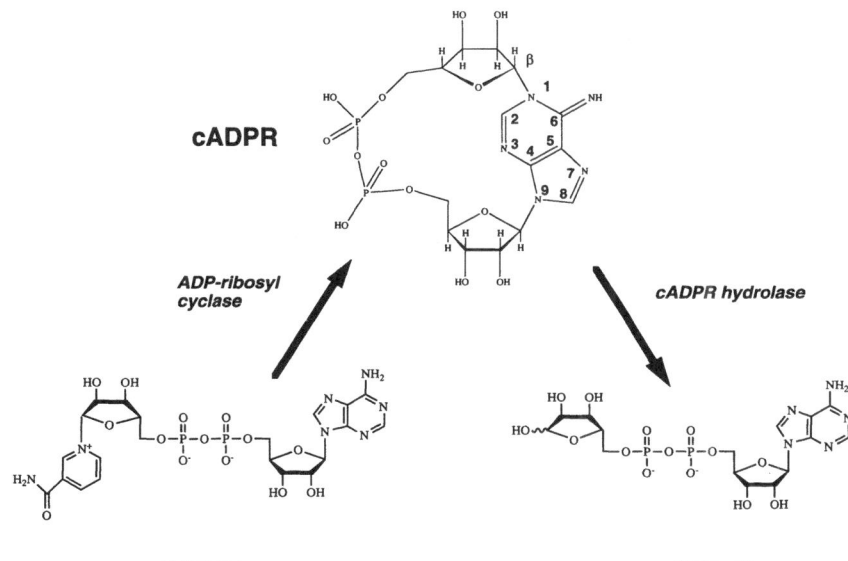

cADPR

ADP-ribosyl cyclase

cADPR hydrolase

β-NAD+   **ADP-ribose**

Fig. 1. Cyclic ADP-ribose is a cyclic β-NAD+ metabolite. The structure of cyclic ADP-ribose was determined by mass spectroscopy and magnetic resonance imaging and confirmed by crystallography. cADPR is produced by the cyclization of β-NAD+ by ADP-ribosyl cyclases. cADPR is hydrolysed to the non-calcium mobilizing metabolite ADP-ribose by cADPR hydrolases. CD38 is an example of a bifunctional protein expressing both cyclase and hydrolase activities thus catalysing the same overall reaction β-NAD+ to ADP-ribose as NAD+ glycohydrolases but with cADPR as a stable intermediate

β-NAD+ and β-NADP+ are also activators of calcium efflux from vesicles previously loaded by Ca^{2+}-ATPases in the presence of an ATP regenerating system (Clapper et al. 1987). While the calcium releasing effects of β-NADP+ were rapid, calcium mobilization by β-NAD+ occurred only after an appreciable delay, perhaps indicating an indirect action on calcium release. Furthermore, in contrast to the effect of β-NADP+, the effect of β-NAD+ did not persist in Percoll-purified microsomal fractions but could be restored if β-NAD+ was previously incubated with supernatant or cytosol fractions from the same Percoll gradients, but only in the presence of additional supernatant added to the microsomes.

Two cytosolic factors were required for β-NAD$^+$-induced calcium release. One of these was later shown to be a novel enzyme termed ADP-ribosyl cyclase, which cyclizes β-NAD$^+$ to a novel metabolite identified by mass spectroscopy as cADPR (Lee et al. 1989; Fig. 1). cADPR was shown to be a potent calcium mobilizing agent, with an EC$_{50}$ of 17 nM in sea urchin egg homogenates (Dargie et al. 1990). The second cytosolic factor necessary for cADPR-induced calcium release was later identified as calmodulin, which confers cADPR sensitivity on its microsomal release mechanism (Tanaka and Tashjian 1995; Lee et al. 1994).

The calcium mobilizing effect of β-NADP$^+$ has been shown to be due to a contaminant of commercially available β-NADP$^+$ identified as NAADP (Lee and Aarhus 1995). Calcium release by both β-NAD$^+$ and β-NADP$^+$ appears to operate via separate calcium release mechanisms which are distinct from that gated by IP$_3$ since each agent shows homologous desensitization without affecting release by activators of the other two mechanisms (Clapper et al. 1987).

8.3   Mechanism of Cyclic ADP-Ribose Induced Calcium Release

The first indication that the β-NAD$^+$ metabolite cADPR mobilizes calcium via a mechanism distinct from IP$_3$-gated calcium release channel came from studies in sea urchin egg homogenates whereby calcium release by β-NAD$^+$ or IP$_3$ made the calcium release mechanism refractory to a second application of the same agent but not to the other. Once cADPR was identified as the active calcium mobilizing metabolite of β-NAD$^+$, similar results were obtained for cADPR and IP$_3$ (Dargie et al. 1990; Fig. 2). Pharmacological analysis has confirmed that cADPR does not activate IP$_3$ receptors (IP$_3$Rs) since the competitive IP$_3$R antagonist heparin blocks IP$_3$-induced calcium release but not that triggered by cADPR.

The identity of the calcium release mechanism activated by cADPR was determined in studies which demonstrated the presence of a RyR mechanism in the sea urchin egg (Galione et al. 1991). Two pharma-

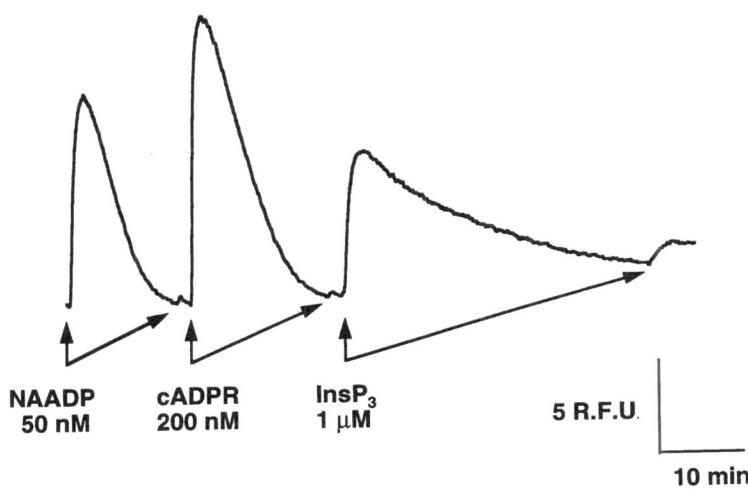

Fig. 2. Homologous desensitization of calcium release mechanisms in sea urchin egg homogenates. Traces are shown of Fluo-3 fluorescence (Ex 490 nm/Em 535 nm) measuring extravesicular calcium during cuvette-based fluorimetry of sea urchin egg homogenates. The homogenates sequester calcium in the presence of an ATP-regenerating system and release calcium in response to calcium mobilizing agents. At least three distinct calcium release mechanisms are present, activated by NAADP, cADPR, or IP$_3$. A feature of calcium release systems in this preparation is that each mechanism undergoes a homologous desensitization, as indicated by the failure of a second administration of each calcium mobilizing agent to produce a second calcium release even after full resequestration of calcium

cological activators of RyRs, caffeine and ryanodine, induced calcium release in both intact eggs and in sea urchin egg homogenates, but precluded a subsequent release of calcium by cADPR but not IP$_3$. Sea urchin egg microsomes which had discharged their calcium contents in response to cADPR were rendered insensitive to caffeine and ryanodine also but not to IP$_3$ (Galione et al. 1991). Furthermore, blockers of RyRs such as ruthenium red and procaine selectively inhibited cADPR-induced calcium release. These later experiments led to the hypothesis that cADPR is an important regulator of RyRs, and hence calcium-induced calcium release (CICR) an important property of RyRs whereby a small rise in cytoplasmic calcium triggers a larger calcium release from internal stores by activating RyRs (Galione 1992). Consistent with this hypothesis was the finding that in sea urchin egg homogenates and in intact cells cADPR potentiates calcium release by the divalent cations Ca^{2+} and Sr^{2+}, and by caffeine (Lee 1993; Guo and Becker 1997), and that cADPR-induced calcium release is inhibited by magnesium ions (Graeff et al. 1995).

Since the RyR hypothesis for cADPR action was formulated, cADPR has been shown to mobilize calcium in many cell types. The majority of studies examining the pharmacology of release have shown similarities to RyRs (Galione and Summerhill 1996). The development of highly selective cADPR analogues, including caged compounds (Aarhus et al. 1995a), competitive antagonists (Walseth and Lee 1993), metabolically resistant agonists and antagonists (Bailey et al. 1996, 1997) and membrane permeable analogues (Sethi et al. 1997) have led to important advances in cADPR research and have been of great benefit in probing the fundamental mechanisms governing cADPR-mediated signalling mechanisms and pathways.

It is probably useful at this point to review briefly the characteristics of RyRs. RyRs are very large structures consisting of homotetramers, with each subunit of around 560 kDa (Sorrentino and Volpe 1993). There are three mammalian isoforms, termed RyR1 (skeletal), RyR2 (cardiac) and RyR3 (brain) denoted by a numerical suffix or by the name of the tissue in which they were first thought to be found predominantly. However, this terminology may be confusing since, for example it seems that the RyR2 or cardiac form is the most widely distributed form in the mammalian CNS. The bulk of the structure is cytoplasmic, which permits multiple sites for interactions with potential regulators. The way in which cADPR modulates RyRs is unknown since its binding site is as yet undefined, nor is it clear whether all RyRs are equally sensitive to regulation by cADPR. Although RyR2 in lipid bilayers have been demonstrated under some circumstances to be activated by cADPR (Meszaros et al. 1993), and expression of RyR2 receptors in PC12 cells have been shown to confer sensitivity of calcium stores to cADPR (Clementi et al. 1996), it is not clear whether cADPR activates RyRs directly, or whether accessory proteins are required. Indeed candidates for cADPR-binding sites include 100- and 140-kDa soluble proteins indicated by photoaffinity labelling of sea urchin egg homogenates with 8-azido-cADPR (Walseth et al. 1993), the ryanodine receptor associated protein FKBP12.6 in pancreatic β-cells (Noguchi et al. 1997) and RyR adenine nucleotide binding sites (Sitsapasen et al. 1995). Recently IP$_3$Rs have been shown to express a novel cADPR-binding site which on binding cADPR leads to inhibition of IP$_3$-induced calcium release (Missiaen et al. 1997).

In addition, other modulatory factors have been shown to regulate the sensitivity of the cADPR-induced calcium release, including calmodulin and calcium (see above) and the enzymes calmodulin-dependent protein kinase II (Noguchi et al. 1997) and cAMP-dependent protein kinase (Morita et al. 1997).

8.4 Enzymology of cADPR Metabolism

The finding that sea urchin egg homogenates contain enzymatic activities to synthesize cADPR from β-NAD$^+$ has been extended to many other animal tissues. The synthetic enzymes, known as ADP-ribosyl cyclases, are widespread in tissues (Rusinko and Lee 1989). Enzymes that hydrolyse cADPR to ADP-ribose are equally widespread (Lee et al. 1993). The first molecularly characterized form was found in *Aplysia* ovotestis granules (Hellmich and Strumwassser 1991; Lee and Aarhus 1991), which on account of its high cyclase activity, monofunctional activity, and loose substrate specificity has been used for the chemoenzymatic synthesis of many cADPR analogues (Ashamu et al. 1995) used to probe cADPR signalling (see Sect. 8.3). The *Aplysia* cyclase has been crystallized and its three-dimensional structure solved, which should help to shed light on its enzymatic functions and mechanisms (Prasad et al. 1996). An intriguing finding is that in many tissues both cyclase and hydrolase activities are expressed on the same bifunctional polypeptide (Kim et al. 1993). The best characterized example of such a protein is the cell surface antigen CD38 (Howard et al. 1993). This transmembrane protein is involved in the regulation of proliferation and differentiation of lymphocytes and other cells, but is an ectoenzyme. The way in which extracellular production of cADPR leads to calcium mobilization from internal stores remains a mystery but influence of extracellular cADPR and β-NAD$^+$ on calcium mobilization in cerebellar granule cells has recently been reported (De Flora et al. 1996). ADP-ribosyl cyclase activities have been reported in cytoplasmic compartments in sea urchin eggs (Sethi et al. 1996) and mammalian brain (Yamauchi and Tanuma 1994) and to be associated with cardiac sarcoplasmic reticulum (Meszaros et al. 1997) and mitochondria (Ziegler et al. 1997).

8.5 cADPR in Stimulus-Response Coupling

The role of cADPR in cell regulation has been elucidated by use of selective cADPR analogues to probe cADPR-mediated signalling and by measurement of ADP-ribosyl cyclase activities and endogenous cADPR levels in response to cellular stimuli.

The finding that cADPR modulates CICR via RyRs in sea urchin eggs (Galione et al. 1991; Lee 1993) has been extended to several mammalian excitable cells. In the NG-108-15 neuroblastoma cell line cytosolic application of cADPR through a patch pipette enhances and globalizes the calcium signals elicited by calcium influx through plasma membrane voltage-sensitive calcium channels (Empson and Galione 1997). RyR2 plays a pivotal role in cardiac excitation-contraction coupling, whereby a small sarcolemma calcium influx is amplified by a larger calcium release from the sarcoplasmic reticulum leading to contraction. An important role for cADPR in regulating contractility has been demonstrated in guinea pig isolated ventricular myocytes. Intracellular administration of the competitive cADPR antagonist 8-amino-cADPR depresses sarcoplasmic reticular calcium release and contractility (Rakovic et al. 1996), whereas exogenous cADPR potentiates both calcium release and cell shortening (Iino et al. 1997). A model has been presented by which too little cADPR leads to failure of excitation contraction coupling whereas too much leads to spontaneous cycles of CICR, which may lead to arrhythmias (Galione et al. 1998).

A key question in cADPR research is how cellular stimuli are translated into changes in ADP-ribosyl cyclase activities and intracellular cADPR levels to allow it to function as an intracellular messenger. This has required the development of sensitive assays for ADP-ribosyl cyclase activities, for example, using NGD^+ as a substrate generating the fluorescent product cGDPR (Graeff et al. 1996), and for determining cADPR levels by thin-layer chromatography (Galione et al. 1993a; Higashida et al. 1997), HPLC (Walseth et al. 1991), sea urchin egg microsome bioassay (Horton et al. 1995) and radioimmunoassay (Takahashi et al. 1995).

The first clue as to how ADP-ribosyl cyclase activities can be regulated came from studies in the sea urchin egg which examined the mechanism of cGMP-induced calcium release in these cells. During fertilization in many different eggs, both IP3 and cADPR have been implicated as mediators of sperm-induced calcium release, but to different degrees depending on the species. In sea urchin eggs, calcium mobilization may be under dual control (Galione et al. 1993b; Lee et al. 1993), but in mouse and ascidian eggs IP3 is the major calcium mobilizing messenger, with cADPR regulating membrane-associated phenomena (Ayabe et al. 1995; Albrieux et al. 1997), while in *Xenopus* eggs IP3Rs may operate alone (Galione et al. 1993b). When microinjected into sea urchin eggs, cGMP induces a large, prolonged calcium transient after a considerable latency (Whalley et al. 1992; Sethi et al. 1996), reminiscent of the calcium transient seen in the fertilizing egg. Pharmacological studies indicate that RyRs are likely to be involved since this effect of cGMP is blocked by the RyR inhibitor ruthenium red (Galione et al. 1993a) but not by the IP3R antagonist heparin (Whalley et al. 1992). Using sea urchin egg homogenates to dissect the cGMP pathway, it was found that cGMP-induced calcium release can be reconstituted only if homogenates are supplemented with the cADPR precursor β-NAD+. In this system it was also found that calcium release by cGMP is blocked by 8-amino-cADPR, a selective competitive antagonist analogue of cADPR (Walseth and Lee 1993) but not by heparin, suggesting that cADPR mediates the effect, and thin-layer chromatography analysis has shown that cGMP stimulates cADPR production from β-NAD+ (Galione et al. 1993a). A role for ADP-ribosyl cyclase activity is suggested by the finding that the sea urchin egg ADP-ribosyl cyclase inhibitor nicotinamide blocks cGMP-induced calcium transients in both sea urchin egg homogenates and in intact cells (Sethi et al. 1996). Furthermore, agents such as nitric oxide (NO) which activate cGMP-synthesizing guanylyl cyclases induce calcium waves in sea urchin eggs via the cADPR-signalling pathway (Willmott et al. 1996). Since cGMP-dependent protein kinase inhibitors block calcium release by both NO and cGMP, a role for this kinase enzyme in stimulating ADP-ribosyl cyclase seems likely. A similar pathway activated by NO has also been described in neurosecretory PC12 cells (Clementi et al. 1996).

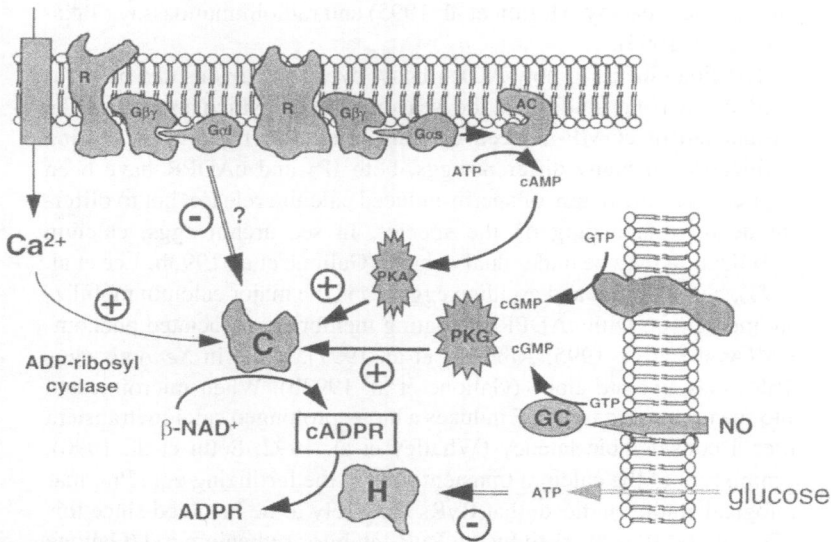

Fig. 3. Possible mechanisms for coupling cell surface receptor activation to ADP-ribosyl cyclase activity. Several mechanisms have been proposed in different cells for regulating cADPR levels by modulating its synthesis or hydrolysis. In sea urchin eggs and PC12 cells, NO and cGMP acting through a cGMP-dependent protein kinase (G-kinase) activates cADPR production (Galione at al. 1993a; Willmot et al. 1996; Clementi et al. 1996). In addition, other receptors coupled to cGMP production including α_1-adrenoceptors in rat lacrimal gland may be coupled to cADPR signalling pathways (Jorgensen et al. 1996). In chromaffin cells acetylcholine-induced increase in cAMP leads to cAMP-dependent protein kinase activation which stimulates cADPR production (Morita et al. 1997). In longitudinal smooth muscle it has been suggested that cholecystokinin receptors stimulate arachidonic acid production, which leads to the opening of dihydropyridine-sensitive plasma membrane calcium channels. ADP-ribosyl cyclase activity is raised by the calcium influx (Kummerle and Maklouf 1995). In NG-108 cells ADP-ribosyl cyclase may be under dual control by stimulatory and inhibitory G proteins coupled to M_1/M_3AChR or M_2/M_4 AChR, respectively (Higashida et al. 1997). Glucose may elevate cADPR levels in pancreatic β-cells by increasing ATP levels. ATP then inhibits cADPR hydrolases, leading to accumulation of cADPR due to basal activity of the ADP-ribosyl cyclase enzyme (Okamoto et al. 1997)

An important role for cADPR has been suggested by Okamoto and his colleagues in stimulus-secretion coupling in pancreatic β-cells (Takasawa et al. 1993). They have postulated that glucose-induced insulin secretion is mediated by cADPR which accumulates due to the inhibition of the cADPR hydrolase activity of a CD38-like enzyme (Fig. 3), leading to the activation of RyR2 receptors and hence calcium release and exocytosis. Interestingly, using a bioassay to measure cADPR production, these authors have shown that glucose-induced increases in cADPR levels occur in normal but not in diabetic pancreatic islets, and that this and other defects in cADPR signalling may play a crucial role in the aetiology of this disease (Okamoto et al. 1997). The origin of pancreatic material may be important and account for the failure of other groups to see glucose-induced cADPR changes by radioimmunoassay for cADPR (Malaisse et al. 1997).

Using the NGD^+ fluorescence assay for ADP-ribosyl cyclase activity, it has been shown in bovine chromaffin cell membranes that acetylcholine stimulates cADPR synthesis (Morita et al. 1997). The proposed mechanism is that cholinergic receptor activation promotes calcium influx which stimulates adenylyl cyclase, and the cAMP formed activates a cAMP-dependent protein kinase which in turn promotes synthesis of cADPR via stimulation of ADP-ribosyl cyclase. A role for calcium influx in the stimulation of cADPR production has also been proposed for cholecystokinin receptor induced calcium release from ryanodine-sensitive stores and contraction in rabbit longitudinal smooth muscle (Kummerle and Maklouf 1995).

As previously described, cADPR promotes CICR in NG108-15 cells (Empson and Galione 1997). In a recent study ADP-ribosyl cyclase has been shown to be under dual control of different muscarinic acetylcholine receptors (AChR), with M_1 and M_3 AChR stimulating the enzyme while M_2 and M_4 AChR inhibit cADPR synthesis (Higashida et al. 1997). Thin-layer chromatography of the products of the enzymatic reaction also indicates that direct stimulation of G proteins by guanine nucleotides leads to the activation or inhibition of the ADP-ribosyl cyclase enzymes in these cells.

Purinergic receptors in macrophages (Ebihara et al. 1997) and α_1-adrenoceptors in rat exocrine glands (Jorgensen et al. 1996) have also been suggested to couple to cADPR-signalling pathways. Other important candidates for receptors coupled to cADPR signalling pathways include those linked to calcium mobilization in the apparent absence of IP$_3$ production. An example of such a receptor is the endothelin B receptor in testicular myoid cells (Tripiciano et al. 1997). Preliminary investigations indicate that these cells express functional ryanodine receptors, and, in contrast to adjacent Sertoli and germ cells, exhibit high ADP-ribosyl cyclase and hydrolase activities (A. Filippini, A. Genazzani, R.M. Empson and A. Galione, unpublished observations). Most recently, cADPR but not IP$_3$ has been proposed as a second messenger for calcium mobilization in plant cells in response to the plant stress hormone abscisic acid (Wu et al. 1997; Pennisi 1997).

In addition to the acute regulation of cADPR levels by the modulation of ADP-ribosyl cyclase activities, modulation of the levels of ADP-ribosyl cyclase enzymes can influence cADPR concentrations in cells. Retinoic acid enhances the expression of CD38 in HL60 cells and leads to increases in cellular cADPR levels as measured by radioimmunoassay (Takahashi et al. 1995). In uterine muscle oestrogens increase the levels of ADP-ribosyl cyclases (Chini et al. 1997), while in smooth muscle thyroid hormones and retinoic acid similarly upregulate ADP-ribosyl cyclase expression (de Toledo et al. 1997).

8.6 NAADP-Gated Calcium Release Channels

ADP-ribosyl cyclases such as CD38 can catalyse two types of reaction, cyclization and base exchange (Fig. 4), and use β-NAD$^+$ and β-NADP$^+$ as alternative substrates (Aarhus et al. 1995b). If β-NADP$^+$ is cyclized, the product is 2-phospho-cADPR (cADPRP). cADPRP appears more potent than cADPR in activating RyRs in brain microsomes (Vu et al. 1996) and has been shown to release calcium in Jurkat cells (Guse et al. 1997) but is ineffective in sea urchin egg homogenates. This raises the intriguing possibility that subtypes of cADPR receptor exist. In the base exchange mode, nicotinamide is exchanged for nicotinic acid, yielding nicotinic acid adenine dinucleotide and NAADP, respectively, depending on whether β-NAD$^+$ or β-NADP$^+$ is used as substrate. NAADP has also been shown to be the calcium mobilizing contaminant of commercially available β-NADP$^+$ first described over 10 years ago in sea urchin egg homogenates (Clapper et al. 1987). It is at least as potent as cADPR, but its mechanism of calcium release is independent of both IP$_3$Rs and

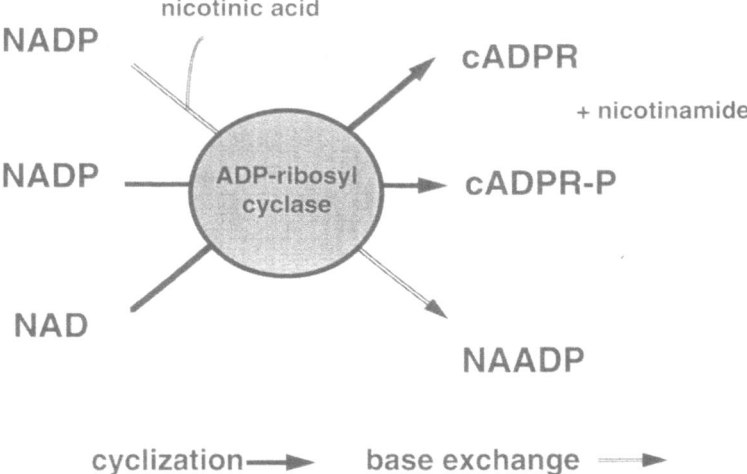

Fig. 4. ADP-ribosyl cyclases can produce several calcium mobilizing agents. ADP-ribosyl cyclases may use different substrates and catalyse two types of reaction to produce several calcium mobilizing messengers. These enzymes can cyclize NAD and NADP to cADPR and cADPRP, respectively (*solid arrows*) In the presence of nicotinic acid it catalyses base exchange (*open arrows*), swapping nicotinamide for nicotinic acid. If NADP is the substrate, NAADP is the product

RyRs and represents a new class of calcium release channel (Genazzani and Galione 1997).

NAADP-gated calcium channels do not appear to be regulated by calcium, and have a remarkable pharmacology for a putative calcium release channel in that they are selectively blocked by potassium and L-type calcium channel blockers (Genazzani et al. 1997). Furthermore, in contrast to calcium stores expressing IP3Rs and RyRs, those sensitive to NAADP are thapsigargin insensitive, suggesting that they are expressed on a different part of the endoplasmic reticulum or even a separate organelle (Genazzani et al. 1996). Perhaps the most unusual feature of the NAADP-gated calcium release mechanism is in its inactivation properties. Unlike the mechanisms regulated by IP3 and cADPR in sea urchin eggs, which after induction of calcium release appear to become refractory to subsequent activation, very low concentrations of

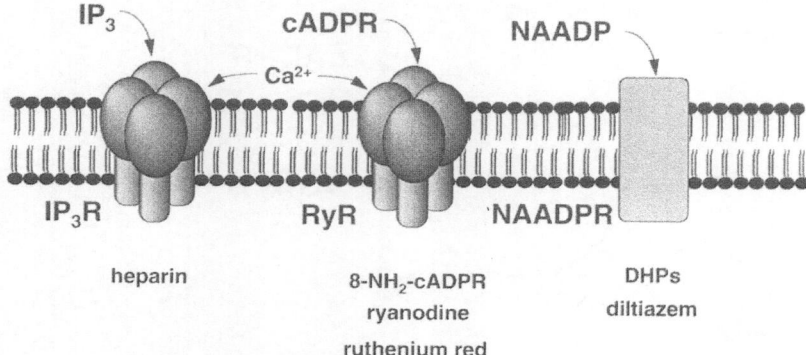

Fig. 5. Multiple mechanisms for calcium mobilization. At least three separate calcium release mechanisms are present on the internal stores of the sea urchin egg. The IP3R is gated by IP3 and blocked by the competitive antagonist heparin. RyRs are modulated by cADPR which is antagonized by 8-amino-cADPR, ryanodine and ruthenium red. Both IP3Rs and RyRs can be activated by calcium, resulting in CICR which is modulated by IP3 and cADPR, respectively. The NAADP-gated calcium release mechanism is distinct, and its pharmacology has not been fully investigated. The mechanism is activated by NAADP but blocked by certain potassium and L-type calcium channel blockers and by non-stimulating concentrations of NAADP itself

NAADP are able to inactivate NAADP-induced calcium release fully at concentrations well below those required to activate calcium release (Genazzani et al. 1996; Aarhus et al. 1996). The mechanism and physiological significance of this most unusual desensitization phenomenon are unclear.

8.7 Summary and Future Prospects

The past decade has seen the emergence of a family of pyridine nucleotides which function as calcium mobilizing agents. cADPR has been shown to be an important regulator of RyR-based CICR in many cells, and the use of selective pharmacological tools to study cADPR-mediated signalling has suggested that cADPR has an important role in many physiological and pathological processes. With the advent of techniques to measure cellular levels of cADPR, information about the way in which receptor activation is coupled to cADPR synthesis is emerging, which suggests that cADPR and IP_3 act as dual calcium mobilizing intracellular messengers. The discovery of the calcium releasing properties of NAADP in sea urchin eggs has defined a novel calcium release mechanism with remarkable properties quite distinct from IP_3Rs and RyRs.

Over the next few years our understanding will improve of the molecular details of both cADPR- and NAADP-induced calcium release and of the cellular responses that these molecules regulate. The discovery of multiple calcium release mechanisms controlled by multiple messengers (Fig. 5) may help in understanding the complexities of intracellular calcium signals widely observed, and how calcium ions can differentially regulate the myriad of calcium-dependent processes that occur in cells.

References

Aarhus R, Gee K, Lee HC (1995a) Caged cyclic ADP-ribose: synthesis and use. J Biol Chem 270:7745–7749

Aarhus R, Graeff RM, Dickey DM, Walseth TF, Lee HC (1995b) ADP-ribosyl cyclase and CD38 catalyze the synthesis of a calcium-mobilizing metabolite from $NADP^+$. J Biol Chem 270:30327–30333

Aarhus R, Dickey DM, Graeff RM, Gee KR, Walseth TF, Lee HC (1996) Activation and inactivation of Ca^{2+} release by $NAADP^+$. J Biol Chem 271:8513–8516

Albrieux M, Sardet C, Villaz M (1997) The two intracellular Ca^{2+} release channels ryanodine receptor and inositol 1,4,5-trisphosphate receptor play different roles during fertilization in ascidians. Dev Biol 189:174–185

Ashamu GA, Galione A, Potter BVL (1995) Chemo-enzymatic synthesis of analogues of the second messenger candidate cyclic adenosine 5'-diphosphate ribose. Chem Commun 1359–1360

Ayabe T, Kopf GS, Schultz RM (1995) Regulation of mouse egg activation: presence of ryanodine receptors and effects of microinjected ryanodine and cyclic ADP ribose on uninseminated and inseminated eggs. Development 121:2233–2244

Bailey V, Summerhill R, Galione A, Potter BVL (1996) Cyclic aristeromycin diphosphate ribose: a potent and poorly hydrolysable Ca^{2+} mobilizing mimic of cyclic adenosine diphosphate ribose. FEBS Lett 379:227–230

Bailey V, Sethi J, Fortt SM, Galione A, Potter BVL (1997) 7-Deaza-cyclic adenosine 5'-diphosphate ribose: first example of a Ca^{2+} mobilizing partial agonist related to cyclic adenosine 5'-diphosphate ribose. Chem Biol 4:51–61

Berridge MJ (1993) Inositol trisphosphate and calcium signalling. Nature 361:315–325

Campbell AK (1983) Intracellular calcium Its universal role as regulator. Wiley, Chichester

Chini EN, de Toledo FGS, Thompson MA, Dousa TP (1997) Effect of estrogen upon cyclic ADP ribose metabolism: beta-estradiol stimulates ADP ribosyl cyclase in rat uterus. Proc Natl Acad Sci USA 94:5872–5876

Clapper D, Walseth T, Dargie P, Lee HC (1987) Pyridine nucleotide metabolites stimulate calcium release from sea urchin egg microsomes desensitized to inositol trisphosphate. J Biol Chem 262:9561–9568

Clementi E, Riccio M, Sciorati C, Nistico G, Meldolesi J (1996) The type 2 ryanodine receptor of neurosecretory PC12 cells is activated by cyclic ADP-ribose. J Biol Chem 271:17739–17745

Dargie PJ, Agre MC, Lee HC (1990) Comparison of calcium mobilizing activities of cyclic ADP-ribose and inositol trisphosphate. Cell Regul 1:279–290

De Flora A, Guida L, Franco L, Zocchi E, Pestarino M, Usai C, Marchetti C, Fedele E, Fontana G, Raiteri M (1996) Ectocellular in-vitro and in-vivo metabolism of cADPR-ribose in cerebellum. Biochem J 320:665–671

de Toledo F, Cheng J, Dousa T (1997) Retinoic acid and triiodothyronine stimulate ADP-ribosyl cyclase activity in rat vascular smooth muscle cells. Biochem Biophys Res Commun 238:847–850

Ebihara S, Sasaki T, Hida W, Kikuchi Y, Oshiro T, Shimura S, Takasawa S, Okamoto H, Nishiyama A, Akaike N, Shirato K (1997) Role of cyclic ADP-ribose in ATP-activated potassium currents in alveolar macrophages. J Biol Chem 272:16023–16029

Empson R, Galione A (1997) Cyclic ADP-ribose enhances coupling between voltage gated Ca^{2+} entry and intracellular Ca^{2+} release. J Biol Chem 272:20967–20970

Galione A (1992) Ca^{2+} induced Ca^{2+} release and its modulation by cyclic ADP-ribose. Trends Pharmacol Sci 13:304–306

Galione A, Summerhill RS (1996) cADP-ribose as an endogenous regulator of ryanodine receptors. In: Sorrentino V (ed) Ryanodine receptors. CRC, Boca Raton, p 52

Galione A, Lee HC, Busa WB (1991) Ca^{2+} induced Ca^{2+} release in sea urchin egg homogenates: modulation by cyclic ADP-ribose. Science 253:1143–1146

Galione A, White A, Willmott N, Turner M, Potter BVL, Watson SP (1993a) cGMP mobilizes intracellular calcium in sea urchin eggs by stimulating cyclic ADP-ribose synthesis. Nature 365:456–459

Galione A, McDougall A, Busa W, Willmott N, Gillot I, Whitaker M (1993b) Redundant mechanisms of calcium-induced calcium release underlying calcium waves during fertilization of sea urchin eggs. Science 261:348–352

Galione A, Cui Y, Empson R, Iino S, Wilson H, Terrar DA (1998) Cyclic ADP-ribose and the regulation of calcium-induced calcium release in eggs and cardiac myocytes. Cell Biochem Biophys 28:19–30

Genazzani AA, Galione A (1997) A new calcium release mechanism gated by the novel pyridine nucleotide NAADP. Trends Pharmacol Sci 18:108–110

Genazzani AA, Empson R, Galione A (1996) Unique inactivation properties of NAADP-induced Ca^{2+} release. J Biol Chem 271:11599–11602

Genazzani AA, Walseth TF, Menza M, Michaelangeli F, Galione A (1997) Pharmacology of NAADP-induced calcium release. Br J Pharmacol 121:1489–1495

Graeff RM, Podein RJ, Aarhus R, Lee HC (1995) Magnesium ions but not ATP inhibit cyclic ADP-ribose-induced calcium release. Biochem Biophys Res Commun 206:786–791

Graeff RM, Walseth TF, Hill HK, Lee HC (1996) Fluorescent analogs of cyclic ADP-ribose: synthesis spectral characterization and use. Biochemistry 35:379–386

Guo X, Becker PL (1997) Cyclic ADP-ribose-gated Ca^{2+} release in sea urchin eggs requires an elevated $[Ca^{2+}]_i$. J Biol Chem 272:16984–16989

Guse AH, da Silva CP, Weber K, Armah CN, Ashamu GA, Schulze C, Potter BVL, Mayr GW, Hilz H (1997) 1-(5-Phospho-β-d-ribosyl)2'-phosphoadenosine 5'-phosphate cyclic anhydride induced Ca^{2+} release in human T-cell lines. Eur J Biochem 245:411–417

Hellmich MR, Strumwasser F (1991) Purification and characterization of a molluscan egg-specific NADase, a second-messenger enzyme. Cell Regul 2:193–202

Higashida H, Yokoyama S, Hashi M, Taketo M, Higashida M, Takayasu T, Ohshima T, Takasawa S, Okamoto H, Noda M (1997) Muscarinic receptor-mediated dual regulation of ADP-ribosyl cyclase in NG-108-15 neuronal cell membranes. J Biol Chem 272:31272–31277

Horton JK, Kalinka S, Martin R, Galione A, Baxindale PM (1995) A mass assay for determining endogenous cyclic ADP-ribose levels in tissues. 9th International Conference on Second Messengers and Phosphoproteins, Nashville, 27 Oct.–1 Nov., p 354

Howard M, Grimaldi JC, Bazan JF, Santos-Argumedo L, Parkhouse RME, Walseth TF, Lee HC (1993) Lymphocyte antigen CD38 catalyzes the formation and hydrolysis of cyclic ADP-ribose. Science 262:1056–1059

Iino S, Cui Y, Galione A, Terrar DA (1997) Actions of cADP-ribose and its antagonists on contraction in guinea-pig isolated ventricular myocytes. Influence of temperature. Circ Res 81:879–884

Jorgensen TD, Dissing S, Gromada J (1996) Cyclic GMP potentiates phenylephrine but not cyclic ADP-ribose-evoked calcium release from rat lacrimal acinar cells. FEBS Lett 391:117–120

Kim H, Jacobson EL, Jacobson MK (1993) Synthesis and degradation of cyclic ADP-ribose by NAD glycohydrolases. Science 261:1330–1333

Kuemmerle JF, Makhlouf GM (1995) Agonist-stimulated Cyclic ADP Ribose: endogenous modulator of Ca^{2+}-induced Ca^{2+} release in intestinal longitudinal muscle. J Biol Chem 270:25488–245494

Lee HC (1993) Potentiation of calcium- and caffeine-induced calcium release by cyclic ADP-ribose. J Biol Chem 268:293–299

Lee HC (1997) Mechanisms of calcium signaling by cyclic ADP-ribose and NAADP. Physiol Rev 77:1134–1164

Lee HC, Aarhus R (1991) ADP-ribosyl cyclase: an enzyme that cyclizes NAD^+ into a calcium-mobilizing metabolite. Cell Regul 2:203–209

Lee HC, Aarhus R (1995) A derivative of NADP mobilizes calcium stores insensitive to inositol trisphosphate and cyclic ADP-ribose. J Biol Chem 270:2152–2157

Lee HC, Walseth TF, Bratt GT, Hayes RN, Clapper DL (1989) Structural determination of a cyclic metabolite of NAD with intracellular calcium-mobilizing activity. J Biol Chem 264:1608–1615

Lee HC, Aarhus R, Walseth TF (1993) Calcium mobilization by dual receptors during fertilization of sea urchin eggs. Science 261:352–355

Lee HC, Aarhus R, Graeff R, Gurnack ME, Walseth TF (1994) Cyclic ADP-ribose activation of the ryanodine receptor is mediated by calmodulin. Nature 370:307–309

Malaisse WJ, Kanda Y, Inageda K, Scruel O, Sener A, Katada T (1997) Cyclic ADP-ribose measurements in rat pancreatic islets. Biochem Biophys Res Commun 231:546–548

Meissner G (1994) Ryanodine receptor Ca^{2+} release channels and their regulation by endogenous effectors. Ann Rev Physiol 56:485–508

Meszaros LG, Bak J, Chu A (1993) Cyclic ADP-ribose as an endogenous regulator of the non-skeletal type ryanodine receptor Ca^{2+} channel. Nature 364:76–79

Meszaros LG, Wrenn R, Varadi G (1997) Sarcoplasmic reticulum-associated and protein kinase C-regulated ADP-ribosyl cyclase in cardiac muscle. Biochem Biophys Res Commun 234:252–256

Missiaen L, Parys JB, de Smedt H, Sienaert I, Sipma H, Vanlingen S, Maes K, Kunzelmann K, Casteels R (1997) Inhibition of inositol trisphosphate-induced calcium release by cyclic ADP-ribose in A7r5 smooth muscle cells and in 16HBE14o-bronchial mucosal cells. Biochem J (in press)

Morita K, Kitayama S, Dohi T (1997) Stimulation of cyclic ADP-ribose synthesis by acetylcholine and its role in catecholamine release in bovine adrenal chromaffin cells. J Biol Chem 272:21002–21009

Noguchi N, Takasawa S, Nata N, Tohgo A, Kato I, Ikehata F, Yonekura H, Okamoto H (1997) Cyclic ADP-ribose binds to FK506-binding protein 126 to release Ca^{2+} from islet microsomes. J Biol Chem 272:3133–3137

Okamoto H, Takasawa S, Nata K (1997) The CD38-cyclic ADP-ribose signalling system in insulin secretion: molecular basis and clinical implications. Diabetologia 40:1485–1491

Pennisi E (1997) Plants decode a universal signal. Science 278:2054–2055

Prasad GS, Levitt DG, Lee HC, Stout CD (1996) Crystallization of ADP-ribosyl cyclase from *Aplysia californica*. Proteins Struct Funct Genet 24:138–140

Rakovic S, Galione A, Ashamu GA, Potter BVL, Terrar DA (1996) A specific cyclic ADP-ribose antagonist inhibits cardiac excitation-contraction coupling. Curr Biol 6:989–996

Ringer S (1882) Concerning the influence exerted by each of the constituents of the blood on the contraction of the ventricle. J Physiol (Lond) 3:380–393

Rusinko N, Lee HC (1989) Widespread occurrence in animal tissues of an enzyme catalyzing the conversion of NAD^+ into a cyclic metabolite with intracellular Ca^{2+} mobilizing activity. J Biol Chem 264:11725–11731

Sethi J, Empson R, Galione A (1996) Nicotinamide inhibits cADPR-mediated calcium signalling in sea urchin eggs. Biochem J 319:613–617

Sethi JK, Empson R, Bailey VC, Potter BVL, Galione A (1997) 7-deaza-8-bromo cyclic adenosine 5'-diphosphate ribose, the first membrane-permeant hydrolysis-resistant cyclic ADP-ribose antagonist. J Biol Chem 272:16358–16363

Sitsapesan R, McGarry SJ, Williams AJ (1995) Cyclic ADP-ribose, the ryanodine receptor and Ca^{2+} release. Trends Pharmacol Sci 16:386–391

Sorrentino V, Volpe P (1993) Ryanodine receptors: how many where and why? Trends Pharmacol Sci 14:98–103

Takahashi K, Kukimoto I, Tokita KI, Inageda K, Inoue SI, Kontani K, Hoshino SI, Nishina H, Kanaho Y, Katada T (1995) Accumulation of cyclic ADP-ribose measured by a specific radioimmunoassay in differentiated human leukemic HL-60 cells with all-trans-retinoic acid. FEBS Lett 371:204–208

Takasawa S, Nata K, Yonekura H, Okamoto H (1993) Cyclic ADP-ribose in insulin secretion from pancreatic beta cells. Science 259:370–373

Tanaka Y, Tashjian AH Jr (1995) Calmodulin is a selective mediator of Ca^{2+}-induced Ca^{2+} release via the ryanodine receptor-like Ca^{2+} channel triggered by cyclic ADP-ribose. Proc Natl Acad Sci USA 92:3244–3248

Tripiciano A, Palombi F, Ziparo E, Filippini A (1997) Dual control of seminiferous tubule contractility mediated by ET_A and ET_B endothelin receptor subtypes. FASEB J 11:276–286

Vu CQ, Lu PJ, Chen CS, Jacobson MK (1996) 2'-Phospho-cyclic ADP-ribose, a calcium-mobilizing agent derived from NADP. J Biol Chem 271:4747–4754

Walseth TF, Lee HC (1993) Synthesis and characterization of antagonists of cyclic-ADP-ribose-induced Ca^{2+} release. Biochim Biophys Acta 1178:235–242

Walseth TF, Aarhus R, Zeleznikar RJJ, Lee HC (1991) Determination of endogenous levels of cyclic ADP-ribose in rat tissues. Biochim Biophys Acta 1094:113–120

Walseth TF, Aarhus R, Kerr JA, Lee HC (1993) Identification of cyclic ADP-ribose-binding proteins by photoaffinity labeling. J Biol Chem 268:26686–26691

Whalley T, McDougall A, Crossley I, Swann K, Whitaker M (1992) Internal calcium release and activation of sea urchin eggs by cGMP are independent of the phosphoinositide signaling pathway. Mol Biol Cell 3:373–383

Willmott N, Sethi J, Walseth TF, Lee HC, White AM, Galione A (1996) Nitric oxide induced mobilization of intracellular calcium via the cyclic ADP-ribose signalling pathway. J Biol Chem 271:3699–3705

Wu Y, Kuzma J, Marechal E, Graeff R, Lee HC, Foster R, Chua NH (1997) Abscisic acid signaling through cyclic ADP-ribose in plants. Science 278:2126–2130

Yamauchi J, Tanuma S (1994) Occurrence of an NAD^+ glycohydrolase in bovine brain cytosol. Arch Biochem Biophys 308:327–329

Ziegler M, Jorke D, Schweiger M (1997) Identification of bovine liver mitochondrial NAD^+ glycohydrolase as ADP-ribosyl cyclase. Biochem J 326:401–405

9 Human Gonadotropin Receptors: Pathophysiology, Pharmacology, and Molecular Mechanisms

Y. Osuga, M. Kudo, and A.J.W. Hsueh

9.1 Gonadotropin and TSH Receptors as Unique Members of the G Protein Coupled Receptor Family

The gonadotropins follicle-stimulating hormone (FSH) and luteinizing hormone (LH) are necessary for the growth and differentiation of mammalian gonads in both sexes. The LH receptor is found in testicular Leydig cells and ovarian theca, granulosa, luteal, and interstitial cells. The FSH receptor is localized on granulosa cells of the ovary and Sertoli cells of the testis. Both types of receptors play a pivotal role in reproduction.

The gonadotropin receptors belong to the large family of G protein coupled receptors characterized functionally by their interaction with guanine nucleotide-binding proteins and structurally by their seven hydrophobic, α-helical transmembrane (TM) domains. The seven-TM, G protein coupled receptors probably represent one of the largest gene families in eukaryotic organisms. Members of this superfamily are functionally diverse and include receptors ranging from the cAMP receptor in slime mold to mammalian neurotransmitter and glycoprotein hormone receptors (Lefkowitz and Caron 1988). Agonist occupancy of these plasma membrane proteins is believed to result in conformational changes of the receptors, leading to the activation of various G proteins which in turn modulate the activity of a number of effector enzymes and ion channels (Gilman 1987). The glycoprotein hormone receptor subfamily, including receptors for LH/choriogonadotropin (CG), FSH, and thyrotropin (TSH), diverges structurally from other G protein coupled receptors in having large extracellular (EC) domains required for interaction with the large glycoprotein hormones (McFarland et al. 1989; Loosfelt et al. 1989; Nagayama and Rapoport 1992). The amino-terminus domains of these glycoprotein hormone receptors confer ligand specificity and are homologous to those of the leucine-rich repeat protein family, including the ribonuclease inhibitor (Kobe and Deisenhofer 1993).

9.2 Gain-of-Function Mutations in the LH Receptor as a Model to Study the Activation of G Protein Coupled Receptors

Although much is known about ligand binding to the G protein coupled receptors (Wess 1997) and the activation of G proteins by activated receptors, the mechanism underlying ligand activation of the receptors is still unclear. Recently, several constitutive activating mutations of these membrane proteins have been found: in rhodopsin (Rao et al. 1994; Robinson et al. 1992) leading to retinitis pigmentosa and congenital night blindness, in melanocyte-stimulating hormone receptor leading to different color coats (Robbins et al. 1993), in parathyroid hormone (PTH)–PTH-related protein receptor leading to Jansen-type metaphyseal chondrodysplasia (Schipani et al. 1995), and in Ca^{2+}-sensing receptor leading to familial hypocalciuric hypercalcemia and neonatal severe hyperparathyroidism (Pollak et al. 1993, 1994). Gain-of-function mutations have also been found for genes in the subfamily of gonadotropin and TSH receptors.

Because these point mutations of the receptors lead to ligand-independent activation of G proteins, they are potentially useful to elucidate the mechanism of receptor activation. In the TSH receptor, mutations in several TM regions, intracellular loop 3 (i3), and the EC loops 2 and 3 are associated with hyperfunctioning thyroid adenoma and congenital hyperthyroidism (Cetani et al. 1996; Parma et al. 1993, 1994; Van Sande et al. 1995), whereas mutations in the TM V and VI and i3 of the LH receptor lead to familial male precocious puberty, which is inherited in an autosomal dominant, male-limited manner (Kosugi et al. 1995; Kremer et al. 1993; Latronico et al. 1995; Laue et al. 1995a, 1996; Shenker et al. 1993; Yano et al. 1994, 1995). Although the FSH receptor shows high homology to LH and TSH receptors, none of the mutations at several conserved amino acids (D567G, D581G, D581Y, and C584R) whose substitution lead to constitutive activation of LH or TSH receptors significantly increases the basal activity of the FSH receptor.

Taking advantage of this difference between the homologous receptors, we designed chimeric FSH/LH receptors with or without a point mutation in i3 to identify the region of the LH receptor that is important for its constitutive activation and to elucidate differences between domains of LH and FSH receptors responsible for constitutive activation (Kudo et al. 1996). We constructed a chimeric receptor containing only the TM V–VI (including i3) from the LH receptor [(FL(V–VI)F; Fig. 1A]. As shown in Fig. 1B, the chimeric receptor retained ligand-binding ability with similar K_d values to that of the wildtype (WT) FSH receptor, whereas incorporation of the D567G mutation further increased its ligand-binding affinity. The expression levels of FL(V–VI)F were comparable to those of the WT FSH receptor, but the mutated receptor had lower expression [WT FSH receptor, 100%; FL(V–VI)F, 90±8%; FL(V–VI)FD567G, 27±4%; $n=3$]. As shown in Fig. 1A, both FL(V–VI)F and its D567G mutant responded to FSH treatment with increases in cAMP production. Of interest, the D567G mutant receptor showed constitutive activation, as demonstrated by 10.5±0.7-fold higher basal cAMP production than that of FL(V–VI)F ($p < 0.01$, $n=6$).

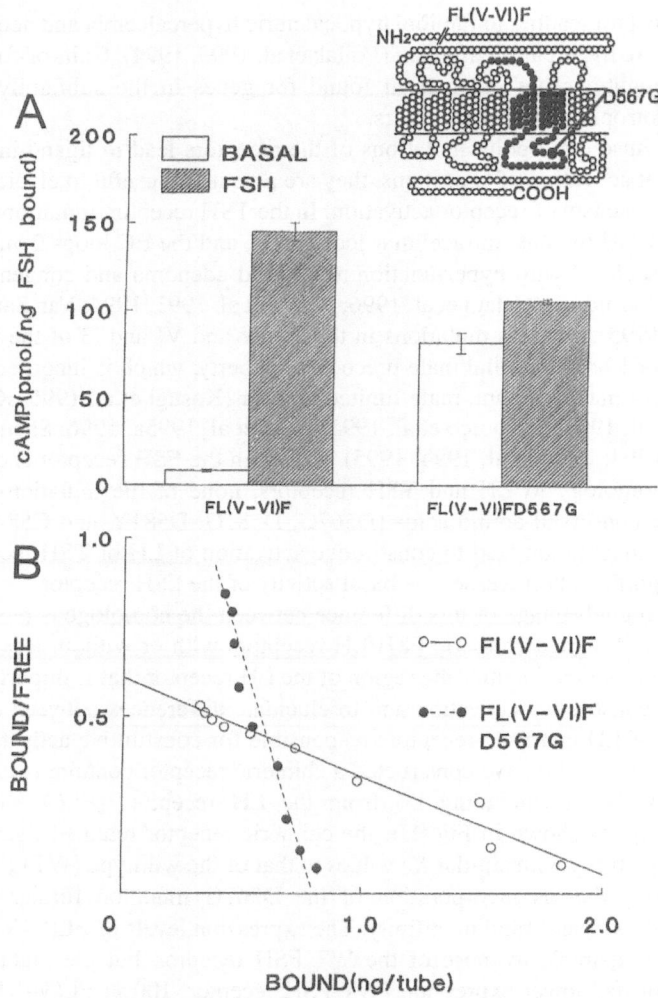

Fig. 1A,B. Legend see p. 157

We further tested the hypothesis that a point mutation in i3 of the FSH receptor alters interactions between TM V and TM VI of the LH receptor. We constructed a chimeric receptor, FL(V/VI)F, in which TM V and TM VI regions are from the LH receptor but i3 and the remaining regions from the FSH receptor (Fig. 2A). A point mutation D567G was also introduced into i3 of the FSH receptor sequence. As shown in Fig. 2B, chimeric receptors with and those without the point mutation were expressed on the cell surface at similar levels comparable to that of WT FSH receptor (100% for WT FSH receptor; 100%±10% for FL(V/VI)F; 110%±10% for FL(V/VI)FD567G; mean±SD, n=3). However, the D567G mutant showed higher affinity to FSH than FL(V/VI)F. As shown in Fig. 2A, FSH treatment stimulated cAMP production in both FL(V/VI)F and its D567G mutant. Of interest, basal cAMP production showed an increase after the introduction of the point mutation (3.6±0.2 times that of FL(V/VI)F; n=3). These results indicate that the EC region of gonadotropin receptors is important for ligand-binding but is not involved in receptor activation, whereas the TM V–VI region of the LH receptor is essential for constitutive activation.

Although i3 of adrenergic receptors has been shown to interact directly with the Gs protein (Cheung et al. 1991; Luttrell et al. 1993; O'Dowd et al. 1988), a chimeric gonadotropin receptor with the mutated i3 derived from the LH receptor and the remaining sequences derived from FSH receptor did not show constitutive activation. Instead, FSH

◀ **Fig. 1A,B.** Constitutive activation of the mutant receptor, FL(V–VI)FD567G, with the TM V, i3, and TM VI regions of the FSH receptor replaced by the LH receptor. **A** Mutagenesis and gene transfer experiments were performed to construct chimeric receptor FL(V–VI)F and its D567G mutant. WT and mutant receptor cDNAs were transfected into 293 cells. After 48 h of incubation the cells were incubated in fresh medium with or without a saturating dose (300 ng/ml) of FSH for 1 h in the presence of 0.25 mM 3-isobutyl-1-methyl xanthine. Total cAMP production by transfected cells was measured by specific radioimmunoassay. Some cells were used for FSH receptor binding analysis to determine K_d and total receptor number. To correct for changes in receptor expression, cAMP production is expressed as pmol cAMP/ng FSH bound. means±SD of three independent transfections with triplicate cultures per experiments are shown. **B** Scatchard plot analysis of chimeric receptor FL(V–VI)F and its mutant, showing an increase in binding affinity after introduction of the point mutation

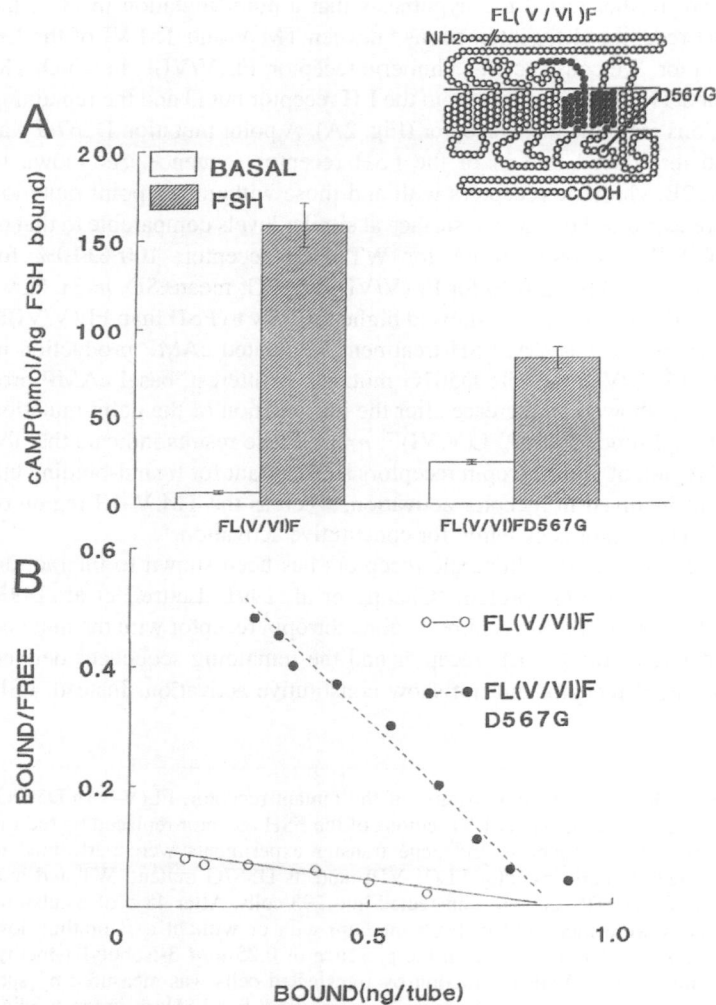

Fig. 2A,B. Legend see p. 159

receptor with the flanking TM V and VI regions replaced by the homologous sequences from the LH receptor, when combined with a mutation in i3, showed ligand-independent increases in basal cAMP production. These data suggest that interactions between specific TM domains and not only the specific site of the point mutation in i3 are responsible for constitutive activation of the LH receptor. The observation that mutations at multiple sites within the region extending from TM V through TM VI of the LH receptor can lead to constitutive activation suggests that these mutations alter interactions between i3 of the receptor and G protein by changing the position of TM V and TM VI relative to each other or to other TM domains. In the FSH receptor, the movement of TM V and TM VI may be more tightly constrained by stronger intramolecular interactions.

A model explaining our findings is shown in Fig. 3. We propose that movement of TM V and TM VI relative to each other would likely alter the conformation of i3. As shown in Fig. 3A, interactions between TM V and TM VI as well as interactions between the amino and carboxyl-terminal ends of i3 maintain the LH receptor in an inactive state. These interactions can be overcome by agonist binding or by mutation of critical amino acids (Fig. 3B). In the FSH receptor the number of stabilizing interactions between TM V and TM VI is greater such that mutation of the amino acids in i3 (or TM VI) is not sufficient to alter the position of TM V relative to TM VI (Fig. 3C,D). Thus one might expect that a chimeric receptor consisting of TM V and TM VI from the LH receptor and the remaining sequence from the FSH receptor would be more susceptible to a mutation in the i3 loop of the FSH receptor (Fig. 3E,F).

◄ **Fig. 2A,B.** Constitutive activation of the mutant receptor FL(V/VI)FD567G with only TM V and TM VI from the LH receptor but the i3 and the remaining parts from the FSH receptor. **A** Mutagenesis and gene transfer experiments were performed to construct a chimeric receptor, FL(V/VI)F, and its D567G mutant with only the TM V and VI from the LH receptor but the flanking i3 and remaining parts from the FSH receptor. Basal and FSH-stimulated cAMP production by transfected 293 cells was determined as described in the legend to Fig. 1. **B** Scatchard plot analysis of chimeric FL(V/VI)F receptor and its D567G mutant, showing an increase in binding affinity after introduction of the point mutation

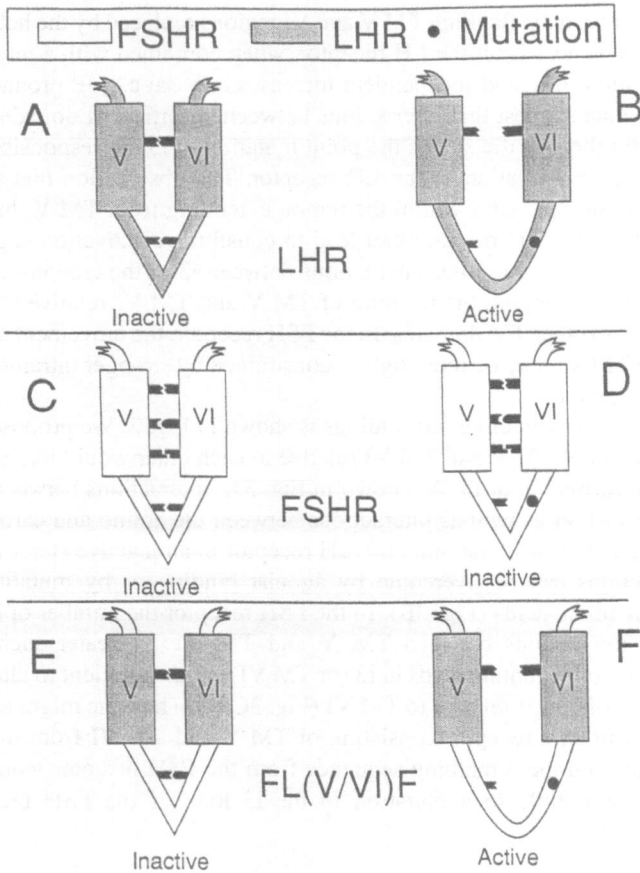

Fig. 3A–F. Models depicting differences between LH and FSH receptors in their susceptibility to constitutive activation. We hypothesize that differences in interactions between TM V and VI of gonadotropin receptors lead to their different susceptibility to constitutive activation by a point mutation in i3. Stronger interactions (*three pairs of black bars*) between TM V and VI of the FSH receptor restrain it in an inactive state, whereas weaker interactions (*one pair of black bars*) between TM V and VI of the LH receptor allow easy activation of the receptor following the i3 mutation. For the chimeric receptor FL(V/VI)F, with TM V and VI from the LH receptor but the remaining parts (including i3) from the FSH receptor, a point mutation in i3 disrupts the weak interactions between the two TM domains of LH receptor

9.3   Loss-of-Function Mutations in LH Receptor and the Use of Complementary Receptor Mutants to Reconstitute Ligand Signaling

Earlier studies showed that the function of truncated β-adrenergic, vasopressin V_2, and muscarinic M_3 receptors can be reconstituted when cotransfected with the missing TM folding domains (Gudermann et al. 1997). These results indicate that the TM regions of these heptahelical molecules are composed of independent functional units. For receptors used in these studies, the TM regions are important for both ligand binding and signal transduction, thus rendering it difficult to separate the two important functions of these proteins.

We have recently found a mutant LH receptor truncated at TM5 in a patient with Leydig cell hypoplasia. The defective receptor retained limited ligand-binding ability but was incapable of mediating cAMP responses (Laue et al. 1995b). Taking advantage of the unique separation of ligand binding and signal transduction domains of gonadotropin receptors, we have studied the interactions between this binding plus signaling minus mutant receptor and several receptor mutants defective in ligand binding but retaining their C-terminal TM endodomain (Osuga et al. 1997a).

An earlier study demonstrated that a mutant rat LH receptor with the EC ligand-binding region deleted can be expressed in transfected cells but requires pharmacological concentrations of hCG for signal transduction (Ji and Ji 1991). Based on this finding we generated a similar mutant LH receptor containing exons 1 and 10 of the human receptor and named it L(TM1–7). As shown in Fig. 4, treatment with up to 1 mg/ml of hCG did not stimulate cAMP production in cells transfected with the plasmid encoding L(TM1–7). However, hCG treatment of cells coexpressing L(TM1–7) and L(EC-TM1–5) led to dose-dependent increases in cAMP production to levels that were 20% of those found in cells expressing WT LH receptors, indicating restoration of ligand signaling. Stimulation of cAMP in cells expressing L(TM1–7) requires high doses (10 mg/ml) of hCG (Ji and Ji 1991). However, cells coexpressing L(TM1–7) and L(EC-TM1–5) respond to 10 ng/ml hCG with significant increases in cAMP production ($p < 0.01$). We further investigated the minimal TM region required for interactions with L(TM1–7). As shown in Fig. 4, hCG treatment induced dose-dependent increases of

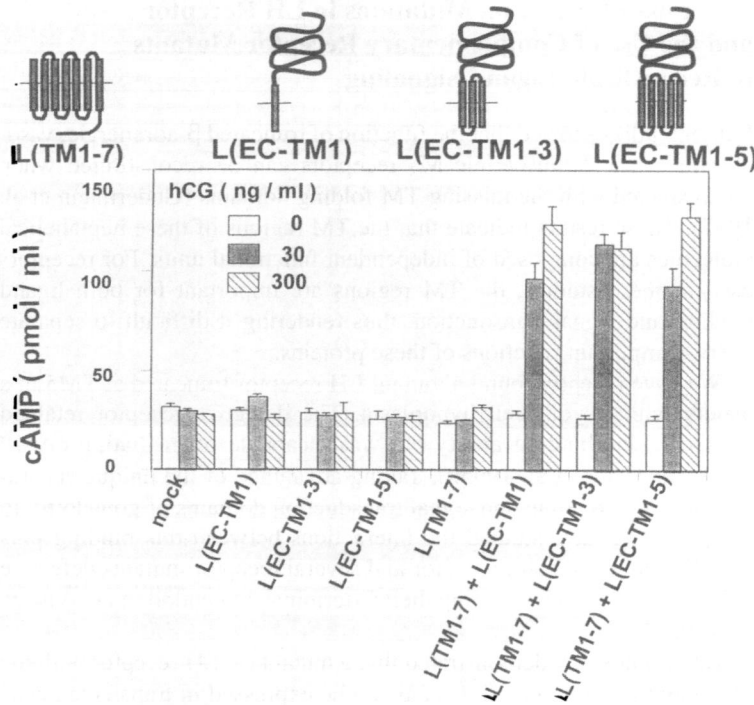

Fig. 4. Coexpression of LH receptors truncated at different TM domains, together with a mutant LH receptor containing only the endodomain L(TM1–7), partially restores ligand signaling. Stimulation of cAMP production by hCG in cells coexpressing different truncated LH receptor mutants together with L(TM1–7)

cAMP production in cells coexpressing L(TM1–7) together with L(EC-TM1) or L(EC-TM1–3). These data suggest that the presence of TM1 is sufficient partially to restore ligand signaling.

Because an earlier report suggested that coexpression of the EC region and endodomain of the porcine LH receptor allows hCG stimulation of cAMP production (Remy et al. 1993), we constructed the plasmid L(EC) encoding the EC region of the human LH receptor but lacking the endodomain. As shown in Fig. 4, treatment with 13/4 μg/ml hCG did not stimulate cAMP production in cells cotransfected with L(EC) together with L(TM1–7), compared with a major stimulation of cAMP by hCG (1003/4 ng/ml) in cells coexpressing L(TM1–7) and L(EC-TM1). Ligand cross-linking experiments were performed to determine whether L(EC) can still bind hCG. As shown in Fig. 4 (left panel), the formation of high molecular mass complexes (873/4 kDa) between labeled hCG and L(EC) was found in the total cell extract from cells cotransfected with plasmids encoding L(EC) and L(TM1–7), and the complex formation was competed by nonlabeled hCG. However, cross-linking of labeled hCG to plasma membrane proteins in the same cells did not lead to complex formation, in direct contrast to the formation of high molecular mass, competable complexes (1303/4 kDa) between labeled hCG and WT LH receptor (Fig. 4, right panel). These data suggest minimal restoration of receptor function when cells are cotransfected with plasmids encoding L(TM1–7) and L(EC) under the present experimental conditions and the importance of TM1 in ligand signaling.

Earlier studies demonstrated that the ligand-binding EC region of the thrombin receptor, anchored on the cell surface through the single TM region of CD8, interacts efficiently with the TM segments (endodomain) of the thrombin receptor to restore ligand signaling (Chen et al. 1994). We also tested whether the anchored receptor approach used for the related thrombin receptor allows restoration of ligand signaling for anchored LH receptors. Our findings suggest that ligand signaling can be partially restored, but no stimulation of cAMP production by hCG is detected in cells coexpressing L(EC)CD8 and L(TM1–7). These data indicate that the LH receptor may differ from the related thrombin receptor in that coexpression of its TM endodomain together with its anchored EC region fused to a foreign TM domain cannot restore ligand signaling.

TM helices of G protein coupled receptors are believed to represent independent folding units and form a tightly packed channel-like structure (Baldwin 1993). Our study shows that cotransfection of cells with LH receptor fragments or chimeric gonadotropin receptors defective in either ligand binding or signal transduction leads to functional complementation and ligand-activated signal generation (Fig. 5). Studies using the EC region of the LH receptor alone, the EC region anchored through the heterologous single TM domain of CD8 to the cell surface or as soluble complexes with its ligand, further suggest that the TM1 region

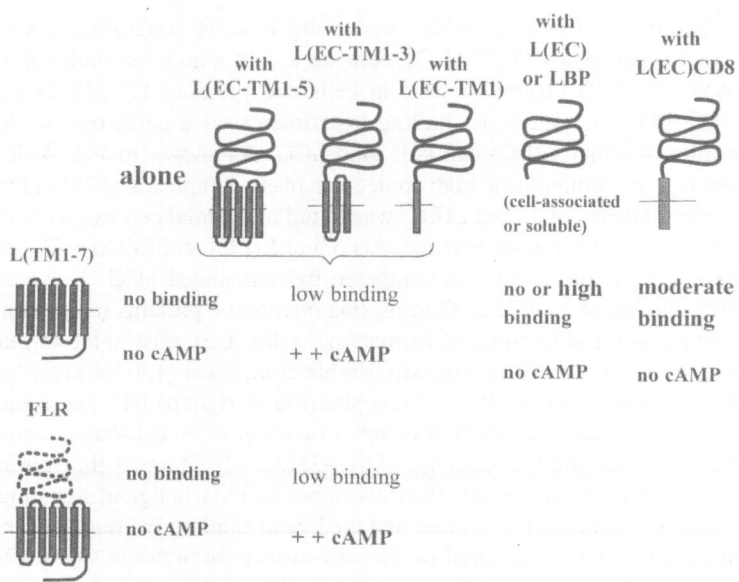

Fig. 5. Coexpression of gonadotropin receptors lacking ligand-binding or signal transduction capability partially restores ligand signaling: diagrammatic summary of interactions between different mutant receptors. Binding of labeled hCG and hCG-induced cAMP production in cells transfected with various mutant receptors is indicated. *Dashed lines*, FSH receptor sequences. L(EC-TM1–5) shows low binding to hCG, whereas L(EC)CD8 shows moderate binding. In cells cotransfected with the endodomain L(TM1–7) together with L(EC-TM1), L(EC-TM1–3), or L(EC-TM1–5), ligand signaling to hCG was partially restored. Likewise, ligand signaling was found in cells coexpressing FLR and L(EC-TM1), L(EC-TM1–3), or L(EC-TM1–5). Although high hCG binding was found for the soluble EC region of the LH receptor (*LBP*), incubation of the hCG-LBP complexes did not activate the endodomain of the receptor. Likewise, expression of the cell-associated EC region of the LH receptor [*L(EC)*] together with the endodomain L(TM1–7) did not allow ligand signaling. Furthermore, no cAMP stimulation by hCG was found in cells coexpressing anchored EC region [*L(EC)CD8*] and the endodomain [*L(TM1–7)*] of the receptor. The requirement of TM1 for interactions between defective receptors suggests the importance of TM1 and/or the EC/TM1 junction in ligand signaling

of the LH receptor is important for receptor function. The large EC region of the LH receptor, when connected to one or several of the TM domains, can be reconstituted into functional proteins after coexpression with its own endodomain. The observed interactions between receptor fragments took place with TM1 connected to the EC region in cells coexpressing L(EC-TM1) together with L(TM1–7) or with FLR. This interaction is receptor-specific, because coexpression of L(EC-TM1–5), together with the WT FSH receptor, was ineffective in restoring ligand signaling. It is likely that the interaction between the endodomain and the ligand-bound EC region is too weak to allow receptor activation without a covalent linkage between the EC and TM1. The present finding that L(EC-TM1) complements L(TM1–7) in functional restoration suggests that conformational changes in the EC/TM junction induced by ligand binding are essential for ligand signaling. Alternatively, these two mutant receptors may interact such that TM1 of L(EC-TM1) displaces TM1 of L(TM1–7) and folds into a functional complex in which the EC region of L(EC-TM1) is in direct contact with the TM domains of L(TM1–7).

Leydig cell hypoplasia is a form of male pseudohermaphroditism, in which affected 463/4XY males show a female phenotype associated with low androgen production by Leydig cells (Laue et al. 1995b). The present findings that cotransfection of L(EC-TM1–5) and L(TM1–7) partially restores ligand signaling suggest that overexpression of L(TM1–7) in testis cells could form the basis of gene therapies to rescue genetic defects found in these patients. A similar approach has allowed the restoration of the function of defective vasopressin V_2 receptors found in patients with nephrogenic diabetes insipidus (Schoneberg et al. 1996). The present finding extends the coexpression strategy in the treatment of diseases caused by inactivating mutations in the seven-TM receptor family.

9.4   The Derivation of Soluble Ectodomain of Gonadotropin and TSH Receptors as Functional Antagonists

Many receptors for hormones of the hematopoietin family have soluble isoforms derived either from alternative mRNA splicing (receptors for granulocyte colony stimulating factor, interleukin-4, leukemia inhibiting factor, etc.) or from proteolytic cleavage of the EC region of the receptor (receptors for interleukin-1, tumor necrosis factor, etc.; Heaney and Golde 1993). Furthermore, the isolation of circulating growth hormone (GH) binding proteins indicated that they are truncated forms of tissue receptors with deletion of the TM region (Leung et al. 1987). Some of these truncated receptors may act as functional antagonists. Although the large EC regions of gonadotropin receptors confer ligand binding, truncated gonadotropin receptors are trapped intracellularly (Tsai-Morris et al. 1990; Xie et al. 1990).

Using an anchored fusion receptor approach followed by proteolytic cleavage, we have generated ligand-binding regions of gonadotropin and TSH receptors as soluble binding proteins to neutralize the action of specific glycoprotein hormones (Osuga et al. 1997b). We fused the EC domains of human FSH and LH receptors to the single TM domain of CD8 through a thrombin cleavage site and termed them FtCD8 and LtCD8, respectively. Human 293 cells transfected with FtCD8 or LtCD8 showed a high-affinity cell surface binding to their specific ligand, with expression levels comparable to those of the WT receptors. For anchored FtCD8, the binding affinity to radiolabeled FSH was three times that of the WT receptor whereas anchored LtCD8 showed a binding affinity comparable to that of the WT receptor (K_d values: FtCD8: 0.31 nM; WT FSH receptor: 1.03 nM; LtCD8: 0.61 nM; WT LH receptor: 0.28 nM).

To solubilize ligand-binding EC regions of these anchored receptors, the cells expressing FtCD8 or LtCD8 were treated with thrombin. The soluble receptor fragments were termed FSH-binding protein (FBP) and LH/hCG-binding protein (LBP), respectively. The addition of FBP prevented binding of labeled FSH to the WT receptors in a dose-dependent manner, reaching a level comparable to nonspecific binding (Fig. 6A). In contrast, inclusion of LBP was ineffective. Furthermore, inclusion of the same preparations of receptor fragments in the hCG-binding assay using WT LH receptors led to a dose-dependent inhibition of binding by

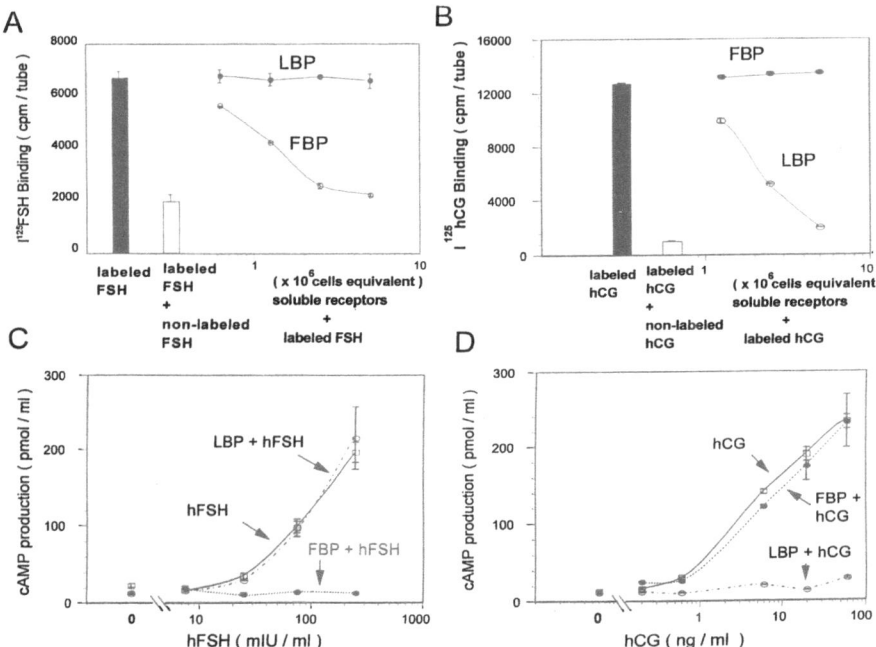

Fig. 6A–D. Competition for receptor binding and neutralization of gonadotropin actions in vitro by solubilized EC regions of FSH and LH receptors. **A** Competition of labeled FSH binding to FSH receptors by solubilized EC regions of FSH receptor (*FBP*) but not LH receptor (*LBP*). Cells expressing human FSH receptors were incubated with labeled FSH with or without increasing amounts of FBP or LBP. **B** Competition of labeled hCG binding to LH receptors by LBP but not FBP. Cells expressing LH receptors were incubated with labeled hCG with or without LBP or FBP. **C** Antagonism of FSH stimulation of cAMP production by FBP but not LBP. Cells expressing FSH receptors were incubated with increasing amounts of FSH in the presence or absence of FBP or LBP (10^7 cells equivalent/well) for 3 h at 37°C before cAMP determination by radioimmunoassay. Concentration of binding proteins was determined based on their ability to inhibit the binding of respective labeled ligands to WT receptors. **D** Antagonism of hCG stimulation of cAMP production by LBP but not FBP. Cells expressing human LH receptors were incubated with hCG with or without LBP or FBP

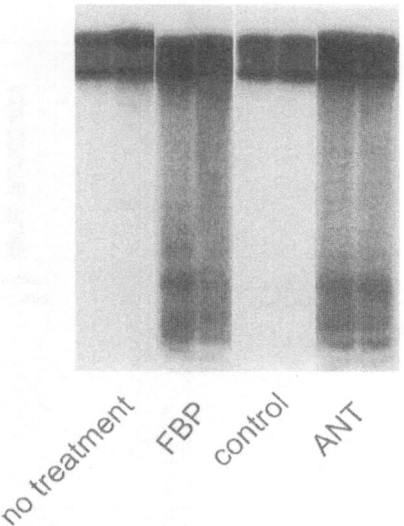

Fig. 7. Induction of testis cell apoptosis following FBP administration in vivo. For expression of FtCD8 in insect cells, recombinant baculovirus was prepared using the Bac-to-Bac baculovirus expression system, and SF9 cells were infected with the recombinant viruses. After a 72-h culture at 27°C in media containing 5% serum and thrombin cells were centrifuged and conditioned media concentrated before filtration with 0.2-µm filters. Immature male rats (21 days of age) were injected (subcutaneously every 6 h) with conditioned media of SF9 cells (10^8 cells equivalent/injection) containing solubilized FBP. Two days later testis weight was determined and testis cell apoptosis quantitated using a 3' end labeling method. Some animals were treated with a potent GnRH antagonist (*ANT*; 50 µg/rat) to suppress pituitary release of LH and FSH whereas others were treated with conditioned media of SF9 cells infected with WT baculovirus. Pattern of apoptotic DNA fragmentation (two samples/group)

LBP but not by FBP (Fig. 6B). Thus, FBP and LBP specifically prevented the binding of their respective ligands. We further evaluated the ability of binding proteins to interfere with signal transduction induced by gonadotropins. We incubated 293 cells expressing WT FSH or LH receptors with increasing concentrations of FSH or hCG for 3 h at 37°C to stimulate cAMP production. As shown in Fig. 6C, the addition of FBP completely blocked cAMP production induced by FSH in FSH receptor expressing cells whereas LBP was ineffective. Conversely, the addition of LBP inhibited cAMP stimulation by hCG in LH receptor-expressing cells whereas FBP was ineffective (Fig. 6D). Thus these binding proteins are capable of selective blockage of gonadotropin-induced signal transduction in vitro.

To test whether FBP can be used as a functional antagonist in vivo, we scaled up the production of FBP using a baculovirus expression system. Experimental data indicate that FBP produced by FtCD8-expressing insect cells retains its ability to inhibit the binding of labeled FSH to WT FSH receptors in vitro. We administered conditioned media from insect cells containing FBP into immature male rats. Treatment with FBP every 6 h for 2 days attenuated testis growth by 33% (untreated: 192±28 mg; FBP-treated: 128±30 mg; $n=14$). Analysis of testis DNA fragmentation using a 3' end-labeling method followed by gel electrophoresis further indicated major increases in testis cell apoptosis in the FBP-treated group, as evidenced by the appearance of internucleosomal DNA fragmentation (Fig. 7). In rats treated with a gonadotropin-releasing hormone (GnRH) antagonist to suppress both LH and FSH secretion we found comparable decreases in testis weight (140±18 mg) and increases in apoptotic DNA fragmentation. In contrast, no retardation of testis growth (201±26 mg) or alteration of testis cell apoptosis was seen in rats treated with conditioned media of insect cells infected with the WT baculovirus. In situ apoptosis analysis further indicated that DNA fragmentation was restricted to primary spermatocytes in rats treated with FBP or the GnRH antagonist and was not found in untreated rats. These results suggest that FBP is capable of neutralizing the action of endogenous FSH, which is essential for testis germ cell survival (Billig et al. 1995; Tapanainen et al. 1993).

This study demonstrated that an anchored fusion receptor approach can be used to generate soluble ligand-binding regions of glycoprotein hormone receptors of the seven-TM protein family. The soluble receptor fragments are capable of binding specific ligands and blocking signal transduction induced by FSH and LH/hCG, thus serving as potent functional antagonists. These receptor antagonists are unlikely to show agonistic activity, in direct contrast to hormone antagonists that interact with target organ receptors and usually exhibit agonistic activity at high concentrations. Furthermore, receptor antagonists do not have to be delivered to the target tissues and, due to their similarity to WT recep-

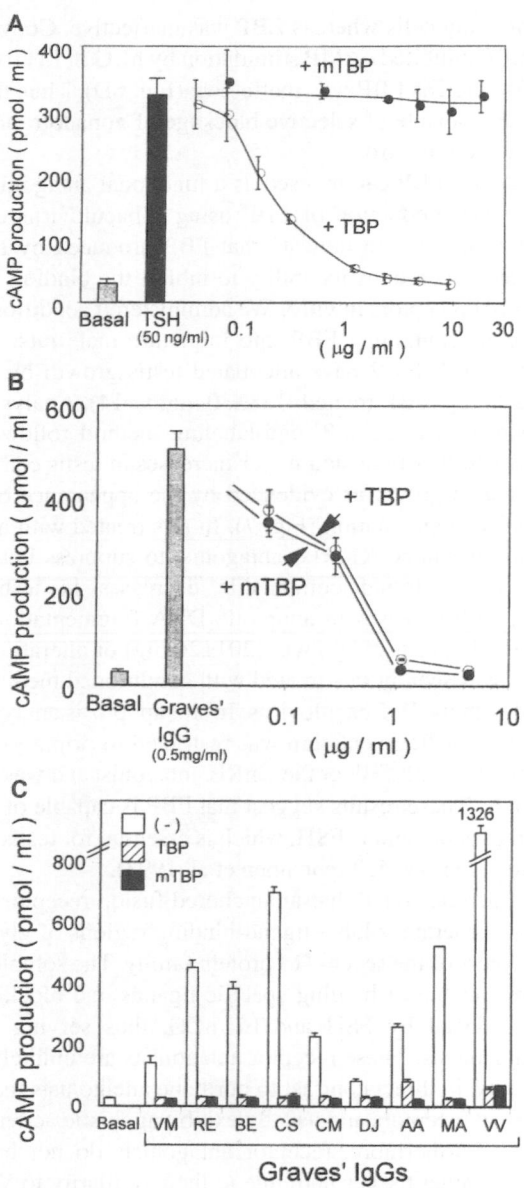

Fig. 8A–C

tors, probably have low antigenicity. If the delivery system is optimized, the present gonadotropin-binding proteins could serve as reversible and reliable contraceptives in both sexes.

We have also constructed TtCD8 and mTtCD8, a mutant of TtCD8 in which nine amino acids (368–376: YTICGDSED; Libert et al. 1989) of the TSH receptor were deleted. The soluble TSH receptor ectodomain (TBP) and its deletion mutant (mTBP) were derived after thrombin cleavage of anchored hybrid receptors (Osuga et al. 1998). Because Flag epitope for monoclonal antibody M1 followed by six histidine residues was fused to the N-terminus of these constructs, two-step affinity chromatography allowed derivation of large quantities of purified TSH-binding proteins and the related mutant for the first time. To study the ability of TBP and mTBP to block signal transduction induced by TSH or Graves' IgGs, 293 cells expressing WT TSH receptors were incubated with 50 ng/ml TSH or 0.5 mg/ml Graves' IgG with or without increasing concentrations of purified TBP or mTBP. As shown in Fig. 8A, treatment with TBP dose-dependently prevented cAMP production induced by TSH with an ED_{50} of 150 ng/ml. At 1 µg/ml TBP the stimulatory effect of TSH was completely blocked. In contrast, treatment with up to 20 µg/ml mTBP did not interfere with TSH action.

Consistent with previous findings using mutant TSH receptors (Kohn et al. 1995; Kosugi and Mori 1995), this study indicated that amino acid residues 368–376 in TBP are important for TSH binding. Graves' disease is a form of hyperthyroidism caused by autoimmune antibodies capable of binding to the ectodomain of TSH receptors and mimicking TSH action in the stimulation of thyroid gland growth and thyroid

◄ **Fig. 8A–C.** Differential ability of TBP and mTBP to block signal transduction induced by TSH and Graves' IgGs. **A** Cotreatment with TBP but not mTBP inhibited cAMP production induced by TSH. Cells expressing the WT TSH receptor were treated with TSH with or without premixing with TBP or mTBP. After 3 h at 37°C total cAMP production was determined by radioimmunoassay. **B** Cotreatment with either TBP or mTBP dose-dependently suppressed cAMP production induced by Graves' IgG. Cells expressing the WT TSH receptor were treated with IgGs with or without premixing with TBP or mTBP. **C** TBP and mTBP blocked cAMP production induced by IgGs from nine different patients with Graves' disease. Cells expressing the WT TSH receptors were treated with Graves' IgGs from individual patients with or without premixing with TBP or mTBP (1 µg/ml) hormone synthesis. The ability of TBP and mTBP to interfere with the action of Graves' IgGs was also tested in a bioassay. As shown in Fig. 8B, treatment with increasing doses of either TBP or mTBP inhibited, with similar potency, cAMP production induced by Graves' IgG. At 1 mg/ml of either TBP or mTBP complete suppression of IgG action was observed. Because IgGs from Graves' patients might show individual variability in their interaction with mTBP, IgGs obtained from nine additional patients were tested. As shown in Fig. 8C, treatment with either TBP or mTBP blocked cAMP production induced by all of the patient IgGs tested.

The present soluble ectodomain approach could be useful for further elucidation of TSH-binding epitopes. In addition, the soluble mTBP may also be of therapeutic value because it lost TSH-binding ability but still blocked signal transduction induced by Graves' IgGs. Because mTBP could, in theory, rapidly block the stimulatory effects of Graves' IgGs without disturbing the normal response to TSH, it might provide rapid alleviation of Graves' symptoms and maintain euthyroidism. Following optimization of its delivery, mTBP could provide an alternative approach to surgery in pregnant patients allergic to antithyroid medications.

Our findings demonstrate the feasibility of generating ligand-binding regions of glycoprotein hormone receptors to selectively neutralize actions of gonadotropins and TSH, thus allowing future design of novel contraceptives and management of various gonadal and thyroid dysfunctions. The present study represents the first successful derivation of soluble, ligand-binding domains from glycoprotein hormone receptors as functional antagonists. Similar approaches could allow generation of EC regions of related receptors to neutralize actions of ligands or receptor antibodies and to facilitate structural-functional analysis.

9.5 Conclusion

Based on gain-of-function mutations of the LH receptor found in precocious puberty patients and a chimeric receptor approach, this study demonstrated the importance of interactions between TM5 and TM6 of the LH receptor in its activation. It is likely that ligand binding also causes similar conformational changes in these receptor domains for its activation. Based on a loss-of-function mutation found in a patient with pseudohermaphroditism and the coexpression of partially defective receptor mutants, we demonstrated the importance of the EC-TM1 junction in receptor complementation for functional restoration of ligand signaling. It is likely that the EC region of the LH receptor, after ligand binding, effects a conformational change in the TM region through the EC/TM1 junction to allow ligand signaling. These studies demonstrated the powerfulness of the human genetic approach in identifying unique receptor functional domains and for elucidating the molecular mechanisms of receptor activation. In addition to these pathophysiological and molecular biology studies, the EC region of gonadotropin and TSH receptors was isolated using a chimeric receptor approach and following insertion of a specific junctional protease cleavage site. The derivation of these pharmacological reagents will allow the future development of drugs with the ability to specifically block the actions of individual glycoprotein hormone and autoimmune antibodies to glycoprotein hormone receptors.

References

Baldwin JM (1993) The probable arrangement of the helices in G-protein-coupled receptors. EMBO J 12:1693–1703

Billig H, Furuta I, Rivier C, Tapanainen J, Parvinen M, Hsueh AJW (1995) Apoptosis in testis germ cells: developmental changes in gonadotropin dependence and localization to selective tubule stages. Endocrinology 136:5–12

Cetani F, Tonacchera M, Vassart G (1996) Differential effects of NaCl concentration on the constitutive activity of the thyrotropin and the luteinizing hormone/chorionic gonadotropin receptors. FEBS Lett 378:27–31

Chen J, Ishii M, Wang L, Ishii K, Coughlin SR (1994) Thrombin receptor activation. Confirmation of the intramolecular tethered liganding hypothesis and discovery of an alternative intermolecular liganding mode. J Biol Chem 269:16041–16045

Cheung AH, Huang RR, Graziano MP, Strader CD (1991) Specific activation of Gs by synthetic peptides corresponding to an intracellular loop of the beta-adrenergic receptor. FEBS Let 279:277–280

Gilman AG (1987) G-proteins: transducers of receptor-generated signals. Annu Rev Biochem 56:615–649

Gudermann T, Schoneberg T, Schultz G (1997) Functional and structural complexity of signal transduction via G-protein-coupled receptors. Annu Rev Neurosci 20:399–427

Heaney ML, Golde DW (1993) Soluble hormone receptors. Blood 82:1945–1948

Ji IH, Ji TH (1991) Human choriogonadotropin binds to a lutropin receptor with essentially no N-terminal extension and stimulates cAMP synthesis. J Biol Chem 266:13076–13079

Kobe B, Deisenhofer J (1993) Crystal structure of porcine ribonuclease inhibitor, a protein with leucine-rich repeats. Nature 366:751–756

Kohn LD, Shimura H, Shimura Y, Hidaka A, Giuliani C, Napolitano G, Ohmori M, Laglia G, Saji M (1995) The thyrotropin receptor. Vitam Horm 50:287–384

Kosugi S, Mori T (1995) TSH receptor and LH receptor. Endocr J 42:587–606

Kosugi S, Van Dop C, Geffner ME, Rabl W, Carel JC, Chaussain JL, Mori T, Merendino JJ Jr, Shenker A (1995) Characterization of heterogeneous mutations causing constitutive activation of the luteinizing hormone receptor in familial male precocious puberty. Hum Mol Genet 4:183–188

Kremer H, Mariman E, Otten BJ, Moll GW Jr, Stoelinga GB, Wit JM, Jansen M, Drop SL, Faas B, Ropers HH, Brunner HG (1993) Cosegregation of missense mutations of the luteinizing hormone receptor gene with familial male-limited precocious puberty. Hum Mol Genet 2:1779–1783

Kudo M, Osuga Y, Kobilka BK, Hsueh AJW (1996) Transmembrane regions V and VI of the human luteinizing hormone receptor are required for constitutive activation by a mutation in the third intracellular loop. J Biol Chem 271:22470–22478

Latronico AC, Anasti J, Arnhold IJ, Mendonca BB, Domenice S, Albano MC, Zachman K, Wajchenberg BL, Tsigos C (1995) A novel mutation of the luteinizing hormone receptor gene causing male gonadotropin-independent precocious puberty. J Clin Endocrinol Metab 80:2490–2494

Laue L, Chan WY, Hsueh AJW, Kudo M, Hsu SY, Wu SM, Blomberg L, Cutler GB Jr (1995a) Genetic heterogeneity of constitutively activating mutations of the human luteinizing hormone receptor in familial male-limited precocious puberty. Proc Natl Acad Sci USA 92:1906–1910

Laue L, Wu SM, Kudo M, Hsueh AJW, Cutler GB Jr, Griffin JE, Wilson JD, Brain C, Berry AC, Grant DB, Chan WY (1995b) A nonsense mutation of the human luteinizing hormone receptor gene in Leydig cell hypoplasia. Hum Mol Genet 4:1429–1433

Laue L, Wu SM, Kudo M, Hsueh AJW, Cutler GB Jr, Jelly DH, Diamond FB, Chan WY (1996) Heterogeneity of activating mutations of the human luteinizing hormone receptor in male-limited precocious puberty. Biochem Mol Med 58:192–198

Lefkowitz RJ, Caron MG (1988) Adrenergic receptors. Models for the study of receptors coupled to guanine nucleotide regulatory proteins. J Biol Chem 263:4993–4996

Leung DW, Spencer SA, Cachianes G, Hammonds RG, Collins C, Henzel WJ, Barnard R, Waters MJ, Wood WI (1987) Growth hormone receptor and serum binding protein: purification, cloning and expression. Nature 330:537–543

Libert F, Lefort A, Gerard C, Parmentier M, Perret J, Ludgate M, Dumont JE, Vassart G (1989) Cloning, sequencing and expression of the human thyrotropin (TSH) receptor: evidence for binding of autoantibodies. Biochem Biophys Res Commun 165:1250–1255

Loosfelt H, Misrahi M, Atger M, Salesse R, Vu Hai-Luu Thi MT, Jolivet A, Guiochon-Mantel A, Sar S, Jallal B, Garnier J, Milgrom E (1989) Cloning and sequencing of porcine LH-hCG receptor cDNA: variants lacking transmembrane domain. Science 245:525–528

Luttrell LM, Ostrowski J, Cotecchia S, Kendall H, Lefkowitz RJ (1993) Antagonism of catecholamine receptor signaling by expression of cytoplasmic domains of the receptors. Science 259:1453–1457

McFarland KC, Sprengel R, Phillips HS, Kohler M, Rosemblit N, Nikolics K, Segaloff DL, Seeburg PH (1989) Lutropin-choriogonadotropin receptor: an unusual member of the G-protein-coupled receptor family. Science 245:494–499

Nagayama Y, Rapoport B (1992) The thyrotropin receptor 25 years after its discovery: new insight after its molecular cloning. Mol Endocrinol 6:145–156

O'Dowd BF, Hnatowich M, Regan JW, Leader WM, Caron MG, Lefkowitz RJ (1988) Site-directed mutagenesis of the cytoplasmic domains of the human beta 2-adrenergic receptor. Localization of regions involved in G-protein-receptor coupling. J Biol Chem 263:15985–15992

Osuga Y, Hayashi M, Kudo M, Conti M, Kobilka B, Hsueh AJW (1997a) Co-expression of defective luteinizing hormone receptor fragments partially reconstitutes ligand-induced signal generation. J Biol Chem 272:25006–25012

Osuga Y, Kudo M, Kaipia A, Kobilka B, Hsueh AJW (1997b) Derivation of functional antagonists using N-terminal extracellular domain of gonadotropin and thyrotropin receptors. Mol Endocrinol 11:1659–1668

Osuga Y, Liang S-G, Dallas J, Wang C, Hsueh AJW (1998) Soluble ecto-domain mutant of thyrotropin receptor incapable of binding thyrotropin neutralizes the action of thyroid stimulating antibodies from Graves' patients. Endocrinology (in press)

Parma J, Duprez L, Van Sande J, Cochaux P, Gervy C, Mockel J, Dumont J, Vassart G (1993) Somatic mutations in the thyrotropin receptor gene cause hyperfunctioning thyroid adenomas. Nature 365:649–651

Parma J, Duprez L, Van Sande J, Paschke R, Tonacchera M, Dumont J, Vassart G (1994) Constitutively active receptors as a disease-causing mechanism. Mol Cell Endocrinol 100:159–162

Pollak MR, Brown EM, Chou YH, Hebert SC, Marx SJ, Steinmann B, Levi T, Seidman CE, Seidman JG (1993) Mutations in the human Ca2+-sensing receptor gene cause familial hypocalciuric hypercalcemia and neonatal severe hyperparathyroidism. Cell 75:1297–1303

Pollak MR, Brown EM, Estep HL, McLaine PN, Kifor O, Park J, Hebert SC, Seidman CE, Seidman JG (1994) Autosomal dominant hypocalcemia caused by a Ca2+-sensing receptor gene mutation. Nat Genet 8:303–307

Rao VR, Cohen GB, Oprian DD (1994) Rhodopsin mutation G90D and a molecular mechanism for congenital night blindness. Nature 367:639–642

Remy JJ, Bozon V, Couture L, Goxe B, Salesse R, Garnier J (1993) Reconstitution of a high-affinity functional lutropin receptor by co-expression of its extracellular and membrane domains. Biochem Biophys Res Commun 193:1023–1030

Robbins LS, Nadeau JH, Johnson KR, Kelly MA, Roselli-Rehfuss L, Baack E, Mountjoy KG, Cone RD (1993) Pigmentation phenotypes of variant extension locus alleles result from point mutations that alter MSH receptor function. Cell 72:827–834

Robinson PR, Cohen GB, Zhukovsky EA, Oprian DD (1992) Constitutively active mutants of rhodopsin. Neuron 9:719–725

Schipani E, Kruse K, Juppner H (1995) A constitutively active mutant PTH-PTHrP receptor in Jansen-type metaphyseal chondrodysplasia. Science 268:98–100

Schoneberg T, Yun J, Wenkert D, Wess J (1996) Functional rescue of mutant V2 vasopressin receptors causing nephrogenic diabetes insipidus by a co-expressed receptor polypeptide. EMBO J 15:1283–1291

Shenker A, Laue L, Kosugi S, Merendino JJ Jr, Minegishi T, Cutler GB Jr (1993) A constitutively activating mutation of the luteinizing hormone receptor in familial male precocious puberty. Nature 365:652–654

Tapanainen JS, Tilly JL, Vihko KK, Hsueh AJW (1993) Hormonal control of apoptotic cell death in the testis: gonadotropins and androgens as testicular cell survival factors. Mol Endocrinol 7:643–650

Tsai-Morris CH, Buczko E, Wang W, Dufau ML (1990) Intronic nature of the rat luteinizing hormone receptor gene defines a soluble receptor subspecies with hormone binding activity. J Biol Chem 265:19385–19388

Van Sande J, Parma J, Tonacchera M, Swillens S, Dumont J, Vassart G (1995) Somatic and germline mutations of the TSH receptor gene in thyroid diseases. J Clin Endocrinol Metab 80:2577–2585

Wess J (1997) G-protein-coupled receptors: molecular mechanisms involved in receptor activation and selectivity of G-protein recognition. FASEB J 11:346–354

Xie YB, Wang H, Segaloff DL (1990) Extracellular domain of lutropin/chorio-gonadotropin receptor expressed in transfected cells binds choriogonadot-ropin with high affinity. J Biol Chem 265:21411–21414

Yano K, Hidaka A, Saji M, Polymeropoulos MH, Okuno A, Kohn LD, Cutler GB Jr (1994) A sporadic case of male-limited precocious puberty has the same constitutively activating point mutation in luteinizing hor-mone/choriogonadotropin receptor gene as familial cases. J Clin Endocrinol Metab 79:1818–1823

Yano K, Saji M, Hidaka A, Moriya N, Okuno A, Kohn LD, Cutler GB Jr (1995) A new constitutively activating point mutation in the luteinizing hor-mone/choriogonadotropin receptor gene in cases of male-limited precocious puberty. J Clin Endocrinol Metab 80:1162–1168

10 Steroidogenic Acute Regulatory Protein and Steroidogenesis

D.M. Stocco

10.1 Introduction

Steroid hormones share a common characteristic in that, regardless of the tissue of origin or the final steroid synthesized, they all arise from a common precursor substrate, cholesterol. Thus the biosynthesis of all steroids begins with the cleavage of cholesterol to form the first steroid synthesized, pregnenolone. This reaction is catalyzed by the cytochrome P450 side chain cleavage enzyme (P450scc), which is located on the matrix side of the inner mitochondrial membrane (Simpson and Boyd 1966, 1967; Farkash et al. 1986). Once formed, pregnenolone can be converted within the mitochondria to progesterone by a mitochondrial form of 3β-hydroxysteroid dehydrogenase (3β-HSD; Cherradi et al. 1997). Exiting the mitochondria, progesterone undergoes further metabolism by microsomal steroid dehydrogenases and cytochrome P450 steroid hydroxylases to form tissue specific steroids.

For many years the action of the P450scc enzyme in converting cholesterol to pregnenolone was considered as the rate-limiting step in steroidogenesis. However, while the action of the P450scc may be the rate-limiting *enzymatic* step in steroidogenesis (Stone and Hechter 1954; Karaboyas and Koritz 1965), many observations indicated that the *true* rate-limiting step is delivery of cholesterol to the inner mitochondrial membrane and the P450scc (Karaboyas and Koritz 1965; Brownie et al. 1972, 1973; Simpson et al. 1979; Mori and Marsh 1982). The major barrier in the translocation of cholesterol to the P450scc is the aqueous space between the outer and inner mitochondrial membranes through which hydrophobic cholesterol must pass, and it is this transfer which is now readily accepted as the rate-limiting step in hormone-regulated steroidogenesis.

10.2 Acute Regulation of Steroidogenesis

Acute steroidogenic responses to trophic hormone share many characteristics. They are usually dose dependent, have similar temporal relationships, and are sensitive to protein synthesis inhibitors. For these and other reasons it is highly likely that the mechanism(s) involved in this acute regulation is similar in all steroidogenically active cell types. While the focus of this Workshop is the testis, the adrenal was the first model system used to study steroid hormone biosynthesis (Hechter et al. 1951; Haynes et al. 1952; Stone and Hechter 1954). In addition to the adrenal, many studies on steroidogenesis were performed in the testis and ovary; therefore the work described in this chapter includes all three organs. One of the first and most fundamental observations concerning steroidogenesis was that acute steroid production in response to hormone stimulation has an absolute requirement for de novo protein synthesis (Ferguson 1962, 1963). Also, Garren and coworkers clearly demonstrated that ACTH stimulated steroidogenesis is highly dependent upon the synthesis of new proteins (Garren et al. 1965, 1966; Davis and Garren 1968; Garren 1968). Importantly, they also observed that while steroid synthesis is dependent upon de novo protein synthesis, the conversion of cholesterol esters to free cholesterol is not (Davis and Garren 1966), indicating that the hormonally controlled step is distal to cholesterol ester hydrolysis but proximal to its side chain cleavage.

Many similar studies have confirmed the need for de novo protein synthesis in the hormone-regulated, acute production of steroids (Karaboyas and Koritz 1965; Farese 1967; Cooke et al. 1975; Paul et al. 1976; Farese and Prudente 1977; Janszen et al. 1976; Janszen et al. 1977; Crivello and Jefcoate 1978; Toaff et al. 1979; Kreuger and Orme-Johnson 1983; Privalle et al. 1983; Solano et al. 1984; Pon and Orme-Johnson 1988; Epstein and Orme-Johnson 1991a; Stocco and Sodeman 1991; Stocco and Chen 1991; Stevens et al. 1993). Importantly, Simpson and Boyd (1966) determined that the cycloheximide sensitive step is located in the mitochondria, but, just as importantly, Arthur and Boyd (1976) showed that protein synthesis inhibitors have no effect on the activity of the P450scc itself. Later studies demonstrated that inhibition of protein synthesis has no effect on the delivery of cellular cholesterol to the outer mitochondrial membrane, but that its delivery to the inner mitochondrial membrane is completely inhibited (Privalle et al. 1983; Ohno et al. 1983). Thus the precise site of the cycloheximide-inhibited regulation had been pinpointed to the transfer of cholesterol to the P450scc enzyme. The major characteristics of this process indicated that acute production of steroids depends upon a *hormone-stimulated, rapidly synthesized, cycloheximide-sensitive,* and *highly labile protein* which mediates the transfer of cholesterol from the outer to the inner mitochondrial membrane and the P450scc enzyme.

10.3 The Steroidogenic Acute Regulatory Protein

This review summarizes the results of studies performed on a protein initially described by Orme-Johnson and colleagues and proposed as the acute regulator of steroid biosynthesis (Krueger and Orme-Johnson 1983; Pon and Orme-Johnson 1986, 1988; Pon et al. 1986a,b; Alberta et al. 1989; Epstein and Orme-Johnson 1991a,b). These careful studies indicated a close relationship between the appearance of cycloheximide-sensitive 30-kDa proteins and steroid hormone biosynthesis in several different steroidogenic tissues. Probably identical proteins have been characterized in hormone-stimulated MA-10 mouse Leydig tumor cells (Stocco and Kilgore 1988; Stocco and Chaudhary 1990; Stocco and Sodeman 1991; Stocco and Chen 1991; Stocco 1992; Stocco and Ascoli 1993; Stocco et al. 1995). These proteins have been localized in mitochondria and consist of several forms of a newly synthesized 30-kDa protein. In addition, 37-kDa precursor forms have also been detected, a common observation with mitochondrial proteins (Epstein and Orme-Johnson 1991b; Stocco and Sodeman 1991).

Since these initial observations many studies have demonstrated correlations between the synthesis of steroids and the 30-kDa proteins. An important, but incomplete, list of these correlations include: (a) Hormone-induced synthesis of the 30-kDa proteins parallel steroid production in both a time- and dose-responsive manner (Krueger and Orme-Johnson 1983; Stocco and Sodeman 1991). (b) Their synthesis is sensitive to cylocheximide (Krueger and Orme-Johnson 1983; Stocco and Sodeman 1991). (c) They are found associated with the mitochondria, the site of the acutely regulated step (Stocco and Kilgore 1988; Alberta et al. 1989; Stocco and Chaudhary 1990; Stocco and Sodeman 1991; Stocco and Chen 1991; Epstein and Orme-Johnson 1991a; Epstein and Orme-Johnson 1991b; Stocco 1992; Stocco and Ascoli 1993; Stocco et al. 1995). (d) The 30-kDa proteins are maximally expressed in the constitutive steroid-producing rat R2C Leydig tumor cell line in which steroidogenesis is also constitutive (Stocco and Chen 1991). However, a direct cause and effect relationship between 30-kDa protein expression and steroidogenesis is lacking, and it was necessary to clone the 30-kDa protein to confirm unequivocally its function in steroidogenesis.

The 30-kDa protein was purified from hormone stimulated MA-10 mouse Leydig tumor cell mitochondria. Microsequence analysis from three tryptic peptides allowed the design of degenerate oligonucleotides which were used to obtain a polymerase chain reaction generated 400-bp product from an MA-10 cell cDNA library. This was used to probe the same cDNA library, and a full length cDNA clone containing an open reading frame of 852 nucleotides encoding a protein of 284 amino acids was obtained (Clark et al. 1994). Comparison of the nucleic acid and protein sequences in the data base indicated the 30-kDa protein represented a novel protein. The full-length cDNA was shown to encode the 37-kDa precursor protein which could be imported and correctly processed and modified by isolated mitochondria to the mature 30-kDa proteins (Clark et al. 1994). Most importantly, expression of the cDNA-derived protein in MA-10 cells resulted in a significant increase in steroid production. Similarly, transfection of COS-1 cells with P450scc, adrenodoxin, and adrenodoxin reductase (Harikrishna et al. 1993) and the cDNA for the 37-kDa protein resulted in a several-fold increase in the conversion of cholesterol to pregnenolone (Sugawara et al. 1995a; Lin et al. 1995; Stocco and Clark 1996). These results extended the previous correlative studies and indicated a direct role for the 30-kDa proteins in hormone-regulated steroid production, and as a result the protein was named the steroidogenic acute regulatory (StAR) protein (Clark et al. 1994).

Many subsequent studies have demonstrated close correlations between the presence of StAR and steroid hormone biosynthesis. The organophosphate diethylumbelliferyl phosphate, a cholesterol ester hydrolase (CEH) inhibitor, which inhibits steroidogenesis by blocking the transfer of cholesterol into the mitochondria, inhibited the synthesis of the StAR protein (Choi et al. 1995). Mice injected with lipopolysaccharide display a 90% reduction in serum testosterone levels within 2 h, and this decrease was found to parallel a decrease in StAR protein found in the Leydig cells of these animals (Bosmann et al. 1996). Ramnath et al. (1997) showed that the level of steroid production and StAR synthesis are tightly correlated in MA-10 cells stimulated with cAMP analog in the presence of low levels of chloride ion, suggesting that the increased steroid production observed is due to an increase in StAR. In primary cultures of both mouse Leydig cells and MA-10 cells, Huang et al. (1995) showed that corticotropic-releasing hormone (CRH) results in a dose- and time-dependent increase in both intracellular cAMP and steroid hormone production. This increase in steroid production in response to CRH exactly paralleled an increase in the levels of StAR protein (Huang et al. 1997). Insulin-like growth factor-1 (IGF-1) acts with trophic hormone to enhance steroidogenesis in cultured Leydig cells. IGF-1 treatment of hCG-stimulated rat Leydig cells results in a significant increase in steroid production over hCG alone and a concomitant increase in synthesis of both StAR mRNA and StAR protein (Lin et al. 1998).

In rabbit corpora lutea (CL) both progesterone and StAR protein were found to be stimulated by estrogen, the luteotropic agent in the rabbit CL, indicating for the first time that the gene for StAR can be regulated by a steroid hormone (Townson et al. 1996). Furthermore, changes in StAR mRNA have been linked to physiological changes in steroid secretion in the sheep and cow (Juengel et al. 1995; Hartung et al. 1995; Pescador et al. 1996). In sheep hypophysectomy results in decreased serum progesterone levels as well as CL StAR mRNA levels, both of which can be restored to control levels by treatment with the luteotropic hormones LH or GH (Juengel et al. 1995). Conversely, prostaglandin $F_{2\alpha}$ ($PGF_{2\alpha}$) and phorbol myristate acetate (PMA), which cause luteal regression, decrease ovine CL StAR transcripts. In the cow Hartung et al. (1995) demonstrated that StAR mRNA increase in the CL during the estrous cycle and concluded that both the cell- and tissue-specific characteristics of the expression of StAR are consistent with a role in steroidogenesis.

In bovine CL it was demonstrated that the synthesis of StAR mRNA and protein are tightly coupled, and that the appearance of StAR is consistent with a role in progesterone production (Pescador et al. 1996), being low during luteal development, elevated in active CL, and absent in regressed CL and in CL treated for 24 h with prostaglandin $F_{2\alpha}$. The latter investigators later demonstrated that both StAR and P450scc expression can be regulated in luteinized porcine granulosa cells by follicle-stimulating hormone (FSH) and cAMP analog, and that this expression is dependent on ongoing protein synthesis (Pescador et al. 1997). Soumano and Price (1997) demonstrated that StAR expression increased in bovine follicular thecal cells after treatment with eCG but not with FSH, establishing that StAR expression is tightly coupled to progesterone production. Pilon and colleagues (1997) demonstrated that in the pig and the cow StAR expression occurs in both adult and fetal tissues. They found that StAR is present in adult testes and ovaries in both species and in fetal testes but not in fetal ovaries, an observation consistent with the steroidogenic capacity of those tissues. They also demonstrated StAR transcripts in both the pig and cow placenta, confirming previous observations made in the cow (Pescador et al. 1996).

Using the rat ovary, Sandhoff and McLean (1996a) demonstrated that serum progesterone levels and StAR expression rise in parallel in response to trophic hormone stimulation whereas P450scc enzyme levels are unchanged. These investigators also demonstrated that treatment of rats with $PGF_{2\alpha}$ results in pronounced inhibition of both progesterone production and StAR expression (Sandhoff and McLean 1996b). In porcine granulosa cells, Balasubramanian et al. (1997) found progesterone synthesis, StAR mRNA, and StAR protein increased in response to a combination of FSH and IGF-1 but not to either agent alone. Subsequently, LaVoie et al. (1997) demonstrated a correlation between progesterone synthesis and the expression of StAR (r=+0.71) and P450sc (r=+0.37) mRNAs during the pig follicular and luteal phases, the steroidogenic life of the follicle and CL. Similarly, Thompson et al. (1997) observed StAR expression in rat ovarian granulosa cells only following stimulation with FSH, a treatment which induces progesterone production. Selvaraj et al. (1996) showed that both progesterone synthesis and StAR expression can be stimulated simultaneously by gonadotropins in SV40 immortalized rat granulosa cells transfected with either LH or FSH receptor genes as well as by isoproterenol in cells transfected with the β_2-adrenergic receptor gene.

Liu et al. (1996) showed that StAR mRNA is expressed abundantly in normal human adrenals and in adrenocortical neoplasms, and further, that the expression of StAR can be stimulated by ACTH and cAMP analog. In addition, Nishikawa et al. (1996) showed a close correlation between ACTH stimulation and StAR protein expression in bovine adrenal fasciculata cells and also suggested that StAR expression is regulated by both protein kinase (PK) A and C signaling pathways. Kiriakidou et al. (1996) demonstrated that StAR messenger RNA is expressed in luteinized granulosa cells in response to the LH surge and that its expression is antagonized by activators of PKC. In a similar study the treatment of immature rats with PMSG resulted in a dramatic increase in StAR expression in both the ovarian theca interna cells and the CL of these animals, further confirming that StAR expression is confined to the steroidogenic cells in this organ (Mizutani et al. 1997).

Behrman's group demonstrated that rat luteal cells respond to temperature-induced heat shock with an induction of heat shock protein 70 and a concomitant cessation of hormone-stimulated progesterone synthesis (Khanna et al. 1994, 1995). They were able to place this inhibition at cholesterol transfer to the P450scc enzyme. Using the same heat shock model, Liu and Stocco (1997) showed in hormone-stimulated, heat-shocked MA-10 cells that heat shock protein -70 is increased, progesterone synthesis completely inhibited, and the synthesis of StAR completely blocked. An extensive study was recently undertaken by

Ronen-Fuhrmann et al. (1998) in which both StAR mRNA and protein levels were measured throughout the follicular phase in the rat. They observed that in response to pregnant mare's serum gonadotropin (PMSG) the first phase of StAR expression occurred mostly in the secondary interstitial and somewhat less in the theca interna cells and lasted for approximately 24 h. In the second phase, i.e., the LH surge as stimulated by hCG, StAR expression was observed in the entire theca interna and interstitial cells as well as in those granulosa cells that were confined to the periovulatory follicles. These results demonstrated that the first phase of StAR expression occurs in nonfollicular androgen-producing cells while the second phase occurs in the granulosa and theca interna cells of the dominant follicles, suggesting a functional collaboration between the different ovarian cell types.

10.4 StAR Expression

Many studies have attempted to determine the role of StAR in regulated steroid production, and for the most part they have demonstrated a close temporal and tissue-specific relationship between steroid biosynthesis and StAR mRNA and protein synthesis. One study demonstrated that StAR mRNA and protein are induced in close coordination via cAMP and display a time frame that parallels that of the acute production of steroid hormones in MA-10 cells (Clark et al. 1995a). The mechanism of hormone action on StAR expression was speculated to be due to a cAMP-induced change in StAR transcription and/or mRNA stability (Sugawara et al. 1995a; Clark et al. 1995a). Clark et al. (1997) have determined that while ongoing translation of the StAR protein does not require new transcription, the continued translation of StAR and steroid hormone production clearly depend on continued transcription of the StAR gene. This study also suggested that the actinomycin D induced stability of the StAR mRNA plays very little role in the observed level of acutely synthesized steroids in MA-10 cells.

Tissue-specific expression of StAR protein and mRNA in the adrenal, testis, and ovary of the mouse and human, respectively, provided a further indication of the specific role of StAR in steroidogenesis (Clark et al. 1995a; Sugawara et al. 1995a). The spatial and temporal relationship between the presence of StAR transcripts and the capacity to produce steroid hormones was also confirmed during mouse embryonic development (Clark et al. 1995a). In situ hybridization studies in embryonic mice clearly demonstrated that StAR is expressed only in the steroid-producing cells of the developing adrenal and testis. Conversely, StAR mRNA was absent in the developing ovary, an organ which is not steroidogenic during development, further indicating the spatial confinement of StAR to steroid-producing tissue. In the adult, StAR transcripts were found in the adrenal, testis, and ovary and were specifically localized to their steroidogenic cells (Clark et al. 1995a).

StAR mRNA has been studied in a number of species and reveals three specific transcripts of 3.4, 2.7, and 1.6 kb in the mouse (Clark et al. 1995a), three transcripts of 7.4, 4.4, and 1.6 kb in the human (Sugawara et al. 1995a), two transcripts of 3.0 and 1.8 kb in the cow (Hartung et al. 1995; Pescador et al. 1996), one transcript of 2.8 kb in the sheep (Juengel et al. 1995), three transcripts of 3.4, 1.7, and 1.2 kb in the rat (Sandhoff and McLean 1996a; Lee et al. 1997; Kim et al. 1997), and three transcripts of 2.7, 1.6, and 0.8 kb in the pig (Pescador et al. 1997). At this time, while the functional significance of the different sizes of the transcripts is not yet known, Kim et al. (1997) have provided some initial discussion on this subject. It was also determined that while steroidogenic cells appear to have a specific level of StAR-independent steroidogenesis equal to approximately 10%–20% of the total, maintenance of optimal steroid synthesis requires not only ongoing translation of the StAR mRNA but active transcription of the StAR gene as well (Clark et al. 1997).

10.5 Description of the StAR Gene

Full-length cDNA clones for StAR have been isolated for the mouse (Clark et al. 1994), human (Sugawara et al. 1995a), bovine (Hartung et al. 1995), hamster (Fleury et al. 1996), rat (Lee et al. 1997; Mizutani et al. 1997), and pig (Pilon et al. 1997), and these have at least 84% homology. In addition to studies characterizing StAR cDNA, the structural gene for StAR has been isolated and characterized for both mouse and human (Clark et al. 1995a; Caron et al. 1997a; Sugawara et al. 1995a,b). The genes span 6.5 kb in the mouse and 8 kb in the human, with the intronic sequences contributing to the increased length ob-

served in the human. Both genes are organized into seven exons and six
introns with exons 3–6 being of identical size. In the human, a StAR
pseudogene has also been identified (Sugawara et al. 1995a), and sequence analysis of the pseudogene indicated that it lacks introns and has
several nucleotide insertions, deletions, and substitutions. The human
StAR structural gene has been mapped to chromosome 8p.11.2 and the
StAR pseudogene to chromosome 13 (Sugawara et al. 1995a).

10.6 Regulation of StAR Expression

To determine the manner in which the StAR gene is regulated approximately 1 and 1.3 kb of the 5' flanking regions of the mouse and human
gene, respectively, have been isolated and sequenced (Clark et al. 1995a;
Sugawara et al. 1995a; Sugawara et al. 1997a,b). While StAR expression is regulated through the cAMP second messenger system, the
murine and human StAR promoters lack a canonical TATA box and also
lack any sequence similar to a consensus cAMP-responsive element.
Sugawara et al. (1995b) demonstrated that a 1.3-kb sequence of the
human promoter confers both basal and cAMP-dependent transcriptional activation of a reporter gene in Y1 mouse adrenal cells. Inspection
of the human StAR promoter sequence demonstrated that it contains
multiple steroidogenic factor 1 (SF-1) binding sites located at positions
–926 to –918, -105 to –95, and –42 to –35 relative to the start site of
transcription (Suguwara et al. 1997a,b). Results obtained by these investigators indicated that SF-1 plays a key role in regulation of both basal
and hormone-stimulated levels of StAR expression, and that interaction
at multiple SF-1 sites is required for maximal StAR promotor activity
and its regulation by cAMP.

   Sequence motifs that match the known requirements for binding
SF-1 have also been found at positions –135 and –42 relative to the
transcriptional start site in the mouse StAR gene (Clark et al. 1995a;
Caron et al. 1997a), and deletion of the distal SF-1 site completely
inhibited StAR promotor activity (Caron et al. 1997a). Similarly, approximately 1 kb of the 5' upstream sequence of the mouse StAR gene
has been shown to drive expression of a human growth hormone reporter in Y1 cells (Caron et al. 1997a). This same study convincingly
demonstrated that in the SF-1 knockout mouse expression of the StAR

gene is not detected in the gonadal ridge during embryonic development whereas it is readily seen in this region in the wild type animal. Lastly, a preliminary report indicates that the rat ovary StAR gene is also subject to regulation by SF-1 (Sandhoff and McLean 1997; Sandhoff et al. 1997).

In addition to SF-1, as indicated above, the StAR gene is regulated by estrogen in rabbit CL (Townson et al. 1996). StAR can also be up-regulated in the sheep by growth hormone (Juengel et al. 1995), a ligand which acts through tyrosine kinases (Argetsinger et al. 1993). StAR is also regulated and/or modified by IGF-1 (Lin et al. 1998). Thus the molecular mechanisms controlling both the cell-specific and hormone-dependent expression of the StAR gene may be quite varied and complex depending on the species and tissue involved.

Some steroidogenic cells can also be regulated by Ca^{2+} second messenger pathways. Elliott et al. (1993) detected the appearance of several 30-kDa mitochondrial proteins in bovine adrenal glomerulosa cells in response to angiotensin II and K^+ which increase aldosterone synthesis through the Ca^{2+} pathway. The physical characteristics of these proteins indicated that they are in all likelihood StAR. Since that time StAR has been observed to be induced by angiotensin II, K^+, tetradecanoylphorbol acetate (TPA) and the calcium channel agonist, BAY K8644 (BAY K) in the H295R human adrenocortical tumor cell line, thereby confirming that StAR expression can be regulated by the Ca^{2+} signaling pathway (Clark et al. 1995b). Furthermore, a dose-dependent inhibition of steroid production has been observed when AII, K^+, or BAY K-stimulated H295R cells are cotreated with a specific inhibitor of Ca^{2+}/CaM-dependent protein kinase II (CaM kinase II) (Pezzi et al. 1996). The agonist effect on increased StAR expression was not inhibited; however, the phosphorylation state of StAR was not addressed in those experiments.

Cherradi et al. (1996, 1997) have demonstrated that Ca^{2+} clamping of bovine glomerulosa cells results in a cycloheximide-sensitive increase in cholesterol transfer through mitochondrial contact sites to the inner mitochondrial membrane. They also demonstrated (Cherradi et al. 1997) that Ca^{2+} results in a cycloheximide-sensitive increase in StAR protein in the inner mitochondrial membrane. Furthermore, StAR was also present in the contact site region of the submitochondrial fractions, as were the first two enzymes of the steroidogenic pathway, P450scc and

3β-HSD. These findings confirmed that 3β-HSD can be found in the mitochondria as well as in the microsomal compartment (Cherradi et al. 1994, 1995). Possible implications of this observation are discussed below. Lastly, the observation that Ca^{2+} second messenger systems can result in steroid hormone biosynthesis and expression of StAR has recently been made by Elliott et al. (1997) and Kim et al. (1997) in both bovine and rat adrenal glomerulosa cells.

Recent observations indicate that the StAR promotor may harbor elements involved in negative regulation as well. The transcription factor DAX-1 (for dosage sensitive sex reversal, adrenal hypoplasia congenita, X chromosome, gene 1) is an unusual member of the nuclear hormone receptor family which has been shown to be involved in the related diseases of adrenal hypoplasia congenita and hypogonadotropic hypogonadism (Zanaria et al. 1994; Muscatelli et al. 1991; Guo et al. 1995; Habiby et al. 1996). Mutations in the human DAX-1 gene have been shown to be responsible for these conditions. In addition, duplication of the X chromosome in the Xp21 region containing the DAX-1 gene results in male to female sex reversal, a condition known as dosage-sensitive sex reversal (Bardoni et al. 1994).

The DAX-1 protein retains homology only with the ligand-binding domain of nuclear hormone receptors. The DNA binding domain lacks canonical zinc finger motifs and consists of three and one half repeats of a 65–67 amino acid sequence in its N-terminus (Zanaria et al. 1994). It has recently been shown that DAX-1 expression can block the synthesis of steroids in Y-1 mouse adrenal tumor cells, and this block can be attributed to an inhibition of the expression of the StAR gene (Zazopoulos et al. 1997). Attempts to demonstrate binding of DAX-1 to double-stranded DNA have been unsuccessful. Zazopoulos et al. (1997) showed that DAX-1 inhibits StAR gene expression by binding to a hairpin structure in single-stranded DNA which is found in the promotor region of the StAR gene. Indeed, the DAX-1 protein has been demonstrated to contain a powerful transcriptional silencing domain in its C-terminal region (Lalli et al. 1997). Thus it is possible that the observed phenotype in dosage-sensitive sex reversal (DSS) is due to the excess levels of DAX-1 protein which would result from duplication of the Xp21 region. If true, this would represent a situation in which the negative regulation of the StAR gene had most serious consequences, somewhat analogous to the synthesis of nonfunctional StAR protein which occurs in lipoid congenital adrenal hyperplasia (CAH).

10.7 Characteristics of the StAR Protein

The StAR protein sequence is highly conserved, with 85%–88% identity and greater than 90% similarity in the species studied to date. The area of greatest divergence appears to be in the putative mitochondrial signal sequence cleavage site described for the mouse sequence. In this region the protein contains an amino acid motif that is highly conserved in presequences that undergo a sequential two-step cleavage (Hendrick et al. 1989). However, this motif is not found in any other species whose StAR cDNA has been sequenced to date. Although the mechanism for StAR import and processing is not known, the submitochondrial localization of StAR has been determined. Protein-A gold labeling of immunoreacted StAR in mouse adrenal zona fasciculata cells and rat ovarian theca cells has determined that StAR protein is concentrated within the mitochondria and is localized to the intermembrane space and the intermembrane space side of the cristae membrane (King et al. 1995; Ronen-Fuhrmann et al. 1998). StAR is synthesized in the cytosol as a larger precursor protein and is imported and processed to its mature form by the mitochondria. The steroidogenically active form of the StAR protein is believed to be the 37-kDa precursor form which is present on the cytosolic side of the outer mitochondrial membrane, a position thought to be required for its activity in cholesterol transfer. This is discussed in further detail below. Import and processing of the 37-kDa form results in the formation of the 30-kDa intramitochondrial mature forms of StAR.

In vitro transcription/translation systems have been used to demonstrate that isolated mitochondria are competent to import and process both mouse and bovine StAR protein. Interestingly, bovine StAR protein can be imported into rat heart mitochondria, indicating that import of StAR is not dependent upon factors specifically present in steroidogenic tissues (Gradi et al. 1995). This is consistent with results obtained from transfection of both murine and human StAR into monkey kidney COS-1 cells which demonstrated that StAR is imported into the mitochondria and processed to its mature form (Sugawara et al. 1995a; Lin et al. 1995; Stocco and Clark 1996). Also, cotransfection of StAR with P450scc and adrenodoxin in COS-1 cells results in a several-fold increase in steroid synthesis (Lin et al. 1995; Sugawara et al. 1995a; Stocco and Clark 1996). The ability of StAR to increase steroid production has also been confirmed in an in vitro reconstituted system by King et al. (1995), who demonstrated that addition of StAR protein to MA-10 cell mitochondria results in a time- and dose-dependent increase in pregnenolone synthesis. In yet another interesting experiment Sugawara et al. (1995b) demonstrated that StAR can stimulate cholesterol metabolism in COS-1 cells cotransfected for expression of the mitochondrial enzyme, cholesterol 27-hydroxylase, a P450 enzyme usually found in high abundance in the liver. Therefore the ability of StAR to translocate cholesterol to the inner mitochondrial membrane does not appear to depend upon the presence of the cytochrome P450scc enzyme.

10.8 The Role of Phosphorylation in StAR Activity

The major signaling pathway in trophic hormone stimulated steroidogenesis involves the activation of protein kinase A (PKA) by increased cAMP accumulation. Chaudhary and Stocco (1991) detected the mitochondrial-localized mature 30-kDa StAR protein in its unphosphorylated state in PMA-treated MA-10 mouse Leydig tumor cells. This study observed, importantly, that while PMA induces StAR protein expression and import, it results in only marginal steroid production, indicating that phosphorylation of the StAR protein, while not required for protein import, is required for maximal steroidogenesis The observation that StAR is not phosphorylated in response to PMA has more recently been confirmed in rat adrenal glomerulosa cells, which are also not steroidogenically active in response to PMA (Hartigan et al. 1995). In contrast, PMA-treated bovine adrenal fasciculata cells do synthesize steroids, and in this case the StAR protein was phosphorylated (Hartigan et al. 1995). These data appear to indicate that phosphorylation of StAR is directly linked to the steroidogenic response of the cell to hormone stimulation.

Analysis and comparison of StAR protein sequences from several species whose sequences are known have identified two putative PKA/Cam kinase II phosphorylation sites and one PKC phosphorylation site. In an attempt to determine the role of phosphorylation on the steroidogenic capacity of the StAR protein Arakane et al. (1997a) mutated the consensus PKA sites which appear at positions 56/57 and 194/195 in the mouse and human StAR proteins, respectively. Both sites are serines, and both were altered by site directed mutagenesis to produce alanine residues. Mutation of either site resulted in a decrease in ^{32}P incorporation into the StAR protein, indicating that these sites were phosphorylated in vivo. Transfection of COS-1 cells with the StAR protein containing the serine 56/57 to alanine mutation had no effect on steroidogenesis. Conversely, transfection with the serine 194/195 to alanine mutation resulted in a 50%–60% inhibition of steroid biosynthesis. These results indicate that phosphorylation of the StAR protein at position 194/195 can significantly increase its biological activity but is not required for full activity.

10.9 Disruption of the StAR Gene

Given the purported role of StAR in steroid hormone biosynthesis, disruption of the StAR gene would be predicted to have most serious consequences. The seriousness of a disordered StAR gene has been demonstrated in studies on lipoid CAH, a potentially lethal condition which results from an almost complete inability of the affected individual to synthesize steroids. The lack of mineralocorticoids and glucocorticoids usually results in death within days to weeks of birth if not detected and treated with adequate steroid hormone and salt-replacement therapy. This condition is manifested by the presence of large adrenals containing high levels of cholesterol and cholesterol esters and also by an increased amount of lipid accumulation in testicular Leydig cells. This condition was originally thought to be due to a mutation of P450scc (20,22 desmolase) enzyme activity which is responsible for the conversion of cholesterol to pregnenolone (Camacho et al. 1968; Degenhart et al. 1972; Koizumi et al. 1977; Hauffa et al. 1985). However, the gene for this enzyme (Lin et al. 1991) and the P450scc protein levels (Sakai et al. 1994) have been shown to be normal in patients afflicted with this disease. Therefore it was deduced that the defect lies upstream of P450scc at the point of cholesterol delivery to the enzyme.

In studies designed to determine whether StAR is involved in lipoid CAH Sugawara et al. (1995a) cloned the human StAR cDNA and demonstrated that StAR mRNA is expressed only in the human adrenal, testis, ovary, and to a lesser extent the kidney of adult tissues. This investigation also demonstrated that StAR is not expressed in the human placenta, an observation consistent with it being a candidate for causing lipoid CAH since placental steroidogenesis persists in lipoid CAH (Saenger et al. 1995). When StAR cDNA was prepared using RNA from testicular tissue of two patients with lipoid CAH, Lin et al. (1995) identified nonsense mutations in the cDNA which were confirmed in the genomic DNA. Expression of the normal human StAR protein in COS-1 cells resulted in an eightfold increase in steroid production while expression of the mutated StAR cDNA indicated that the protein produced is completely inactive in promoting steroidogenesis.

A patient suffering from a milder form of lipoid CAH was also shown to have a mutation in the StAR gene (Tee et al. 1995). In this patient cloned genomic DNA was found to have a T to A transversion in intron 4, 11 bp from the splice acceptor site of exon 5 in the StAR gene. This transversion resulted in the finding that most of the StAR mRNA was abnormally spliced and nonfunctional, but a small percentage was normal and resulted in a milder form of the disease. Many additional examples of mutations in StAR resulting in this disease are being reported (Bose et al. 1996, 1997; Fujieda et al. 1997; Nakae et al. 1997; Okuyama et al. 1997), and lipoid CAH may prove more prevalent than previously believed. This disease seems to affect persons of Japanese and Palestinian ancestry disproportionately, and a summary of these data has recently been compiled (Bose et al. 1996). This report also indicates that several of the more common mutations in the StAR gene leading to lipoid CAH can be diagnosed using specific restriction endonucleases, a contribution which is certain to have a significant clinical impact.

Interestingly, the same report discusses the possibility that steroidogenic cells possess both StAR-dependent and StAR-independent steroid production, a concept also raised by other investigators (Clark et al. 1997; Caron et al. 1997b). This hypothesis seems to be borne out clinically in that several 46,XX lipoid CAH patients who underwent spontaneous puberty have been described, indicating that some degree of StAR-independent ovarian steroidogenesis can occur (Bose et al. 1996; Fujieda et al. 1997). Interest has been rekindled in this condition, which is essentially a human StAR knockout model, and a number of reviews on the subject have appeared (Miller 1997, 1998; Arakane et al. 1997b; Saenger 1997). To date, with only one exception (patient 14 in Bose et al. 1996), mutations in the StAR gene are the only reported causes of this potentially lethal disease and have clearly demonstrated the indispensable role of StAR in the production of steroids.

The observation that mutations in the StAR gene result in lipoid CAH produced compelling evidence for its essential role in steroidogenesis. However, many potentially interesting studies on this syndrome cannot be performed since the disease occurs only in humans, limiting the availability of tissue and experimental procedures which can be performed. An obvious strategy was to produce a knockout of the StAR gene in an animal system with the goal of having a model system to study this interesting protein. With this goal in mind, Caron et al. (1997b) used targeted disruption of the StAR gene in mice to produce StAR knockout mice. Initial observations of these mice have indicated that regardless of genotype all mice have female external genitalia, as seen in the human. Following birth the pups failed to grow normally, and death occurred within a short period of time, presumably as a result of adrenocortical insufficiency. This was confirmed by the observation that serum levels of corticosterone and Ialdosteronealdosterone were depressed while levels of ACTH and CRH were elevated. These observations indicated an impairment in the production of adrenal steroids with an accompanying loss of feedback regulation at the level of the hypothalamus or pituitary. Microscopic inspection of the adrenal gland revealed a normal medulla but an abnormal cortex, having a disrupted fascicular zone. Specific staining procedures revealed elevated lipid deposits in the adrenal cortex region of the StAR knockout mouse. While the StAR knockout mice were all phenotypically sex reversed, the testes of these animals appeared normal upon gross inspection. However, once again, specific staining indicated the presence of elevated levels of lipid within this organ. In contrast, the ovaries of the StAR knockout mice were essentially indistinguishable from wild-type animals, a similar situation as that found with human StAR mutations (Bose et al. 1996, 1997; Fujieda et al. 1997). The availability of the StAR knockout mouse should greatly expedite important studies which can be performed on this protein within the milieu of an intact endocrine system.

10.10 How Does StAR Work?

A model was earlier proposed whereby StAR acts in the transfer of cholesterol to the P450scc and has appeared in a previous review (Stocco and Clark 1996). It was proposed that in response to hormone stimulation the StAR 37-kDa precursor is rapidly synthesized and targeted to the mitochondria. As the precursor protein is imported into the mitochondria, contact sites between the inner and outer membranes are formed. This model proposes that import of the protein with the accompanying formation of contact sites collapses the aqueous intermembrane space and allows cholesterol to transfer to the inner mitochondrial membrane for pregnenolone synthesis (Jefcoate et al. 1992; Epstein and Orme-Johnson 1991b; Stocco and Sodeman 1991). Once imported, the membranes separate, and no further cholesterol transfer can occur without additional synthesis and processing of StAR precursor proteins. The half-life of the StAR precursor proteins is very short (Epstein and Orme-Johnson 1991b), which would explain the rapid decay in steroidogenesis in the absence of new protein synthesis. The observation that import of mitochondrial proteins occurs at contact sites made this a viable model (Vestweber and Schatz 1988; Rassow et al. 1989; Pon et al. 1989; Pfanner et al. 1990; Hwang et al. 1991). A model similar to the above was first suggested by Stevens et al. (1985).

However, recent reports by Strauss and colleagues (Arakane et al. 1996), have indicated that a revision of this model is necessary. It has been shown that N-terminal truncations of the StAR protein which remove as many as 62 amino acids have no inhibitory effect on steroid production when expressed in COS-1 cells. Western analysis and immunostaining for StAR protein indicate that the truncated StAR protein is not imported into the mitochondria. On the other hand, truncation of the C-terminus by 10 amino acids resulted in a 50% decrease in steroid production while a 28 amino acid truncation resulted in a complete loss of steroid production (Arakane et al. 1996). Thus it appears that the C-terminal region of the StAR protein is extremely important in cholesterol transfer. This observation could have perhaps been predicted from the observation that all mutations in lipoid CAH have been shown to be in the C-terminal region of the StAR protein (Bose et al. 1996, 1997; Fujieda et al. 1997; Nakae et al. 1997; Okuyama et al. 1997).

The importance of the C-terminal region of the StAR protein in cholesterol transfer can be seen in findings by Watari et al. (1997) that report the steroidogenic properties of a protein known as MLN64, which has significant homology to the C-terminal region of StAR. This protein was originally described as a gene product of unknown function which was highly expressed in specific breast tumors (Bieche et al. 1996; Moog-Lutz et al. 1997). Importantly, expression of the MLN64 protein in COS-1 cells results in a twofold increase in steroid production, and removal of N-terminal sequences results in a further increase. The relationship between StAR and MLN64 as well as the role of MLN64 in the cell remain to be determined, and hopefully useful information concerning sterol trafficking in the cell will be obtained. Yet another gene, termed CAB1, was recently isolated from gastric and esophageal cancer cell lines and shown to have considerable homology to the StAR gene (Akiyama et al. 1997). The significance of the homology between the StAR and CAB1 genes is presently unknown, but it has been speculated that CAB1 is involved in tumor development through estrogen or some other steroid, and that overexpression of the CAB1 gene facilitates steroid production in these cancer cells (Akiyama et al. 1997).

While the mechanism of action of the StAR protein is still unknown, it is becoming increasingly clear that cholesterol transfer requires that it interact with as yet unknown proteins and/or other factors on the outside of the outer mitochondrial membrane and produce alterations which result in cholesterol transfer. This model could still incorporate the formation of contact sites between the two membranes. It is also possible that the import of StAR into the inner mitochondrial compartments which is known to occur with "normal" StAR is the "off switch" for steroidogenesis by removing StAR from its position on the outer membrane and cutting off the flow of cholesterol (Arakane et al. 1996; Stocco 1997). Therefore much remains to be determined concerning the mechanism whereby StAR mediates cholesterol transfer to the inner mitochondrial membrane. Identification of the components with which StAR interacts on the outer mitochondrial membrane is of critical importance in understanding its mechanism of action.

Although import of StAR does not appear to be an absolute requirement for cholesterol transfer, the findings that import of other mitochondrial proteins does not induce steroidogenesis, and that expression of StAR can directly increase steroid output suggest a specificity between

StAR import and cholesterol transport. It is especially intriguing that earlier observations demonstrated that mitochondrial contact sites in bovine adrenocortical cells contain the first two enzymes in the steroido-genic pathway, P450scc and 3β-HSD (Cherradi et al. 1994). Thus it is tempting to speculate that interaction of StAR with the mitochondria causes the formation of a protein complex consisting of P450scc and 3β-HSD, the enzymes required for the first two steps in steroidogenesis. In this manner cholesterol which enters the inner mitochondrial mem-brane via the action of StAR can quickly be converted to progesterone, as speculated in an earlier study (Cherradi et al. 1995). The possibility that P450scc, 3β-HSD, and StAR are all associated in the same contact sites in steroidogenic cells is supported by the observations of Cherradi et al. (1997) which demonstrate by immunoblot analysis that all three proteins, P450scc, 3β-HSD, and StAR, are found in contact sites iso-lated from mitochondria of hormone-stimulated bovine glomerulosa cells.

It is also possible that the outer mitochondrial membrane protein, the peripheral benzodiazepine receptor (PBR), which has been shown to play a key role in steroidogenesis, is also involved in the recognition of StAR by the outer mitochondrial membrane (reviewed in Papadopoulos 1993; Papadopoulos et al. 1996). Also, the role of the steroidogenesis activator polypeptide (SAP) in this process must be taken into consid-eration, given its reported characteristics (Pedersen and Brownie 1983, 1987). However, at this time these hypotheses are purely speculative, and further studies are necessary to confirm the exact relationship be-tween StAR, P450scc, 3β-HSD, PBR, SAP, and perhaps additional proteins in the mitochondrial membranes.

10.11 Conclusions

In summary, the demonstrated characteristics of the StAR protein make it the most attractive candidate available for the long-sought, hormone-stimulated protein factor responsible for acutely regulating the transfer of cholesterol from the outer to the inner mitochondrial membrane, and thus acutely regulating steroid hormone biosynthesis. Additional pro-teins are unquestionably involved and required in this transfer, but no strong evidence indicates that any of them are regulatory in nature.

Therefore perhaps the most interesting studies concerning StAR will be to determine the highly specific mechanism whereby StAR is able to effect the transfer of cholesterol to the inner mitochondrial membrane and the P450scc. The mechanism of action of StAR in transferring cholesterol to the inner mitochondrial membrane and the potential roles of other proteins such as P450scc, 3β-HSD, SAP, PBR, and perhaps as yet unidentified mitochondrial proteins remain to be determined and as such should prove to be some of the most interesting questions for the future as the picture of the acute regulation of steroidogensis continues to unfold. A number of the players appear to be known. Now the challenge is to determine how they work in concert with one another.

Acknowledgements. The author acknowledges the support of NIH grant HD 17481. He also thanks Drs. Barbara Clark, Xing Jia Wang, and Zhiming Liu and Ms. Deborah Alberts and Mr. Steven King for their contributions during the course of this work.

References

Akiyama N, Sasaki H, Ishizuka T, Kishi T, Sakamoto H, Onda M, Hirai H, Yazaki Y, Sugimura T, Terada M (1997) Isolation of a candidate gene, CAB1, for cholesterol transport to mitochondria from the c-ERBB-2 amplicon by a modified cDNA selection method. Cancer Res 57:3548–3553

Alberta JA, Epstein LF, Pon LA, Orme-Johnson NR (1989) Mitochondrial localization of a phosphoprotein that rapidly accumulates in adrenal cortex cells exposed to adrenocorticotropic hormone or to cAMP. J Biol Chem 264:2368–2372

Arakane F, Sugawara T, Nishino H, Liu Z, Holt HA, Pain D, Stocco DM, Miller WL, Strauss JF (1996) Steroidogenic acute regulatory protein (StAR) retains activity in the absence of its mitochondrial import sequence: implications for the mechanism of StAR action. Proc Natl Acad Sci USA 93:13731–13736

Arakane F, King SR, Du Y, Kallen KB, Walsh LP, Watari H, Stocco DM, Strauss III JF (1997a) Phosphorylation of steroidogenic acute regulatory protein (StAR) modulates steroidogenic activity. J Biol Chem (in press)

Arakane F, Sugawara T, Kiriakidou M, Kallen CB, Watari H, Christenson LK, Strauss III JF (1997b) Molecular insights into the regulation of steroidogenesis from laboratory to clinic and back. Hum Reprod [Natl Suppl] 12:46–50

Argetsinger LS, Campbell GS, Yang X, Witthuhn BA, Silvennoinen O, Ihle, JN, Carter-Su C (1993) Identification of JAK2 as a growth hormone receptor-associated tyrosine kinase. Cell 74:237–244

Arthur JR, Boyd GS (1976) The effect of inhibitors of protein synthesis on cholesterol side-chain cleavage in the mitochondria of luteinized rat ovaries. Eur J Biochem 49:117–127

Balasubramanian K, LaVoie HA, Garmey JC, Stocco DM, Velduis JD (1997) Regulation of porcine granulosa cell steroidogenic acute regulatory protein (StAR) by insulin-like growth factor I: synergism with follicle-stimulating hormone or protein kinase A agonist. Endocrinology 138:433–439

Bardoni B, Zanaria E, Guioli S, Floridia G, Worley KC, Tonini G, Ferrante E, Chiumello G, McCabe ERB, Fraccaro M, Zuffardi O, Camerino G (1994) A dosage sensitive locus at chromosome Xp21 is involved in male to female sex reversal. Nat Gen 7:497–501

Bieche I, Tomasetto C, Regnier CH, Moog-Lutz C, Rio MC, Lidereau R (1996) Two distinct amplified regions at 17q11-q21 involved in human primary breast cancer. Cancer Res 56:3886–3890

Bose HS, Sugawara T, Strauss III JF, Miller WL (1996) The pathophysiology and genetics of congenital lipoid adrenal hyperplasia. N Engl J Med 335:1870–1878

Bose HS, Pescovitz OH, Miller WL (1997) Spontaneous feminization in a 46,XX female patient with congenital lipoid adrenal hyperplasia due to a homozygous frameshift mutation in the steroidogenic acute regulatory protein. J Clin Endocrinol Metab 82:1511–1515

Bosmann HB, Hales KH, Li X, Liu Z, Stocco DM, Hales DB (1996) Endotoxemia causes a dramatic and abrupt decrease in circulating testosterone levels. Endocrinology 137:4522–4525

Brownie AC, Simpson ER, Jefcoate CR, Boyd GS, Orme-Johnson WH, Beinert H (1972) Effect of ACTH on cholesterol side-chain cleavage in rat adrenal mitochondria. Biochem Biophys Res Commun 46:483–490

Brownie AC, Alfano J, Jefcoate CR, Orme-Johnson W, Beinert H, Simpson ER (1973) Effect of ACTH on adrenal mitochondrial cytochrome P-450 in the rat. Ann NY Acad Sci 212:344.-360

Camacho AM, Kowarski A, Migeon CJ, Brough AJ (1968) Congenital adrenal hyperplasia due to a deficiency of one of the enzymes involved in the biosynthesis of pregnenolone. J Clin Endocrinol Metab 28:153–161

Caron KM, Ikeda Y, Soo SC, Stocco DM, Parker KL, Clark BJ (1997a) Characterization of the promoter region of the mouse gene encoding the steroidogenic acute regulatory protein. Mol Endocrinol 11:138–147

Caron KM, Soo SC, Wetsel WC, Stocco DM, Clark BJ, Parker KL (1997b) Targeted disruption of the mouse gene encoding steroidogenic acute regulatory protein provides insights into congenital lipoid adrenal hyperplasia. Proc Natl Acad Sci USA 94:11540–11545

Chaudhary LR, Stocco DM (1991) Effect of different steroidogenic stimuli on protein phosphorylation in MA-10 mouse Leydig tumor cells. Biochim Biophys Acta 1094:175–184

Cherradi N, Defaye G, Chambaz EM (1994) Characterization of the 3β-hydroxysteroid dehydrogenase activity associated with bovine adrenocortical mitochondria. Endocrinology 134:1358–1364

Cherradi N, Chambaz EM, Defaye G (1995) Organization of 3β-Hydroxysteroid dehydrogenase/isomerase and cytochrome P-450scc into a catalytically active molecular complex in bovine adrenocortical mitochondria. J Steroid Biochem Mol Biol 55:507–514

Cherradi N, Rossier MF, Vallotton MB, Capponi AM (1996) Calcium stimulates intramitochondrial cholesterol transfer and StAR protein in bovine adrenal glomerulosa cells. J Biol Chem 271:25971–25975

Cherradi N, Rossier MF, Vallotton MB, Timberg R, Friedberg I, Orly J, Wang XJ, Stocco DM, Capponi AM (1997) Submitochondrial distribution of three key steroidogenic proteins (steroidogenic acute regulatory protein, P450 side-chain cleavage and 3β-hydroxysteroid dehydrogenase isomerase enzymes) upon stimulation by intracellular calcium in adrenal glomerulosa cells J Biol Chem 272:7899–7907

Choi YS, Stocco DM, Freeman DA (1995) Diethylumbelliferyl phosphate inhibits steroidogenesis by interfering with a long-lived factor acting between protein kinase A activation and induction of the steroidogenic acute regulatory (StAR) protein. Eur J Biochem 234:680–685

Clark BJ, Wells J, King SR, Stocco DM (1994) The purification, cloning, and expression of a novel LH-induced mitochondrial protein in MA-10 mouse Leydig tumor cells: characterization of the steroidogenic acute regulatory protein (StAR). J Biol Chem 269:28314–

Clark BJ, Soo SC, Caron KM, Ikeda Y, Parker KL, Stocco DM (1995a) Hormonal and developmental regulation of the steroidogenic acute regulatory (StAR) protein. Mol Endocrinol 9:1346–1355

Clark BJ, Pezzi V, Stocco DM, Rainey WE (1995b) The steroidogenic acute regulatory protein is induced by angiotensin II and K$^+$ in H295R adrenocortical cells. Mol Cell Endocrinol 115:215–219

Clark BJ, Combs R, Hales KH, Hales DB, Stocco DM (1997) Inhibition of transcription affects the synthesis of the steroidogenic acute regulatory protein (StAR) and steroidogenesis in MA-10 mouse Leydig tumor cells. Endocrinology 138:4893–4901

Cooke BA, Janszen FHA, Clotscher WF, van der Molen HJ (1975) Effect of protein-synthesis inhibitors on testosterone production in rat testis interstitial tissue and Leydig-cell preparations. Biochem J 150:413–418

Crivello JF, Jefcoate CR (1978) Mechanism of corticotropin action in rat adrenal cells. 1. Effect of inhibitors of protein synthesis and of microfilament formation on corticosterone synthesis. Biochim Biophys Acta 542:315–329

Davis WW, Garren LD (1966) Evidence for the stimulation by adrenocorticotropic hormone of the conversion of cholesterol esters to cholesterol in the adrenal, in vivo. Biochem. Biophys Res Commun 24:805–810

Davis WW, Garren LD (1968) On the mechanism of action of adrenocorticotropic hormone. The inhibitory site of cycloheximide in the pathway of steroid biosynthesis. J Biol Chem 243:5153–5157

Degenhart HJ, Visser HKA, Boon H, O'Doherty NJ (1972) Evidence for deficient 20α-cholesterol-hydroxylase activity in adrenal tissue of a patient with lipoid adrenal hyperplasia. Acta Endocrinol 71:512–518

Elliott ME, Goodfriend TL, Jefcoate CR (1993) Bovine adrenal golmerulosa and fasciculata cells exhibit 28.5-kilodalton proteins sensitive to angiotensin, other agonists, and atrial natriuretic peptide. Endocrinology 133:1669–1677

Elliott ME, Goodfriend TL, Ball DL, Jefcoate CR (1997) Angiotensin-responsive adrenal glomerulosa cell proteins: characterization by protease mapping, species comparison, and specific angiotensin receptor antagonists. Endocrinology 138:2530–2536

Epstein LF, Orme-Johnson NR (1991a) Acute action of luteinizing hormone on mouse Leydig cells: accumulation of mitochondrial phosphoproteins and stimulation of testosterone biosynthesis. Mol Cell Endocrinol 81:113–126

Epstein LF, Orme-Johnson NR (1991b) Regulation of steroid hormone biosynthesis: identification of precursors of a phosphoprotein targeted to the mitochondrion in stimulated rat adrenal cortex cells. J Biol Chem 266:19739–19745

Farese RV (1967) Adrenocorticotrophin-induced changes in the steroidogenic activity of adrenal cell-free preparations. Biochemistry 6:2052–2065

Farese RV, Prudente WJ (1977) On the requirement for protein synthesis during corticotropin-induced stimulation of cholesterol side chain cleavage in rat adrenal mitochondrial and solubilized desmolase preparations. Biochim Biophys Acta 496:567–570

Farkash Y, Timberg R, Orly J (1986) Preparation of antiserum to rat cytohrome P-450 cholesterol side chain cleavage, and its use for ultrastructural localization of the immunoreactive enzyme by protein A-gold technique. Endocrinology 118:1353–1365

Ferguson JJ (1962) Puromycin and adrenal responsiveness to adrenocorticotropic hormone. Biochim Biophys Acta 57:616–617

Ferguson JJ (1963) Protein synthesis and adrenocorticotropin responsiveness. J Biol Chem 238:2754–2759

Fleury A, Cloutier M, Ducharme L, Lefebvre A, LeHoux J, LeHoux JG (1996) Hamster adrenal acute regulatory rotein cDNA: its characterization and regulation of its expression be ACTH. Endocr Res 22:515–520

Fujieda K, Tajima T, Nakae J, Sageshima S, Tachibana K, Suwa S, Sugawara T, Strauss III JF (1997) Spontaneous puberty in 46,XX subjects with congenital lipoid adrenal hyperplasia. J Clin Invest 99:1265–1271

Garren LD (1968) The mechanism of action of adrenocorticotropic hormone. Vitam Horm 29:119

Garren LD, Ney RL, Davis WW (1965) Studies on the role of protein synthesis in the regulation of corticosterone production by ACTH in vivo. Proc Natl Acad Sci USA 53:1443–1450

Garren LD, Davis WW, Crocco RM (1966) Puromycin analogs: action of adrenocorticotropic hormone and the role of glycogen. Science 152:1386–1388

Gradi A, Tang-Wai R, McBride HM, Chu LL, Shore GC, Pelletier J (1995) The human steroidogenic acute regulatory (StAR) gene is expressed in the urogenital system and encodes a mitochondrial polypeptide. Biochim Biophys Acta 1258:228–233

Guo W, Mason JS, Stone CG, Morgan SA, Madu SI, Baldini A, Lindsay EA, Biesecker LG, Copeland KC, Horlick MNB, Pettigrew AL, Zanaria E, and McCabe ERB (1995) Diagnosis of X-linked adrenal hypoplasia congenita by mutation analysis of the DAX-1 gene. JAMA 274:324–330

Habiby RL, Boepple P, Nachtigall L, Sluss PM, Crowley Jr WF, Jameson JL (1996) Adrenal hypoplasia congenita with hypogonadotropic hypogonadism. Evidence that DAX-1 mutations lead to combined hypothalamic and pituitary defects in gonadotropin production. J Clin Invest 98:1055–1062

Harikrishna JA, Black SM, Szklarz GD, Miller WL (1993) Construction and function of fusion enzymes of the human cytochrome P450scc system. DNA Cell Biol 12:371–379

Hartigan JA, Green EG, Mortensen RM, Menachery A, Williams GH, Orme-Johnson NR (1995) Comparison of protein phosphorylation patterns produced in adrenal cells by activation of cAMP-dependent protein kinase and Ca-dependent protein kinase. J Steroid Biochem Mol Biol 53:1–6

Hartung S, Rust W, Balvers M, Ivell R (1995) Molecular cloning and in vivo expression of the bovine steroidogenic acute regulatory protein. Biochem Biophys Res Comm 215:646–653

Hauffa PT, Miller WL, Grumbach MM, Conte FA, Kaplan SL (1985) Congenital adrenal hyperplasia due to deficient cholesterol side-chain cleavage activity (20,22-desmolase) in a patient treated for 18 years. Clin Endocrinol 23:481–493

Haynes R, Savard K, Dorfman RI (1952) An action of ACTH on adrenal slices. Science 116:690–691

Hechter O, Zaffaroni A, Jacobsen RP, Levy H, Jeanloz RW, Schenker V, Pincus G (1951) The nature and the biogenesis of the adrenal secretory product. Rec Prog Horm Res 6:215–246

Hendrick JP, Hodges PE, Rosenberg LE (1989) Survey of amino-terminal proteolytic cleavage sites in mitochondrial precursor proteins: leader peptides cleaved by two matrix proteases share a three amino acid motif. Proc Natl Acad Sci USA 86:4056–4060

Huang BM, Stocco DM, Hutson JC, Norman RL (1995) Corticotropin-releasing hormone (CRH) stimulates steroidogenesis in mouse Leydig cells. Biol Reprod 53:620–626

Huang BM, Stocco DM, Li PH, Yang HY, Wu CM, Norman, RL (1997) Corticotropin-releasing hormone stimulates the expression of the steroidogenic acute regulatory protein in MA-10 cells. Biol Reprod 57:547–551

Hwang ST, Wachter C, Schatz G (1991) Protein import into the yeast mitochondrial matrix: a new translocation intermediate between the two mitochondrial membranes. J Biol Chem 266:21083–21089

Janszen FHA, Cooke BA, van Driel MJA, van der Molen HJ (1976) LH induction of a specific protein (LH-IP) in rat testis Leydig cells. FEBS Lett 71:269–272

Janszen FHA, Cooke BA, van der Molen HJ (1977) Specific protein synthesis in isolated rat testis Leydig cells. Influence of luteinizing hormone and cycloheximide. Biochem J 162:341–346

Jefcoate CR, McNamara BC, Artemenko I, Yamazaki T (1992) Regulation of cholesterol movement to mitochondrial cytochrome P450scc in steroid hormone synthesis. J Steroid Biochem Mol Biol 43:751–767

Juengel JL, Meberg BM, Turzillo AM, Nett TM, Niswender GD (1995) Hormonal regulation of messenger ribonucleic acid encoding steroidogenic acute regulatory protein in ovine corpora lutea. Endocrinology 136:5423–5429

Karaboyas GC, Koritz SB (1965) Identity of the site of action of cAMP and ACTH in corticosteroidogenesis in rat adrenal and beef adrenal cortex slices. Biochemistry 4:462–468

Khanna A, Aten, RF, Behrman HR (1994). Heat shock protein induction blocks hormone-sensitive steroidogenesis in rat luteal cells. Steroids 59:4–9

Khanna A, Aten RF, Behrman HR (1995) Physiological and pharmacological inhibitors of luteinizing hormone-dependent steroidogenesis induce heat shock protein-70 in rat luteal cells. Endocrinology 136:1775–1781

Kim YC, Ariyoshi N, Artemenko I, Elliott ME, Bhattacharyya KK, Jefcoate CR (1997) Control of cholesterol access to cytochrome P450scc in rat adrenal cells mediated by regulation of the steroidogenic acute regulatory protein. Steroids 62:10–20

King SR, Ronen-Fuhrmann T, Timberg R, Clark BJ, Orly J, Stocco DM (1995) Steroid production after in vitro transcription, translation, and mitochondrial processing of protein products of complementary deoxyribonucleic acid for steroidogenic acute regulatory protein. Endocrinology 136:5165–5176

Kiriakidou M, McAllister JM, Sugawara T, Strauss JF (1996) Expression of steroidogenic acute regulatory protein (StAR) in the human ovary. J Clin Endocrin Metab 81:4122–4128

Koizumi S, Kyoya S, Miyawaki T, Kidani H, Funabashi T. Nakashima Y, Ohta, G, Itagaki E, Katagiri M (1977) Cholesterol side-chain cleavage enzyme activity and cytochrome P450 content in adrenal mitochondria of a patient with congenital lipoid adrenal hyperplasia (Prader disease). Clin Chim Acta 77:301–306

Krueger RJ, Orme-Johnson NR (1983) Acute adrenocorticotropic hormone stimulation of adrenal corticosteroidogenesis. J Biol Chem 258:10159–10167

Lalli E, Bardoni B, Zazopoulos E, Wurtz JM, Strom TM, Moras D, Sassone-Corsi P (1997) A transcriptional silencing domain in DAX-1 whose mutation causes adrenal hypoplasia congenita. Mol Endocrinol (in press)

LaVoie HA, Benoit AM, Garmey JC, Dailey RA, Wright DJ, Veldhuis JD (1997) Coordinate developmental expression of genes regulating sterol economy and cholesterol side-chain cleavage in the porcine ovary. Biol Reprod 57:402–407

Lee HK, Ahn RS, Kwon HB, Soh J (1997) Nucleotide sequence of rat steroidogenic acute regulatory protein complementary DNA. Biochem Biophys Res Comm 230:528–532

Lin D, Gitelman SE, Saenger P, Miller WL (1991) Normal genes for the cholesterol side chain cleavage enzyme, P450scc, in congenital lipoid adrenal hyperplasia. J Clin Invest 88:1955–1962

Lin D, Sugawara T, Strauss III JF, Clark BJ, Stocco DM, Saenger P, Rogol A, Miller WL (1995) Role of steroidogenic acute regulatory protein in adrenal and gonadal steroidogenesis. Science 267:1828–

Lin T, Wang D, Hu J, Stocco DM (1998) Up-regulation of steroidogenic acute regulatory protein by insulin-like growth factor-1 in rat Leydig cells. Endocrine (in press)

Liu J, Heikkila P, Kahri AI, Voutilainen R (1996) Expression of the steroidogenic acute regulatory protein mRNA in adrenal tumors and cultured adrenal cells. J Endocrinol 150:43–50

Liu Z, Stocco DM (1997) Heat shock-induced inhibition of acute steroidogenesis in MA-10 cells is associated with inhibition of the synthesis of the steroidogenic acute regulatory (StAR) protein. Endocrinology 138:2722–2728

Miller W (1997) Congenital lipoid adrenal hyperplasia: the human gene knockout of the steroidogenic acute regulatory protein. J Mol Endocrinol 19:227–240

Miller W (1998) Congenital lipoid adrenal hyperplasia. In: Chrousos GP, Margioris AN (eds) Adrenal disorders. Humana, Totowa (in press)

Mizutani T, Sonoda Y, Minegishi T, Wakabayashi K, Miyamoto K (1997) Molecular cloning, characterization and cellular distribution of rat steroidogenic acute regulatory protein (StAR) in the ovary. Life Sci 61:1497–1506

Moog-Lutz C, Tomasetto C, Regnier CH, Wendling C, Lutz Y, Muller D, Chenard MP, Basset P, Rio MC (1997) MLN64 exhibits homology with the steroidogenic acute regulatory protein (StAR) and is overexpressed in human breast carcinomas. Int J Cancer (in press)

Mori M, Marsh JM (1982) The site of luteinizing hormone stimulation of steroidogenesis in mitochondria of the rat corpus luteum. J Biol Chem 257:6178–6183

Muscatelli F. Strom TM, Walker AP, Zanaria E. Recan D, Meindl A, Bardoni B, Guioll S, Zehetner G, Rabl W, Schwarz HP, Kaplan JC, Camerino G, Meitinger T, Monaco AP (1991) Mutations in the DAX-1 gene give rise to both X-linked adrenal hypoplasia congenita and hypogonadotropic hypogonadism. Nature 372:672–676

Nakae J, Tajima T, Sugawara T, Arakane F, Hanaki K, Hotsubo T, Igarashi N, Igarashi Y. Ishii T, Koda N, Kondo T. Kohno H, Nakagawa Y, Tachibana, K, Takeshima Y, Tsubouchi K, Strauss III JF, Fujieda K (1997) Analysis of the steroidogenic acute regulatory protein (StAR) gene in Japanese patients with congenital lipoid adrenal hyperplasia. Human Mol Gen 6:571–576

Nishikawa T. Sasano H, Omura M, Suematsu S (1996) Regulation of expression of the steroidogenic acute regulatory (StAR) protein by ACTH in bovine adrenal fasciculata cells. Biochem. Biophys Res Comm 223:12–18

Ohno Y, Yanagibashi K, Yonezawa Y, Ishiwatari S, Matsuba M (1983) A possible role of "steroidogenic factor" in the corticoidogenic response to ACTH; effect of ACTH, cycloheximide and aminoglutethimide on the content of cholesterol in the outer and inner mitochondrial membrane of rat adrenal cortex. Endocrin J 30:335–338

Okuyama E, Nishi N, Onishi S, Itoh S, Ishii Y, Miyanake H, Fujita K, Ichikawa Y (1997) A novel splicing junction mutation in the gene for the steroidogenic acute regulatory protein causes congenital lipoid adrenal hyperplasia. J Clin Endocrinol Metab 82:2337–2342

Papadopoulos V (1993) Peripheral-type benzodiazepine/diazepam binding inhibitor receptor: biological role in steroidogenic cell function. Endocr Rev 14:222–240

Papadopoulos V, Amri H, Boujrad N, Cascio C, Culty M, Garnier M, Hardwick M, Li H, Vidic B, Brown AS, Reversa JL, Bernassau JM, Drieu K (1996) Peripheral benzodiazepine receptor in cholesterol transport and steroidogenesis. Steroids 62:21–28

Paul DP, Gallant S, Orme-Johnson NR, Orme-Johnson WH, Brownie AC (1976) Temperature dependence of cholesterol binding to cytochrome P-450scc of the rat adrenal. Effect of adrenocorticotropic hormone and cycloheximide. J Biol Chem 251:7120–7126

Pedersen RC, Brownie AC (1983) Cholesterol side-chain cleavage in the rat adrenal cortex: isolation of a cycloheximide-sensitive activator peptide. Proc Natl Acad Sci USA 80:1882–1886

Pedersen RC, Brownie AC (1987) Steroidogenesis activator polypeptide isolated from a rat Leydig cell tumor. Science 236:188–190

Pescador N, Korian Soumano S, Stocco DM, Price CA, Murphy BD (1996) Steroidogenic acute regulatory protein in bovine corpora lutea. Biol Reprod 55:485–491

Pescador N, Houde A, Stocco DM, Murphy BD (1997) Follicle stimulating hormone and intracellular second messengers regulate steroidogenic acute regulatory protein messenger ribonucleic acid in luteinized porcine granulosa cells. Biol Reprod 57:660–668

Pezzi V, Clark BJ, Ando S, Stocco DM, Rainey WE (1996) Role of calmodulin-dependent protein kinase II in the acute stimulation of aldosterone production. J Steroid Biochem Mol Biol 58:417–424

Pfanner N, Rassow J, Wienhues U, Hergersberg C, Sollner Becker K, Neupert, W (1990) Contact sites between inner and outer membranes: structure and role in protein translocation into the mitochondria. Biochim Biophys Acta 1018:239–242

Pilon N, Daneau I, Brisson C, Ethier JF, Lussier JG Silversides DW (1997) Porcine and bovine steroidogenic acute regulatory protein (StAR) gene expression during gestation. Endocrinology 138:1085–1091

Pon LA, Orme-Johnson NR (1986) Acute stimulation of steroidogenesis in corpus luteum and adrenal cortex by peptide hormones: rapid induction of a similar protein in both tissues. J Biol Chem 261:6594–6599

Pon LA, Hartigan JA, Orme-Johnson NR (1986a) Acute ACTH regulation of adrenal corticosteroid biosynthesis: rapid accumulation of a phosphoprotein. J Biol Chem 261:13309–13316

Pon LA, Epstein LF, Orme-Johnson NR (1986b) Acute cAMP stimulation in Leydig cells: rapid accumulation of a protein similar to that detected in adrenal cortex and corpus luteum. Endocr Res 12:429–

Pon LA, Orme-Johnson NR (1988) Acute stimulation of corpus luteum cells by gonadotropin or adenosine 3' 5'-monophosphate causes accumulation of

a phosphoprotein concurrent with acceleration of steroid synthesis. Endocrinology 123:1942–1948

Pon L, Moll T, Vestweber D, Marshallsay B, Schatz G (1989) Protein import
into mitochondria: ATP-dependent protein translocation activity in a submitochondrial fraction enriched in membrane contact sites and specific proteins. J Cell Biol 109:2603–2616

Privalle CT, Crivello J, Jefcoate CR (1983) Regulation of intramitochondrial
cholesterol transfer to side-chain cleavage cytochrome P450scc in rat adrenal gland. Proc Natl Acad Sci USA 80:702–706

Ramnath HI, Peterson S, Michael AE, Stocco DM, Cooke BA (1997) Modulation of steroidogenesis by chloride ions in MA-10 mouse tumor Leydig
cells: roles of calcium, protein synthesis and the steroidogenic acute regulatory (StAR) protein. Endocrinology 138:2308–2314

Rassow J, Guiard B, Weinhues U, Herzog V, Hartl FU, Neupert W (1989)
Translocation arrest by reversible folding of a precursor protein imported
into mitochondria. A means to quantitate translocation contact sites. J Cell
Biol 109:1421–1428

Ronen-Fuhrmann T, Timberg R, King SR, Hales K, Hales DB, Stocco DM,
Orly J (1998) Spatio-temporal expression patterns of steroidogenic acute
regulatory protein (StAR) during follicular development in the rat ovary.
Endocrinology (in press)

Saenger P, Klonari Z, Black SM, Compagnone N, Mellon SH, Fleischer A,
Abrams CAL, Shackelton CHL, Miller WL (1995) Prenatal diagnosis of
congenital lipoid adrenal hyperplasia. J Clin Endocrinol Metab 80:200–205

Saenger P (1997) New developments in congenital lipoid adrenal hyperplasia and
steroidogenic acute regulatory protein. Pediatric Endocrinol 44:397–421

Sakai Y, Yanase T, Okabe Y, Hara T, Waterman MR, Takayanagi R, Haji M,
Nawata H (1994) No mutation in cytochrome P450 side chain cleavage in a
patient with congenital lipoid adrenal hyperplasia. J Clin Endocrinol Metab
79:1198–1201

Sandhoff TW, McLean MP (1996a) Hormonal regulation of steroidogenic
acute regulatory (StAR) protein messenger ribonucleic acid expression in
the rat ovary. Endocrine 4:259–267

Sandhoff TW, McLean MP (1996b) Prostaglandin F2α reduces steroidogenic
acute regulatory (StAR) protein messenger ribonucleic acid expression in
the rat ovary. Endocrine 5:183–190

Sandhoff TW, McLean MP (1997) Identification and functional characterization multiple steroidogenic factor-1 elements in the rat steroidogenic
acute regulatory protein (StAR) gene. J Soc Gynecol Invest (in press)

Sandhoff TW, Hales DB, McLean MP (1997) Steroidogenic factor-1 confers
cAMP responsiveness to the rat steroidogenic acute regulatory (StAR) protein gene promoter. J Soc Gynecol Invest (in press)

Selvaraj N, Israeli D, Amsterdam A (1996) Partial sequencing of the rat steroidogenic acute regulatory protein message from immortalized granulosa cells: regulation by gonatropins and isoproterenol. Mol Cell Endocrinol 123:171–177

Simpson ER, Boyd GS (1966) The cholesterol side-chain cleavage system of the adrenal cortex: a mixed function oxidase. Biochem Biophys Res Commun 24:10–17

Simpson ER, Boyd GS (1967) The cholesterol side-chain cleavage system of the adrenal cortex. Eur J Biochem 2:275–285

Simpson ER, McCarthy JL, Peterson JA (1979) Evidence that the cycloheximide-sensitive site of ACTH action is in the mitochondrion. J Biol Chem 253:3135–3139

Solano AR, Neger R, Podesta EJ (1984) Rat adrenal cycloheximide-sensitive factors and phospholipids in the control of acute steroidogenesis. J Steroid Biochem 21:111–116

Soumano K, Price CA (1997) Ovarian follicular steroidogenic acute regulatory protein, low-density lipoprotein receptor, and cytochrome P450 side-chain cleavage messenger ribonucleic acids in cattle undergoing superovulation. Biol Reprod 56:516–522

Stevens VL, Tribble DL, Lambeth JD (1985) Regulation of mitochondrial compartment volumes in rat adrenal cortex by ether stress. Arch Biochem Biophys 242:324–327

Stevens VL, XuT, Lambeth JD (1993) Cholesterol trafficking in steroidogenic cells: reversible cycloheximide-dependent accumulation of cholesterol in a pre-steroidogenic pool. Eur J Biochem 216:557–563

Stocco DM (1992) Further evidence that the mitochondrial proteins induced by hormone stimulation in MA–mouse Leydig tumor cells are involved in the acute regulation of steroidogenesis. J Steroid Biochem Mol Biol 43:319–

Stocco DM (1997) A StAR search: implications in controlling steroidogenesis. Biol. Reprod. 56:328–336

Stocco DM, Ascoli M (1993) The use of genetic manipulation of MA-Leydig tumor cells to demonstrate the role of mitochondrial proteins in the acute regulation of steroidogenesis. Endocrinology 132:959–967

Stocco DM, Chaudhary LR (1990) Evidence for the functional coupling of cAMP in MA-10 mouse Leydig tumor cells. Cell Signal 2:161–170

Stocco DM, Chen W (1991) Presence of identical mitochondrial proteins in unstimulated constitutive steroid-producing R2C rat Leydig tumor and stimulated nonconstitutive steroid-producing MA-10 mouse Leydig tumor cells. Endocrinology 128:1918–1926

Stocco DM, Clark BJ (1996) Regulation of the acute production of steroids in steroidogenic cells. Endocr Rev 17:221–244

Stocco DM, Kilgore MW (1988) Induction of mitochondrial proteins in MA-
10 Leydig tumour cells with human choriogonadotropin. Biochem J
249:95–103

Stocco DM, Sodeman TC (1991) The 30-kDa mitochondrial proteins induced
by hormone stimulation in MA-10 mouse Leydig tumor cells are processed
from larger precursors. J Biol Chem 266:19731–19738

Stocco DM, King S, Clark BJ (1995) Differential effects of dimethylsulfoxide
on steroidogenesis in mouse MA and rat R2C Leydig tumor cells. Endocrinology 136:2993–

Stone D, Hechter O (1954) Studies on ACTH action in perfused bovine adrenals: site of action of ACTH in corticosteroidogenesis. Arch Biochem
Biophys 51:457–469

Sugawara T, Holt JA, Driscoll D, Strauss III JF, Lin D, Miller WL, Patterson
D, Clancy KP, Hart IM, Clark BJ, Stocco, DM (1995a) Human steroidogenic acute regulatory protein: functional activity in COS – cells, tissue –
specific expression, and mapping of the gene to 8p11.2 and a pseudogene to
chromosome 13. Proc Natl Acad Sci USA 92:4778–

Sugawara T, Lin D, Holt JD, Martin KO, Javitt NB, Miller WL, Strauss III JF
(1995b). Structure of the human steroidogenic acute regulatory protein
(StAR) gene: StAR stimulates mitochondrial cholesterol 27-hydroxylase
activity. Biochemistry 34:12506–12512

Sugawara T, Kiriakidou M, McAllister JM, Kallen CB, Strauss III JF (1997a)
Multiple steroidogenic factor 1 binding elements in the human steroidogenic acute regulatory protein gene 5'-flanking region are required for
maximal promoter activity and cyclic AMP responsiveness. Biochemistry
36:7249–7255

Sugawara T, Kiriakidou M, McAllister JM, Holt JA, Arakane F, Strauss III JF
(1997b) Regulation of expression of the steroidogenic acute regulatory protein (StAR) gene: a central role for steroidogenic factor 1. Steroids 62:5–9

Tee M, Lin D, Sugawara T, Holt JA, Guiguen Y, Buckingham B, Strauss III JF,
Miller WL (1995) T-A transversion 11 bp from a splice acceptor site in the
human gene for steroidogenic acute regulatory protein causes congenital
lipoid adrenal hyperplasia. Hum Mol Gen 4:2299–2305

Thompson WE, Sanbuissho A, Lee GY, Anderson E (1997) Steroidogenic
acute regulatory (StAR) protein (p25) and prohibitin (p28) from cultured rat
ovarian granulosa cells. J Reprod Fertil 109:337–348

Toaff ME, Strauss III JF, Flickinger GL, Shattil SJ (1979) Relationship of cholesterol supply to luteal mitochondrial steroid synthesis. J Biol Chem
254:3977–3982

Townson DH, Wang XJ, Keyes PL, Kostyo JL, Stocco DM (1996) Expression
of the steroidogenic acute regulatory protein (StAR) in the corpus luteum of

the rabbit: dependence upon the luteotrophic hormone, 17β-estradiol. Biol Reprod 55:868–874

Vestweber D, Schatz G (1988) A chimeric mitochondrial precursor protein with internal disulphide bridges blocks import of authentic precursors into mitochondria. A means to quantitate translocation contact sites. J Cell Biol 107:2037–2043

Watari H, Arakane F, Moog-Lutz C, Kallen CB, Tomasetto C, Gerton GL, Rio M, Baker ME, Strauss III JF (1997) MLN64 contains a domain with homology to the steroidogenic acute regulatory protein (StAR) that stimulates steroidogenesis. Proc Natl Acad Sci 94:8462–8467

Zanaria E, Muscatelli F, Bardoni B, Strom TM, Guioli S, Guo W, Lalli E, Moser C, Walker AP, McCabe ERB, Meitinger T, Monaco AP Sassone-Corsi P, Camerino G (1994) An unusual member of the nuclear hormone receptor superfamily responsible for X-linked adrenal hypoplasia congenita. Nature 372:635–641

Zazopoulos E, Lalli E, Stocco DM, Sassone-Corsi P (1997) Binding of DAX-1 to hairpin structures and regulation of steroidogenesis. Nature 390:311–314

11 Pem: *an Androgen-Dependent Homeodomain Gene Expressed in the Testis and Epididymis*

C.M. Wayne and M.F. Wilkinson

11.1 Introduction

Homeobox genes encode DNA-binding proteins that regulate the transcription of subordinate downstream genes and thereby control a wide range of developmental events. We have isolated a novel homeobox gene, *Pem*, that is expressed selectively in reproductive tissue. In the testis Pem protein is present specifically in the nuclei of Sertoli cells during the androgen-dependent stages of the seminiferous epithelium cycle. In the epididymis Pem transcripts are found in the region thought to be involved in the final stages of sperm maturation. An androgen-regulated "male-specific" proximal promoter (P_p) is responsible for transcription in testis and epididymis whereas a "female" distal promoter (P_d) is transcriptionally active in ovary and placenta. Experiments in mice and rats have demonstrated that Pp transcription in the testis and the epididymis is dependent on testosterone. To our knowledge, no known or putative transcription factors have previously been shown to depend on androgens for expression in Sertoli cells or the epididymis in vivo. The *cis* elements responsible for the regulation of *Pem* transcription have begun to be defined. Understanding Pem function and regulation is important because Pem may regulate androgen-regulated secondary response and delayed primary response genes.

11.1.1 A Good Model System
for Studying Androgen-Dependent Events

Androgens are of paramount importance to spermatogenesis. Testosterone alone maintains spermatogenesis in gonadotropin-deficient animals, including hypophysectimized rats and mutant hypogonadal (*hpg*) mice (Zirkin 1993; Singh et al. 1995). Testosterone may drive spermatogenesis by acting on Sertoli cells in the testis, which express androgen receptors (AR). Sertoli cells, which are in intimate contact with differentiating germ cells within the seminiferous tubule, perform numerous functions critical for spermatogenesis (Bardin et al. 1988; Sar et al. 1993). In the epididymis androgen regulates the proliferation and differentiation of somatic cells that line the lumen of the epididymal tubule. Androgens control the microenvironment of maturing spermatozoa by regulating the synthesis of adhesion proteins on epididymal somatic cells, the luminal secretion of proteins that are in contact with the spermatozoa, and the transport of ions and small organic molecules across the epididymal epithelium (Robaire and Hermo 1988; Orgebin-Crist 1996).

Although it is clear that spermatogenesis in the testis and sperm maturation in the epididymis are androgen-dependent processes, the molecular mechanisms by which these biological processes occur are only beginning to be elucidated. One critical issue under investigation is how androgens regulate the gene-expression events that direct these biological processes. A seminal discovery was the finding that androgens bind to AR, forming a complex, which in turn binds and activates the transcription of genes bearing androgen-responsive elements (AREs; Dean and Sanders 1996). Androgen-regulated genes can be grouped into three categories. The first category is primary response genes that contain AREs and therefore respond directly to androgens. These genes are transcriptionally activated very rapidly in response to steroids in a manner that does not require de novo protein synthesis. The second category is secondary response genes that do not contain functional AREs, but respond instead to secondary factors that are regulated directly by androgens. The expression of secondary response genes is delayed compared to that of primary response genes and requires ongoing protein synthesis. The third category is delayed primary response genes that contain AREs and thus are regulated, in part, by direct AR action. However, maximal induction of these genes is delayed and requires ongoing protein synthesis, presumably because of the need for secondary factors (Dean and Sanders 1996).

The existence of secondary response and delayed primary response genes implies that transcription factors in addition to AR are important in activating androgen-regulated genes. However, surprisingly few such candidate transcription factors have been identified. Most of the transcription factors known to be present in the testis have been localized to germ cells rather than the androgen-responsive Sertoli cells. These germ cell transcription factors include c-mos, c-jun, jun B, c-fos, c-myc, Zfy, sperm-1, hoxa-4, and the X-linked homeodomain protein Esx/Spx1 (Wolgemuth et al. 1991; Xin et al. 1992; Anderson et al. 1993; Fickenscher et al. 1993; Watrin and Wolgemuth 1993; DeRobertis 1994; Hecht 1996; Lindsey and Wilkinson 1996a; Brandford et al. 1997; Li et al. 1997). In this report we describe a putative transcription factor, Pem, that is expressed in Sertoli cells in an androgen-dependent manner and therefore may regulate androgen-dependent events during spermatogenesis. This androgen-dependent expression contrasts with the expression of all other transcription factors known to be expressed in Sertoli cells, including GATA-1 and CREB (Lindsey and Wilkinson 1996a). We describe the *Pem* gene in detail and present evidence consistent with the notion that it encodes an androgen-regulated transcription factor.

11.2 *Pem* Sequence and Chromosomal Location

Pem contains a homeodomain and is therefore a member of a large family of transcription factors that all have this 60 amino acid DNA-binding motif. All homeodomain transcription factors that have been studied in detail have been shown to regulate subordinate downstream genes important for developmental events (Duboule 1994). The best understood homeodomain proteins are those encoded by the *hox/hom*, *prd/pax*, and *POU* gene families. Studies in null mutant mice have demonstrated that the *Pax-6* gene activates a regulatory cascade necessary for eye development (Gruss and Walther 1992), the *Oct-2 POU* homeobox gene promotes late stages of B-cell maturation (Corcoran et al. 1993), and *Hox* genes specify axial identity during embryogenesis (Krumlauf 1994).

Unlike most homeobox family members, which were isolated by their sequence similarity with other homeobox genes, the original *Pem* cDNA clone was isolated in a screen for developmentally regulated mouse genes using the subtraction hybridization technique (MacLeod et al. 1990). The Pem homeodomain, which is in the C-terminus of Pem (Fig. 1), is sufficiently different from other homeodomains to warrant classification of *Pem* as an orphan homeobox gene (Sasaki et al. 1991; Rayle 1991). Two lines of evidence suggest that the *Pem* gene probably evolved from a primordial member of the *prd/pax* homeobox gene. First, the Pem homeodomain is more related to prd/pax homeodomains (up to 35% sequence identity) than to those from any other homeobox gene family. Second, the positions of the two introns that interrupt the Pem homeodomain-coding region (Maiti et al. 1996a) are the same as those in the *Drosophila melanogaster prd* class homeobox gene *aristaless* (Schneitz et al. 1993). Several other *prd/pax* genes also contain an intron at the same position as the second *Pem* homeodomain intron (Duboule 1994). These observations are significant because other homeobox gene families either lack introns in the homeodomain region or their introns are at other positions within the homeodomain (Duboule 1994).

Both the mouse and rat *Pem* genes are on the X-chromosome (Lin et al. 1994; Maiti et al. 1996a). Recently we localized the mouse *Pem* gene to the *Hprt* region in the proximal end of the mouse X-chromosome (Sutton and Wilkinson 1997a). From its position relative to other nearby genes that we mapped we concluded that the region that contains the

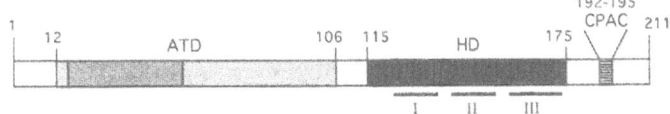

Fig. 1. The three conserved regions of the Pem homeodomain protein. The N-terminus contains a conserved domain (amino acids 12–106) of unknown function (*ATD*). Within this ATD is a highly conserved subdomain (amino acids 16–50). The C-terminus has a homeodomain (amino acids 115–175), with three α-helices. The third helix (helix III) is highly conserved and has been shown to mediate base-specific contacts with DNA in structurally defined homeodomains. The C-terminus contains a conserved CPAC motif (amino acids 192–195) similar to the catalytic centers of oxidoreductases

Pem gene is probably conserved between mice and humans, unlike many other regions of the X-chromosome which have undergone rearrangement during mammalian evolution. The tight linkage between the mouse *Ant2* and *Pem* loci suggests that the human *ANT2* gene may be a useful marker for isolating the human *PEM* gene, which has been impervious to cloning by conventional hybridization methods because of its rapid evolution (see Sect. 11.5).

11.3 *Pem* Expression and Regulation

As with most other homeodomain proteins, Pem is expressed in a stage- and tissue-specific manner during embryogenesis. Pem transcripts and protein are primarily confined to the extraembryonic compartment, including trophoectoderm and descendant cells in the placenta (Wilkinson et al. 1990; Lin et al. 1994). Pem's regulated expression in early embryonic cells in vivo is mimicked in stem cells lines that undergo differentiation in vitro (Sasaki et al. 1991; Lin et al. 1994).

More recently we discovered that Pem is also expressed specifically in reproductive tissues in postnatal and adult mice and rats. We found that *Pem* gene expression is primarily restricted to the testis, epididymis, and ovary (Lindsey and Wilkinson 1996a,b; Maiti et al. 1996a,b; Sutton et al. 1998). Several lines of evidence suggest that in the testis Pem is expressed in Sertoli cells. First, RNase protection analysis showed that the seminiferous fraction of the mouse testis (containing Sertoli and germ cells) contain *Pem* mRNA, whereas *Pem* transcripts cannot be detected in the interstitial cell fraction (enriched for Leydig cells; Lindsey and Wilkinson 1996a). Second, purified mouse Sertoli cells express higher levels of *Pem* transcripts than does whole testis; the increased level in purified Sertoli cells is comparable to that of the Sertoli-specific gene *SGP-1* (Sutton et al. 1998). Third, the testes from dominant white spotting mutant (W^v/W^v) mice, which lack germ cells, express two to three times more *Pem* mRNA than do testes from nonmutant animals (Lindsey and Wilkinson 1996a). This level of increase is expected for a Sertoli-specific gene, based on the relative proportion of RNA in testes contributed by Sertoli cells in mutant W^v/W^v and nonmutant animals. Fourth, in situ hybridization analyses of wild-type and W^v/W^v seminiferous tubules showed that *Pem* transcripts displayed a hybridization pattern expected of the distribution of Sertoli cell cytoplasm (Lindsey and Wilkinson 1996a). Finally, immunohistochemical analysis with a rabbit polyclonal antibody prepared against recombinant mouse Pem (Lin et al. 1994) revealed that Pem protein is present specifically in Sertoli nuclei and is not detectable in any other testicular cell type (Sutton et al. 1998).

11.3.1 P_p and P_d: Two Independently Regulated Promoters

The *Pem* gene has two different promoter regions that are regulated independently (Fig. 2). The testosterone-dependent P_p is responsible for Pem transcription in testis and epididymis whereas the P_d transcribes the *Pem* gene in placenta and ovary (Maiti et al. 1996b). Both the P_p and P_d use multiple clustered transcription start sites (Maiti et al. 1996b; Sutton et al. 1998), as do many other promoters that lack TATA boxes.

Several lines of evidence indicate that the P_p is regulated by androgen. First, hypophysectimized animals that secrete reduced levels of luteinizing hormone (LH), a factor necessary for androgen production by Leydig cells, have greatly depressed levels of P_p-derived *Pem* transcripts in testis than do control animals (Lindsey and Wilkinson 1996b; Sutton et al. 1998). Treatment with either LH or testosterone raises the expression levels to those of control mice. In contrast, follicle-stimulating hormone (FSH) has no detectable effect on P_p *Pem* mRNA levels. Second, similar results were obtained in hypogonadal (*hpg/hpg*) mice,

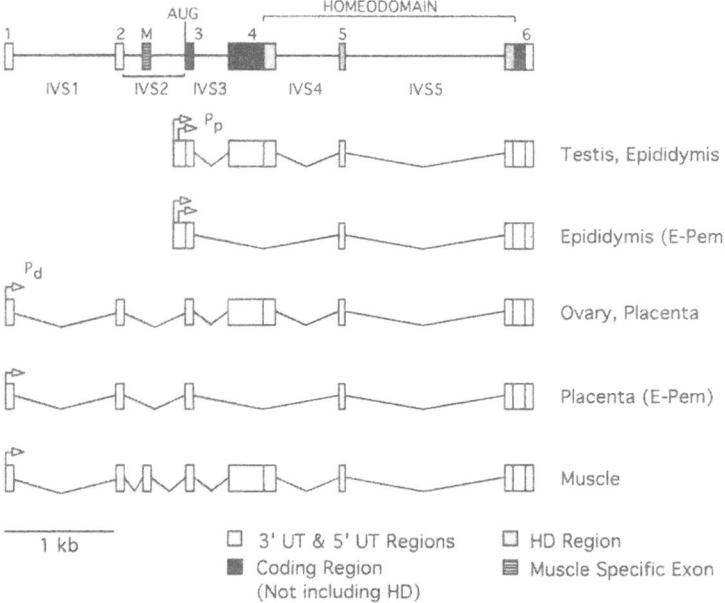

Fig. 2. The *Pem* gene. Shown are the two promoters, the P_p and P_d, which drive Pem transcription in a tissue specific manner. The alternatively spliced mRNAs transcribed from these promoters are also shown with the names of the *major* tissues that express each transcript. Note that the P_p is upstream of the initiator ATG within the second intron

which have a primary defect in the *GnRH* gene that severely depresses endogenous LH, FSH, and androgen levels (Lindsey and Wilkinson 1996a). Unlike hypophysectimized animals, homozygous *hpg* mice develop rudimentary testis in the absence of gonadotropins. Thus the ability of either testosterone or LH to activate *Pem* gene expression in *hpg* mice indicates that androgen can induce Pem transcripts under conditions in which the rudimentary testis has not previously been exposed to gonadotropins. Third, testicular feminization (*tfm*) mutant mice, which have a defect in the AR, lack detectable *Pem* transcripts in the testis (Lindsey and Wilkinson 1996b). Fourth, rats with impaired testosterone production (as a result of hypophysectomy or ethane dimethane sulfonate treatment) express reduced levels of P_p *Pem* transcripts (Lindsey and Wilkinson 1996b; Sutton et al. 1998). Administration of testosterone to ethane dimethane sulfonate treated rats permits Pp *Pem* expression to be sustained (Sutton et al. 1998).

In agreement with the observation that *Pem* gene expression is androgen dependent, we found that Pem is expressed in the androgen-dependent stages of the seminiferous epithelium cycle (Parvinen 1993). In situ hybridization analysis revealed that *Pem* transcripts are preferentially expressed during stages VII and VIII (Lindsey and Wilkinson 1996a). Although some earlier tubules (at stages IV-VI) also expressed *Pem*, virtually no *Pem* transcripts were detected in other stages of the seminiferous epithelium cycle. The *Pem* transcripts in Sertoli cells during these stages are translated, as demonstrated by immunohistochemical analysis with a rabbit polyclonal antibody prepared against recombinant mouse Pem (Sutton et al. 1998). The Pem protein was localized to Sertoli nuclei, consistent with Pem's role as a transcription factor.

11.3.2 Pp *Cis* Elements

We have begun to define the *cis* elements important for controlling the transcriptional activity of the P_p. A fragment of DNA that contained the mouse P_p transcription start site and approx. 1.5 kb of upstream sequence was ligated to the luciferase gene and transfected transiently into four cell lines. This −1548 construct was transcribed in the TM4 Sertoli and PS-1 prostate cell lines (Fig. 3). In contrast, the Rat-1 cell line, which does not detectably express transcripts from the endogenous P_p (but has a highly active endogenous P_d; (Maiti et al. 1996b), did not transcribe from the P_p-containing DNA fragment. The COS-1 kidney cell line also exhibited virtually no transcription of the −1548 construct.

We have begun deletion analysis to dissect the *cis*-regulatory elements in the P_p. Constructs with deletions to nt −807 or −567 had virtually no transcriptional activity suggesting that an upstream element drives the P_p (Fig. 3). A construct lacking −1246 to −904 (Δ1246–904) had low transcriptional activity, indicating that at least one regulatory element exists within this region. Several consensus binding sites for the zinc-finger protein GATA-1 and the homeodomain protein Nkx-3.1 are within this region (Fig. 3). Importantly, these sites are conserved in the

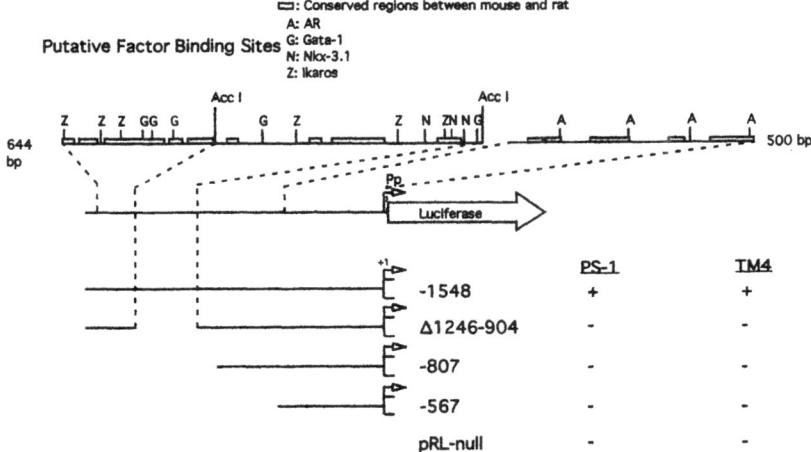

Fig. 3. Deletion analysis of the P_p male-specific Pem promoter. The map shows the region upstream of the mouse *Pem* P_p, including putative transcription factor binding sites that contain core sequences conserved between the mouse and rat *Pem* genes. The mouse Pem genomic fragments shown (which contain sequences up to the *Pem* initiator ATG) were ligated upstream of the *Renilla* luciferase gene in the vector pRL-null (Promega). The nucleotide numbers are with respect to the Pem initiator ATG. Luciferase activity from the longest construct (–1548) was assigned a (+) value; all (–) values represent at least fivefold less activity than from the –1548 construct. Variations in transfection efficiency were corrected for by cotransfection with the plasmid pGL3 control, which contains the firefly luciferase gene driven by the CMV promoter. The firefly and *Renilla* luciferase activities were assayed independently by using the Dual Luciferase Reporter Assay System (Promega)

mouse and rat *Pem* genes (Maiti et al. 1996a,b). Based on their expression pattern, both GATA-1 and Nkx-3.1 are reasonable candidates to regulate Pem gene expression. GATA-1 is selectively expressed in Sertoli cells during the same stages of the seminiferous epithelium cycle as Pem (Yomogida et al. 1994). Nkx-3.1 has been shown to be dependent on androgens for expression (in the prostate) and is known to be expressed in the testis (Bieberich et al. 1996; Sciavolino et al. 1997). We also found six consensus Ikaros-binding sites in the P_p regulatory region (Fig. 3). Although it is not known whether Ikaros is expressed in testis or epididymis (Georgopoulos et al. 1992), the presence of six consensus binding sites suggests that Ikaros or a related zinc-finger protein regulates P_p transcription. Experiments are in progress to identify whether any or all of these transcription factors are responsible for regulating *Pem* transcription.

11.3.3 P_d Regulation

The *cis* elements responsible for regulating the P_d are probably different from those that regulate the P_p, as these two promoters are regulated independently in different reproductive tissues in vivo. The P_d is expressed in a broader range of tissues than the P_p (female reproductive tissues and low levels in testis, skeletal muscle, and other tissues) and does not depend on androgens for transcription (Lindsey and Wilkinson 1996b; Maiti et al. 1996b; Sutton et al. 1998). Our recent transfection experiments suggest that a region between nt −69 and −55 from the major rat P_d transcription initiation site is critical for P_d transcription (S. Maiti and M.F. Wilkinson, manuscript in preparation). This *cis* element contains consensus Ets, nuclear factor (NF) κB, and Sp-1 transcription factor-binding sites. Specific mutations within this element virtually abolish transcription from the P_d. The likelihood that members of the Ets or NFκB transcription factor families play a key role in P_d transcription has several implications. First, Ets family members have been shown to be critical for female reproductive development (Chen et al. 1990; Schulz et al. 1993; McKnight et al. 1995), consistent with their activating *Pem* gene transcription in female reproductive tissue. Second, regulation of *Pem* transcription by either Ets or NFκB family members may explain why *Pem* is expressed in a large proportion of tumor cell lines, regardless of lineage (Wilkinson et al. 1990). Members of both of these transcription factor families are commonly expressed in tumors and have been implicated in causing malignancy.

11.3.4 Post-transcriptional Regulation

Pem transcripts are regulated not only at the promoter-usage level but also at the post-transcriptional level (Maiti et al. 1996b). We have identified several different *Pem* transcripts derived by alternative splicing. One alternatively spliced transcript skips an internal coding exon and therefore encodes a novel protein, E-Pem, that has a portion of the conserved N-terminal domain present in classical Pem, but also contains a novel C-terminus instead of the Pem homeodomain (Fig. 2). Because the N-terminal region of Pem is the most conserved region of this protein in mouse and rat Pem (Maiti et al. 1996a; Sutton and Wilkinson 1997b), the N-terminus may have functional attributes.

Other alternative transcripts differ in the 5' untranslated (UT) region, as a result of alternative splice acceptor use within two of the *Pem* 5' UT exons (Maiti et al. 1996b). In addition, another 5' UT exon (the M exon) is selectively included in *Pem* transcripts in skeletal muscle, where Pem is expressed at trace levels (Maiti et al. 1996b). There is no difference in the relative expression levels of transcripts with and without the M exon in skeletal muscle from male and female animals (Maiti et al. 1996b). Our preliminary transfection studies suggest that the inclusion of the M exon by alternative splicing was regulated by nearby *cis* elements in a tissue-specific manner (T. Cooper, S. Maiti, and M.F. Wilkinson, unpublished observations).

11.3.5 Pem Regulation in Epididymis

The epididymis requires androgen for the expression of many of the genes active in this tissue (see Sect. 11.1.1). With the exception of the AR, the transcription factors that mediate this regulation have not been identified. Few transcription factors have been identified in the epididymis, and those that have, such as Hoxc-8, Pax-2, and PEA-3, have either not been analyzed for androgen regulation or are expressed independently of androgen (Xin et al. 1992; Fickenscher et al. 1993; Lindsey and Wilkinson 1996b). We believe that Pem is a good candidate to regulate a subset of androgen-dependent genes in the epididymis because *Pem* expression is positively regulated by androgen in the epididymis, just as it is in the testis. Hypophysectimized rats have greatly depressed *Pem* mRNA levels in the epididymis, and these levels are restored to control levels by administration of exogenous testosterone (Lindsey and Wilkinson 1996b). Furthermore, we found that the temporal pattern of *Pem* expression in both the rat and mouse epididymis is correlated with the known increase of testosterone levels that occurs postpartum (Lindsey and Wilkinson 1996a,b). These results suggest that androgen limits Pem expression in the epididymis.

A unique feature of the epididymis is the regional localization of gene expression. Many epididymal gene products under androgen control are expressed in discrete regions of the epididymis (Cornwall and Hann 1995; Orgebin-Crist 1996). Because regional transcription factors probably dictate this expression pattern, we determined whether Pem is itself regionally restricted. In situ hybridization analysis revealed that *Pem* transcripts are expressed in the proximal cauda of the rat epididymis (Lindsey and Wilkinson 1996b). RNase protection analysis of sections of the rat epididymis suggested that *Pem* transcripts are also expressed in the corpus but not in the initial segment. This regional localization appeared to be conserved in mice, based on in situ hybridization analysis that showed that mouse epididymis contains *Pem* transcripts in the proximal cauda and distal corpus (Lindsey and Wilkinson 1996a). We therefore hypothesize that Pem regulates a subset of androgen-regulated secondary response and delayed primary response genes expressed in these regions of the epididymis. By analogy, other regional transcription factors, including many homeodomain proteins, dictate the specification of cellular compartments during embryogenesis (Kimble 1994).

11.3.6 Differences in P_p Expression in Mice and Rats

Although the androgen-dependence of the P_p is conserved in mice and rats, some other aspects of *Pem* regulation are unique to each species. Most strikingly, mice express much higher levels of P_p-derived transcripts in the testis than in epididymis, whereas the converse is true for rats (Sutton et al. 1998). We considered the possibility that androgen-binding protein (ABP) is responsible for this reciprocal regulation. ABP is thought to transport androgens away from the testis to other sites, including the epididymis (Robaire and Hermo 1988). ABP levels are at least 20-fold lower in mice than in rats (Wang et al. 1989), and we hypothesized that this explains the high *Pem* expression in mouse testis and low levels in mouse epididymis. However, our results with ABP transgenic mice did not conform with this hypothesis. We found that expression from the P_p in testis and epididymis was virtually identical in ABP transgenic mice and their control littermates (Sutton et al. 1998). There are several explanations for this observation, including the possibility that ABP does not increase sufficiently the concentration of biologically active (free) androgen to modulate P_p transcription.

What are the functional consequences of the reduced expression from the P_p in the rat testis compared with the mouse testis? Not only are P_p transcript levels low in adult rats; there is also a delay in expression. While mouse P_p transcripts first appear on day 8 to 9 postpartum (Lindsey and Wilkinson 1996a; Sutton et al. 1998), rat P_p transcripts are not expressed significantly until after day 30 postpartum (Maiti et al. 1996b). It is possible that this deficit in rat P_p expression is compensated for by the expression of transcripts from the other promoter, the P_d, which are known to be present as early as day 5 postpartum (Maiti et al. 1996b). Experiments are in progress to elucidate whether these P_d transcripts are expressed by rat Sertoli cells or other testicular cell types. Determining why two different strategies, involving differential usage of the P_p and P_d, to control *Pem* gene expression in the testis of postnatal mice and rats will require future investigation.

11.4 Conserved Domains in the Pem Protein

A notable feature of the *Pem* homeobox gene is its unusually rapid rate of evolution. The rat and mouse Pem proteins have only 73% amino acid sequence identity (Maiti et al. 1996a). Many of the amino acid substitutions occur in specific regions of the Pem protein; evidence suggests that this resulted from adaptive selection (see Sect. 11.5). Other regions of the Pem protein have remained relatively conserved in mice, rats, and related rodent species (Sutton and Wilkinson 1977b). One highly conserved domain of Pem is located in the amino terminal domain (ATD). This 95 amino acid domain is 87% identical in rats and mice. A 35 amino acid central subdomain within the ATD is 97% identical in rats and mice, and 89%–97% identical in eight other Old World rodent species (Maiti et al. 1996a; Sutton and Wilkinson 1997b). A portion of the ATD (amino acids 1–42 of Pem) has modest sequence identity with the so-called "death domain" that mediates protein-protein interactions (Cleveland and Ihle 1995), suggesting that the Pem ATD is a protein-binding domain. Another region of the ATD (amino acids 48–64 of Pem) has considerable sequence identity with the membrane-association domain [including the highly conserved (G/A)E(D/Q)LN motif] in the Prospero homeodomain protein and the Numb protein (Hirata et al. 1995; Knoblich et al. 1995). The functional significance of the sequence similarities between the Pem ATD and functional domains in other proteins remains to be determined.

The C-terminus of Pem is also conserved in Old World rodent species. Most strikingly, we found within this C-terminal region a CPAC motif, which is similar to the CPHC motif that comprises the catalytic center in the oxidoreductases DsbA and DnaJ (Grauschopf et al. 1995) and to the CXXC consensus sequence present in thioredoxin, and in mammalian protein disulfide isomerases, which generate disulfide bonds in proteins in the endoplasmic reticulum (Chivers et al. 1996). The CPAC motif is conserved in Pem in all 13 rodent species and subspecies that we have cloned and sequenced (while adjacent residues exhibit divergence), with the exception of *Stochomys longicaudatus*, which has a similar CPVC motif (Sutton and Wilkinson 1997b). Given the need for protection from oxygen-radical formation in the testis and epididymis, it is possible that this cysteine-rich motif acts as a redox catalytic center, which is of interest because no transcription factor has previously been shown to possess reducing or oxidizing activity. Alternatively, the CPAC motif may act as a redox sensor, by analogy with known transcription factors that are regulated by redox conditions (Kambe et al. 1996; Hidalgo et al. 1997).

11.5 Evidence for Adaptive Selection Acting Upon the Pem Homeodomain

A hallmark of homeodomains is their extremely high degree of conservation. Orthologous homeodomain transcription factors in mammals and *D. melanogaster* can have as few as one amino acid substitution in the 60 amino acid homeodomain (Duboule 1994). This conservation may result in part from the constraints of maintaining DNA-binding specificity. We observed a high degree of conservation in the third α-helix of the Pem homeodomain (Fig. 4), which supports this hypothe-

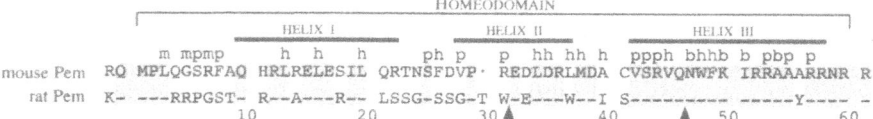

Fig. 4. Comparison of the Pem homeodomain in mouse and rat. *Above the mouse Pem sequence*, positions of the three α-helices and the known functional amino acids of other homeodomains (Duboule 1994): *m*, minor groove binding; *p*, phosphate-sugar backbone binding; *b*, base-specific binding; *h*, hydrophobic core. *Arrowheads*, positions of the two introns that interrupt the Pem homeodomain; *shading*, conserved amino acids between mouse and rat

sis because helix III mediates most of the base-specific contacts with DNA in structurally defined homeodomains (Duboule 1994).

In marked contrast to the strong conservation of helix III, the amino terminal portion of the Pem homeodomain contains many amino acid substitutions among rodent species (Fig. 4). In fact, the Pem homeodomain as a whole is only 62% identical in mice and rats (Maiti et al. 1996a; Sutton and Wilkinson 1997b). The sequence divergence is most marked in the extreme N-terminal portion of the homeodomain and the linker region between the α-helices but is also evident at selected residues within helices I and II (Fig. 4). The amino acid substitutions probably do not disrupt the basic structure of the Pem homeodomain because most of the key hydrophobic residues required for correct folding (labeled "h" in Fig. 4) are conserved. This sequence divergence in the Pem homeodomain is striking because other known homeodomains are subject to strong selection against sequence variation.

What is the significance of the rapid evolution of the Pem homeodomain? Our analysis of the ratio of synonymous to nonsynonymous codon substitutions in different rodents species implies that the divergence of the Pem homeodomain has been driven by adaptive selection (Maiti et al. 1996a; Sutton and Wilkinson 1997b). Why has there been selection for amino acid substitutions in the N-terminal region of the Pem homeodomain? Because the N-termini of many other homeodomains, including the HOX homeodomains, bind and regulate other proteins (Lai et al. 1992; Chan et al. 1994; van Dijk and Murre 1994; Pomerantz et al. 1992; Zappavigna et al. 1994; Grueneberg et al. 1995; Knoepfler and Kamps 1995; Lu et al. 1995; Phelan et al. 1995), we hypothesize that the variation in the Pem homeodomain N-terminus permits novel interactions with different transcription factors or cofactor proteins in different species. Alternatively, Pem-interacting proteins may have coevolved with Pem and thus retained Pem-binding capabilities across species.

We further hypothesize that the biological basis for the amino acid substitutions in specific regions of the Pem homeodomain is the role played by Pem in reproduction, a process that varies considerably between species and is known to be regulated by rapidly evolving proteins (Wachtel 1994). Some other transcription factors in the reproductive system have high levels of sequence divergence (Whitfield et al. 1993; Tucker and Lundrigan 1993; Shimmin et al. 1994; Kamper et al. 1995). Most notably, the Y-chromosome encoded sex determination gene *SRY*, as with *Pem*, encodes a protein that contains domains that have evolved rapidly (Whitfield et al. 1993; Tucker and Lundrigan 1993). Although the central DNA-binding domain, the HMG box, is conserved, the N- and C-terminal regions of the SRY protein are highly divergent in sequence between different mammalian species. Furthermore, a high frequency of nonsynonymous substitutions is evident in these N- and C-terminal domains, suggesting that adaptive selection has driven these amino acid alterations in SRY (Whitfield et al. 1993; Tucker and Lundrigan 1993). Because SRY is a key transcription factor that dictates sexual phenotype in mammals, it will be important to determine the factors that drove this apparent species-specific adaptive selection. Our comparison of the ratio of nonsynonymous and substitutions in SRY and Pem suggested that Pem has been even more strongly selected for amino acid substitutions than SRY has (Sutton and Wilkinson 1997b). It will be intriguing to elucidate the forces that have driven the rapid selection for alterations in the N-terminal region of the Pem homeodomain.

11.6 The *r.Pem2* Gene

During our analysis of *Pem* transcripts in rat male reproductive tissue we detected high levels of epididymis-specific transcripts that partially anneal with rat *Pem* probes. We determined that these transcripts are from a second rat *Pem*-like gene, *r.Pem2* (Nhim et al. 1997). This gene is a processed gene on rat chromosome 4 that lacks the introns of the rat

Pem gene and contains a vestigial poly(A) tail. We originally thought that *r.Pem2* is a pseudogene because it has three premature terminations codons within its coding sequence (Maiti et al. 1996a). However, we later found that *r.Pem2* has evolved one set of splice donor and acceptor sequences that permits these premature termination codons to be spliced-out as a single intron (Nhim et al. 1997).

There are several processed genes that encode functional proteins, including *pgk-2*, *Zfa*, and *Pdha-2*. Like *r.Pem2*, these genes are all autosomally processed genes derived from genes on the X-chromosome (Salehi-Ashtianai and Goldberg 1996). Interestingly, *r.Pem2* and these three processed genes are all expressed specifically in the male reproductive tract, but while *pgk-2*, *Zfa*, and *Pdha-2* are testis specific (Salehi-Ashtianai and Goldberg 1996), *r.Pem2* is expressed specifically in epididymis, not in testis or any other tissues tested (Nhim et al. 1997).

The function of the *r.Pem2* gene is not known. One possibility is that *r.Pem2* is a nonfunctional gene that is transcriptionally active in epididymis merely because it is near an epididymis-specific enhancer that drives the transcription of another gene on chromosome 4. Alternatively, *r.Pem2* may encode a functional protein. The spliced *r.Pem2* message has the potential to encode a 57 amino acid protein very similar to the C-terminus of rat Pem and including the conserved cysteine residues that may be functionally important (see Sect. 11.4). The r.Pem2 protein may function in the intermediate to late stages of epididymal development because *r.Pem2* transcripts are dramatically induced between days 23 and 30 postpartum (Nhim et al. 1997). The classic rat Pem protein (r.Pem) may also function at earlier stages in epididymal development, as *r.Pem* transcripts are evident in rat epididymis as early as day 10 postpartum (Lindsey and Wilkinson 1996b). More studies are required to elucidate the factors responsible for the differential regulation of the *r.Pem* and *r.Pem2* genes, and the functional relevance of their encoded products to the male reproductive system.

11.7 Future Studies

The expression pattern of the Pem gene suggests that it encodes a transcription factor that regulates male reproductive development or function. Our future studies will be directed towards determining the precise biological events in the testis, epididymis, or both that are regulated by the Pem homeodomain protein. We hypothesize that Pem regulates germ cell maturation by controlling the transcription of a defined set of downstream genes in somatic cells in the testis and epididymis. Because Pem is positively regulated by androgen in Sertoli cells and epididymal somatic cells, it may control androgen-regulated secondary response and primary-delayed response genes in these tissues. We predict that these downstream genes will have the same stage- and region-specific expression pattern as Pem. In addition to defining the downstream targets of Pem, our future studies will be directed towards identifying the *cis*- and *trans*-acting factors that regulate Pem transcription. This is an important aim because it may lead to a better understanding of the regulatory networks that dictate androgen-dependent events in male reproductive tissues.

References

Anderson B, Pearse R II, Schlegel P, Cichon Z, Schonemann M, Bardin C, Rosenfeld M (1993) Sperm 1: a *POU*-domain gene transiently expressed immediately before meiosis I in the male germ cell. Proc Natl Acad Sci USA 90:11084–11088

Bardin C, Cheng C, Musto N, Gunsalus G (1988) The Sertoli cell. In: Knobil E, Neill J (eds) The physiology of reproduction. Raven, New York, p 933

Bieberich C, Fujita K, He W-W, Jay G (1996) Prostate-specific and androgen-dependent expression of a novel homeobox gene. J Biol Chem 271:31779–31782

Branford WW, Zhao GQ, Valerius MT, Weinstein M, Birkenmeier, EH, Rowe LB, Potter S (1997) Spx1, a novel X-linked homeobox gene expressed during spermatogenesis. Mech Dev 65:87–98

Chan S-K, Jaffe L, Capovilla M, Botas J, Mann RS (1994) The DNA binding specificity of ultrabithorax is modulated by cooperative interactions with extradenticle, another homeoprotein. Cell 78:603–615

Chen Z-Q, Burdett L, Seth A, Lautenberger J, Papas T (1990) Requirement of *ets-2* expression for *Xenopus* oocyte maturation. Science 250:1416–1418

Chivers PT, Laboissière MCA, Raines RT (1996) The CXXC motif: imperatives for the formation of native disulfide bonds in the cell. EMBO J 15:2659–2667

Cleveland J, Ihle J (1995) Contenders in FasL/TNF death signaling. Cell 81:479–482

Corcoran L, Karvelas M, Nossal G, Ye Z-S, Jacks T, Baltimore D (1993) *Oct-2*, although not required for early B-cell development, is critical for later B-cell maturation and for postnatal survival. Genes Dev 7:570–582

Cornwall G, Hann S (1995) Specialized gene expression in the epididymis. J Androl 16:379–386

Dean D, Sanders M (1996) Ten years after: reclassification of steroid-responsive genes. Mol Endocrinol 10:1489–1495

DeRobertis E (1994) The homeobox in cell differentiation and evolution. In: Duboule D (ed) Guidebook to the homeobox genes. Oxford University Press, Oxford, p 11

Duboule D (1994) Guidebook to the homeobox genes. Oxford University Press, Oxford

Fickenscher H, Chalepakis G, Gruss P (1993) Murine Pax-2 protein is a sequence-specific trans-activator with expression in the genital system. DNA Cell Biol 12:381–391

Georgopoulos K, Moore D, Derfler B (1992) Ikaros, an early lymphoid-specific transcription factor and a putative mediator for T cell commitment. Science 258:808–812

Grauschopf U, Winther JR, Korber P, Zander T, Dallinger P, Bardwell JCA (1995) Why is DsbA such an oxidizing disulfide catalyst? Cell 83:947–955

Grueneberg D, Simon K, Brennan K, Gilman M (1995) Sequence-specific targeting of nuclear signal transduction pathways by homeodomain proteins. Mol Cell Biol 15:3318–3326

Gruss P, Walther C (1992) Pax in development. Cell 69:719–722

Hecht N (1996) Gene expression during male germ cell development. In: Desjardins C (ed) Cellular and molecular regulation of testicular cells. Springer, Berlin Heidelberg New York, p 400

Hidalgo E, Ding H, Demple B (1997) Redox signal transduction: mutations shifting [2Fe-2S] centers of the SoxR sensor-regulator to the oxidized form. Cell 88:121–129

Hirata J, Nakagoshi H, Nabeshima Y-I, Matsuzaki F (1995) Asymmetric segregation of the homeodomain protein Prospero during *Drosophila* development. Nature 377:627–630

Kambe F, Nomura Y, Okamoto T, Seo H (1996) Redox regulation of thyroid-transcription factors, Pax-8 and TTF-1, is involved in their increased DNA-binding activities by thyrotropin in rat thyroid FRTL-5 cells. Mol Endocrinol 10:801–812

Kamper J, Reichmann M, Romeis T, Bolker M, Kahmann K (1995) Multiallelic recognition nonself-dependent dimerization of bE and bW homeodomain proteins in *Ustilago maydis*. Cell 81:73–83

Kimble J (1994) An ancient molecular mechanisms for establishing embryonic polarity? Science 266:577–578

Knoblich JA, Jan LY, Jan YN (1995) Asymmetric segregation of Numb and Prospero during cell division. Nature 377:624–627

Knoepfler P, Kamps M (1995) The pentapeptide motif of Hox proteins is required for cooperative DNA binding with Pbx1, physically contacts Pbx1, and enhances DNA binding by Pbx1. Mol Cell Biol 15:5811–5819

Krumlauf R (1994) Hox genes in vertebrate development. Cell 78:191–201

Lai J, Cleary M, Herr W (1992) A single amino acid exchange transfers VP-16-induced positive control from the *Oct-1* to the *Oct-2* homeodomain. Genes Dev 6:2058–2065

Li Y, Lemaire P, Behringer RR (1997) Esx1, a novel X chromosome-linked homeobox gene expressed in mouse extraembryonic tissues and male germ cells. Dev Biol 188:85–95

Lin T-P, Labosky P, Grabel L, Kozak C, Pitman J, Kleeman J, MacLeod C (1994) The *Pem* homeobox gene is X-linked and exclusively expressed in extraembryonic tissues during early murine development. Dev Biol 166:170–179

Lindsey J, Wilkinson M (1996a) *Pem*: a testosterone- and LH-regulated homeobox gene expressed in mouse Sertoli cells and epididymis. Dev Biol 179:471–484

Lindsey J, Wilkinson M (1996b) An androgen-regulated homeobox gene expressed in rat testis and epididymis. Biol Reprod 55:975–983

Lu Q, Knoepfler P, Scheele J, Wright D, Kamps M (1995) Both Pbx1 and E2A-Pbx1 bind the DNA motif ATCAATCAA cooperatively with the products of multiple murine *Hox* genes, some of which are themselves oncogenes. Mol Cell Biol 15:3786–3795

MacLeod C, Fong A, Seal B, Walls L, Wilkinson M (1990) Isolation of novel complementary DNA clones from T lymphoma cells: one encodes a putative multiple membrane-spanning protein. Cell Growth Differ 1:271–279

Maiti S, Doskow J, Sutton K, Nhim R, Lawlor D, Levan K, Lindsey J, Wilkinson M (1996a) The Pem homeobox gene: rapid evolution of the homeodomain, X chromosomal localization, and expression in reproductive tissue. Genomics 34:304–316

Maiti S, Doskow J, Li S, Nhim R, Lindsey J, Wilkinson M (1996b) The Pem homeobox gene: androgen-dependent and -independent promoters and tissue-specific alternative RNA splicing. J Biol Chem 271:17536–17546

McKnight R, Spencer M, Dittmer J, Brady J, Wall R, Hennighausen L (1995) An Ets site in the whey acidic protein gene promoter mediates transcriptional activation in the mammary gland of pregnant mice but is dispensable during lactation. Mol Endocrinol 9:717–724

Nhim R, Lindsey J, Wilkinson M (1997) A processed homeobox gene expressed in a stage-, tissue-, and region-specific manner in epididymis. Gene 185:271–276

Orgebin-Crist M-C (1996) Androgens and epididymal function. In: Bhasin S, Gabelinck H, Spieler J, Swerdloff R, Wang C (eds) Pharmacology, biology and clinical application of androgens. Wiley, New York, p 27

Parvinen M (1993) Cyclic function of Sertoli cells. In: Russel L, Griswold M (eds) The Sertoli cell. Cache River, Clearwater, p 331

Phelan M, Rambaldi I, Featherstone M (1995) Cooperative interactions between HOX and PBX proteins mediated by a conserved peptide motif. Mol Cell Biol 15:3989–3997

Pomerantz J, Kristie T, Sharp P (1992) Recognition of the surface of a homeodomain protein. Genes Dev 6:2047–2057

Rayle R (1991) The oncofetal gene Pem specifies a divergent paired class homeodomain. Dev Biol 146:255–257

Robaire B, Hermo L (1988) Efferent ducts, epididymis, and vas deferens: structure, functions and their regulation. In: Knobil E, Neill J (eds) The physiology of reproduction. Raven, New York, p 999

Salehi-Ashtiani K, Goldberg E (1996) Testis-specific gene transcription. In: Desjardins C (ed) Cellular and molecular regulation of testicular cells. Springer, Berlin Heidelberg New York, p 127

Sar M, Hall S, Wilson E, French F (1993) Androgen regulation of Sertoli cells. In: Russell L, Griswold M (eds) The Sertoli cell. Cache River, Clearwater, p 509

Sasaki A, Doskow J, MacLeod C, Rogers M, Gudas L, Wilkinson MF (1991) The oncofetal gene Pem encodes a homeodomain and is regulated in primordial and pre-muscle stem cells. Mech Dev 34:155–164

Schulz R, The S, Hogue D, Galewsky S, Guo Q (1993) Ets oncogene-related gene *Elg* functions in Drosophila oogenesis. Proc Natl Acad Sci USA 90:10076–10080

Schneitz K, Spielmann P, Noll M (1993) Molecular genetics of *aristaless*, a *prd*-type homeobox gene, involved in the morphogenesis of proximal and distal pattern elements in a subset of appendages in *Drosophila*. Genes Dev 7:114–129

Sciavolino P, Abrams E, Yang L, Austenberg L, Shen M, Abate-Shen C (1997) Tissue-specific expression of murine Nkx3.1 in the male urogenital system. Dev Dyn 209:127–138

Shimmin L, Chang B, Li W (1994) Contrasting rates of nucleotide substitutions in the X-linked and Y-linked zinc finger genes. J Mol Evol 39:569–578

Singh J, O'Neill C, Handelsman DJ (1995) Induction of spermatogenesis by androgens in gonadotropin-deficient (*hpg*) mice. Endocrinology 136:5311–5321

Sutton KA, Wilkinson MF (1997a) The rapidly evolving *Pem* homeobox gene and *Agtr2*, *Ant2*, and *Lamp2* are closely linked in the proximal region of the mouse X chromosome. Genomics 45:447–450

Sutton KA, Wilkinson MF (1997b) Rapid evolution of a homeodomain: evidence for positive selection. J Mol Evol 45:579–588

Sutton KA, Maiti S, Tribley WA, Lindsey JS, Meistrich ML, Bucana CD, Sanborn BM, Joseph DR, Griswold MD, Cornwall GA, Wilkinson MF (1998) Regulation of the *Pem* homeodomain gene in mice and rat Sertoli and epididymal cells. J Androl 19(1) (in press)

Tucker P, Lundrigan B (1993) Rapid evolution of the sex determining locus In Old World mice and rats. Nature 364:715–717

van Dijk M, Murre C (1994) *extradenticle* raises the DNA binding specificity of homeotic selector gene products. Cell 78:617–624

Wachtel SS (1994) Molecular genetics of sex determination. Academic, San Diego

Wang Y, Sullivan P, Petrusz P, Yarbrough W, Joseph D (1989) The androgen-binding protein gene is expressed in CD1 mouse testis. Mol Cell Endocrinol 63:85–92

Watrin F, Wolgemuth D (1993) Conservation and divergence of patterns of expression and lineage-specific transcripts in orthologues and paralogues of the mouse *Hox-1.4* gene. Dev Biol 156:136–145

Whitfield LS, Lovell-Badge R, Goodfellow P (1993) Rapid sequnce evolution of the mammalian sex-determining gene *SRY*. Nature 364:713–715

Wilkinson MF, Kleeman J, Richards J, MacLeod C (1990) A novel oncofetal gene is expressed in a stage-specific manner in murine embryonic development. Dev Biol 141:451–455

Wolgemuth D, Viviano C, Watrin F (1991) Expression of homeobox genes during spermatogenesis. Ann NY Acad Sci 637:300–312

Xin J-H, Cowie A, Lachance P, Hassell J (1992) Molecular cloning and characterization of PEA3, a new member of the Ets oncogene family that is differentially expressed in mouse embryonic cells. Genes Dev 6:481–496

Yomogida K, Ohtani H, Harigae H, Ito E, Nishimune Y, Engel J, Yamamoto M (1994) Developmental stage- and spermatogenic cycle-specific expression of transcription factor GATA-1 in mouse Sertoli cells. Development 120:1759–1766

Zappavigna V, Sartori D, Mavilio F (1994) Specificity of HOX protein function depends on DNA-protein and protein-protein interactions, both mediated by the homeodomain. Genes Dev 8:732–744

Zirkin B (1993) Regulation of spermatogenesis in the adult mammal: Gonadotropins and androgens. In: Desjardins C, Ewing L (eds) Cellular and molecular biology of the testis. Oxford Univerity Press, Oxford, p 166

12 Studies on the Mechanism of Sperm Production

H. Tanaka, M. Okabe, M. Ikawa, J. Tsuchida, Y. Yoshimura,
K. Yomogida, and Y. Nishimune

12.1 Introduction

Producing functional sperm in mammals requires two steps that take place in two different organs: the production of sperm in the testis and the maturation of sperm in the epididymis. The germ cell differentiation that produces sperm in males involves numerous morphological and physiological changes that are timed precisely. These complex processes, referred to as spermatogenesis, comprise: the proliferation and differentiation of spermatogonia, meiotic prophase of spermatocytes, and substantial morphological changes from postmeiotic haploid spermatids to sperm.

Germ cell differentiation from spermatogonial stem cells into sperm is completed in the mouse in seminiferous tubules in approximately 1 month under the complex regulation of many different molecules, including hormones and growth factors. To determine the mechanism of spermatogenesis we used three different approaches to identify and isolate a number of germ cell specific molecules. First, we isolated monoclonal antibodies (mAb) recognizing specific antigens of mouse germ cells and then characterized and analyzed these specific antigen molecules (Watanabe et al. 1992; Koshimizu et al. 1993, 1995; Tanaka et al. 1998a; Pereira et al. 1998). Second, using specific polyclonal antibodies raised in our laboratory we identified differentiation-specific macromolecules expressed during mouse testicular development (Tsuchida et al. 1995). Third, if the amount of antigens was insufficient or the antigenicity was low, we isolated cDNA clones specifically expressed in testicular germ cells from a subtracted cDNA library generated by subtracting cDNAs derived from supporting cells of germ cell-less mutant testis from wild-type testis cDNAs. We have carried out their characterizations (Tanaka et al. 1994).

Recent progress in molecular biology has stimulated the investigation of many complex biological processes. The isolation of genes specifically expressed in testes and also in various steps of germ cell development has provided new insights into spermatogenesis. Progress in molecular biological techniques has been instrumental in understanding the regulation of specific molecules in germ cell differentiation, the physiological roles of gene products, and their morphological effects in cell differentiation.

Embryological technology has also helped in analyzing the function of genes involved in cell differentiation and the normal development of embryos. By introducing specific genes into fertilized eggs (transgenic animals) we are able to analyze both the function of genes and the regulatory mechanisms of specific gene expression. The method of gene targeting to produce knockout animals has also become a powerful technique in the study of in vivo gene functions.

The combined use of these techniques is continually providing new knowledge of spermatogenesis, as in other fields of biology.

12.2 Isolation and Characterization of Testis-Specific Molecules

12.2.1 Monoclonal Antibodies

In studying germ cell differentiation at the molecular level the use of certain lectins is more effective for isolation of the specific receptor molecules on the germ cell surface (Millette and Scott 1984; Schopperle et al. 1992). However, the use of specific antibodies is much more powerful in identifying germ cell specific molecules. As indicated by the autoallergic orchitis and by the frequent induction of sperm-specific antibodies in both males and females, testicular germ cells are unique and differ from other somatic cells immunologically. Since the germ cells are outside the immunological surveillance mechanism (Welber et al. 1988), it is easy to induce antibodies capable of reacting with germ cells when testicular germ cells are immunized. Furthermore, the specific antibodies are induced to react exclusively with testicular germ cells when immunized to isogenic or autogenic animals. These antibodies can recognize many kinds of antigen molecules that appear or disappear in association with germ cell differentiation.

mAbs recognizing germ cells can also be isolated (Millette and Bellve 1977; Millette 1979; Millette and Moulding 1981; Fenderson et al. 1984; O'Brien and Millette 1984; Head and Kresge 1985; Kallajoki 1986; O'Brien et al. 1988; Anakwe and Gerton 1990; Escalier et al. 1991; Ohsako et al. 1991, 1994; Tanii et al. 1992, 1994; Enders and May 1994; Toshimori et al. 1995). We have isolated many mAbs recognizing specific antigens of mouse germ cells and have performed the characterization and analysis of these specific antigen molecules. The female rat was immunized with mouse germ cell lysates, and hybridoma clones were prepared by fusing the rat spleen cells and myeloma cells. We screened the culture supernatant of the hybridoma reacting with testicular germ cells.

The antigen recognized by mAbs BC7 and CA12 is a 95-kDa plasma membrane protein expressed on zygotene and early pachytene spermatocytes (Koshimizu et al. 1993). The mAb EE2 reacted with type A and B spermatogonia and early meiotic cells. The antigen recognized by EE2 is a glycoprotein with a molecular weight of 114 kDa (Koshimizu et al. 1995). Calmegin (Meg 1), of 93 kDa by sodium dodecyl sulfate

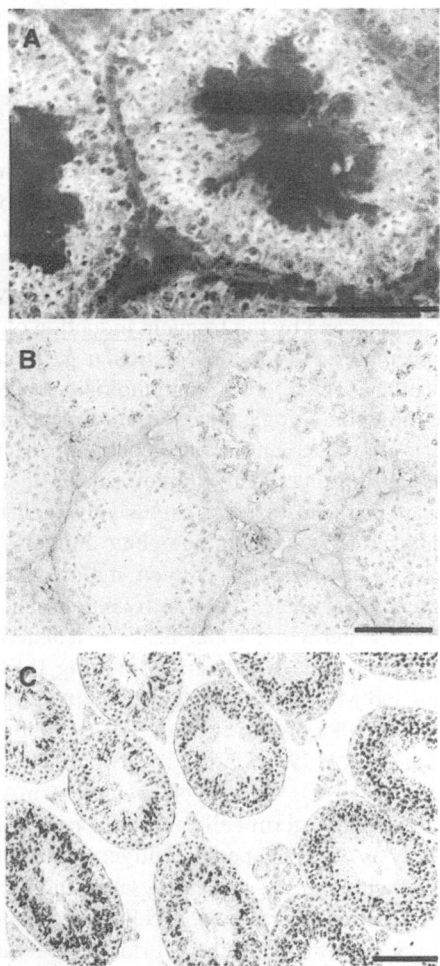

Fig. 1A–C. Immunohistochemical staining of testicular cross-sections with mAbs. **A** TRA 369: paraformaldehyde fixation, fluorescein isothiocyanate staining. (From Watanabe et al. 1992). **B** TRA 104: methanol fixation, frozen section, peroxidase-diaminobenzidine staining. (From Tanaka et al. 1998a). **C** TRA 54: Bouin's fixation, peroxidase-diaminobenzidine staining, and counterstained with hematoxylin (Pereira et al. 1998). *Bar*, 100 μm

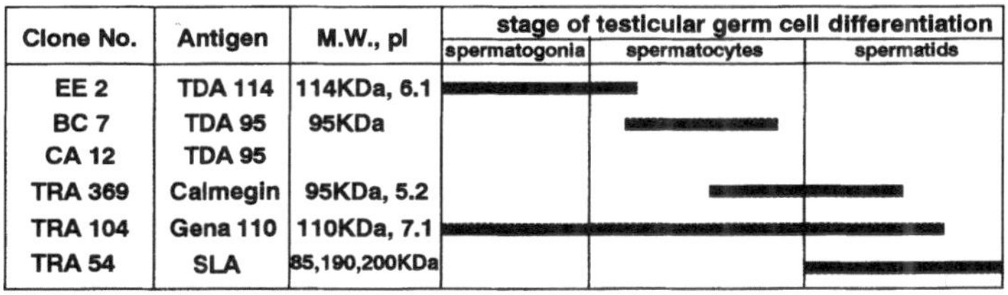

Clone No.	Antigen	M.W., pI	stage of testicular germ cell differentiation		
			spermatogonia	spermatocytes	spermatids
EE 2	TDA 114	114KDa, 6.1	▬▬▬▬	▬▬	
BC 7	TDA 95	95KDa		▬▬▬	
CA 12	TDA 95				
TRA 369	Calmegin	95KDa, 5.2		▬	▬▬
TRA 104	Gena 110	110KDa, 7.1	▬▬▬▬▬▬▬	▬▬▬▬	▬
TRA 54	SLA	85,190,200KDa			▬▬▬

Fig. 2. Schematic presentation of the expression of testicular germ cell specific antigens reacted with monoclonal antibodies. *Solid bar*, detection of each antigen

polyacrylamide gel electrophoresis was identified in male meiotic-germ cells with mAb TRA 369. Calmegin was strongly expressed in specific steps of meiotic germ cells from pachytene spermatocytes to early spermatids (Watanabe et al. 1992; Fig. 1A).

The mAbs TRA 104 and TRA 98 stained nuclei of testicular germ cells in the seminiferous tubules, i.e., spermatogonia, spermatocytes, and spermatids, but elongated spermatids and mature sperms were not stained (Fig. 1B; Tanaka et al. 1998a). Although all types of the spermatogonia and spermatocytes were stained, the strongest staining was observed in round spermatids, especially at steps 1 and 2. During further differentiation the positive signal diminished gradually and finally disappeared in elongated spermatids at steps 15 and 16. Western blotting analysis of various adult tissues with TRA 104 showed positive bands only in testis. These bands were detected at 60–110 kDa exclusively in nuclear fraction of testicular germ cells and have been termed germ cell specific nuclear antigens (GENAs). GENAs exist not only in adult testicular germ cells but also in primordial germ cells and in embryo ovary. GENAs are considered to be unique molecules existing in the nuclei of germ cell lineage.

The mAb TRA 54 recognized specific organelles in germ cell cytoplasm from spermatocytes to spermatids, i.e., a large granule of middle to late pachytene, diplotene, and secondary spermatocytes and of round spermatids at stage 1 stained positively as well as the acrosome of spermatids at steps 2 and 3 to step 12 (Fig. 1C; Pereira et al. 1998). The antigens then disappeared from the spermatids of more advanced stages of differentiation. Immunoblots using TRA 54 revealed broad bands with molecular weights greater than 200, 190, and 85 kDa in the testis. We are interested in the expression of these antigen molecules during testicular germ cell development because they appear to be involved in the biogenesis of organelles such as chromatoid body and acrosome.

These mAbs may serve as a useful maker for germ cell development and differentiation (Fig. 2). Furthermore, cross-reacting antigens have also been detected exclusively in germ cells of other animals such as rat and human by these mAbs. The conservation of these antigens in many mammalian species implies that they are important molecules for germ cell differentiation. The use of mAbs TRA 104 and TRA 54 will lead to improved understanding of the physiological roles of the molecule in testicular germ-cell differentiation, and study is now in progress to purify the protein and isolate the cDNA clones coding for these antigens.

12.2.2 Polyclonal Antibodies

To identify testis-specific molecules we have developed polyclonal antibodies specifically recognized by all of the testicular germ cells (Maekawa and Nishimune 1985). Rabbits were extensively immunized with mouse germ cell antigens using complete Freund's adjuvant. The rabbit antiserum obtained was absorbed in castrated adult male mice by injection of the rabbit serum into the abdominal cavity to remove nonspecific anti-mouse antibodies (in vivo absorption). The mouse sera obtained by bleeding were mixed with the homogenate of mouse liver and centrifuged, and the clear upper layer in the centrifuge tube was used as the specific anti-germ cell antiserum. Under our experimental conditions this antiserum identified more than 20 antigens of molecular weights ranging from 26 to 110 kDa in intact mature testes. Some of the antigens expressed in prepubertal testes increased quantitatively, and a number of newly detectable antigens appeared upon the differentiation of germ cells (Fig. 3; Tsuchida et al. 1995).

These results indicate that the four antigens are the products of differentiated spermatogonia such as intermediate and/or type B. The other two groups of germ cell specific molecules, p31, p55, p80, p85, p93, and p35, p48, p71, appeared first when germ cell differentiation had proceeded to the stages of spermatocytes and spermatids, respec-

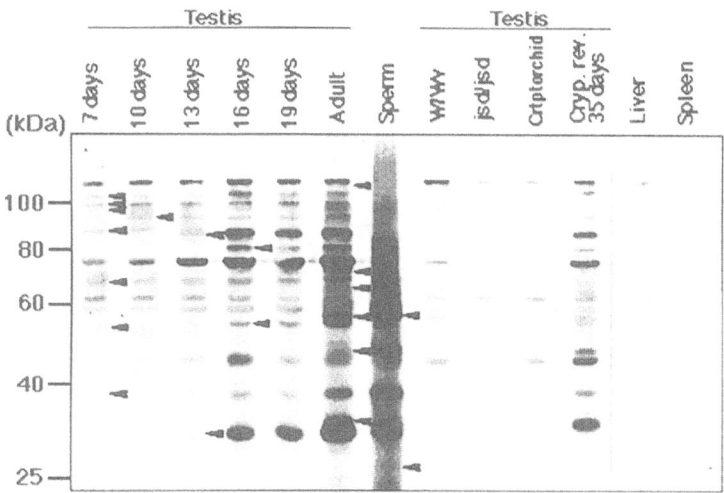

Fig. 3. Immunoblot analysis using anti-germ cell specific polyclonal antibodies. Proteins were extracted from testes of W/Wv, jsd/jsd, cryptorchid, aged 7, 10, 13, 16, and 19 days, and testes 35 days after the surgical reversal of the cryptorchid and from the liver, spleen, and sperm. These were separated by sodium dodecyl sulfate polyacrylamide gel electrophoresis, transferred to a filter, and immunostained with the anti-germ cell antiserum absorbed by in vivo and in vitro methods (described in Sect. 12.2.2). *Arrowheads*, antigens appearing first during testicular germ cell differentiation. *Left margin*, molecular weights. (From Tsuchida et al. 1995)

tively. Some of the germ cell specific antigens (i.e., p67, p71, p80, p88, p93, p100, p105) disappeared and were not present in the sperm although they existed in mature testis. These may be processed or degraded to certain sizes of molecules or abolished with residual bodies during spermiogenesis. In contrast, antigens p26 and p58 were detected as sperm-specific ones, and they did not exist in the testis. These may be the molecules processed in the epididymis. Western blotting analysis showed that expression of the p38 is enhanced in the testis after 16 days of age. Some of the others (p38, p53, p57, and p96) were also identified in the sperm. These antigens may have been expressed not only in testicular somatic cells but also in differentiated germ cells. Another group of the above antigens (p57, p65, p108) were induced following the development of testicular maturation. Thus the expression of some of the testicular germ cell specific or somatic antigens was developmentally controlled.

Understanding the mechanisms controlling the expression of these molecules would require further confirmatory studies, such as testicular germ cell separation and isolation of cDNA clones encoding those antigens [by expression cloning; for example, direct submission in DDBJ D88539 (Kondoh et al. 1997), and D88453 to D88454]. These studies will provide more information on the physiological roles of the molecules expressed specifically in testicular germ cell differentiation.

12.2.3 Subtraction Cloning of Germ Cell Specific cDNAs

We have isolated cDNA clones using antibodies against germ cell specific antigens from expression libraries of bacteriophage in *Escherichia coli* and have characterized some antigens (Watanabe et al. 1994). In this way, however, we cannot isolate cDNA when epitope of antibody is not on polypeptides but on sugar moieties of glycoproteins, or when the avidity of antibody is not strong enough to isolate the corresponding cDNA clone from expression libraries. More systematic screening methods must be designed if we do not wish to lose these clones. A subtracted cDNA library was generated by subtracting cDNAs derived from supporting cells of germ cell-less mutant testis from wild-type testicular cDNAs (Tanaka et al. 1994). Detailed analysis of mRNA expression revealed that the genes corresponding to the cloned cDNAs are expressed exclusively in the testis and are developmentally controlled (Fig. 4).

Computer-assisted sequence analysis indicated that gsg3, for example, which we have isolated, is a novel actin capping protein which would regulate actin polymerization. We have also identified phosphoprotein haspin, which has some unique motifs, such as a part of protein kinase consensus sequences, a homologous region to the myocyte-specific enhancer factor 2B (mef 2B), the nuclear localization signal (KKKRK), and basic amino acid sequence domain in the central region, the leucine zipper in the C-terminal region, and many phosphorylation sites (CK2, PKC, PKA; Fig. 5; Tanaka et al. 1998b). By raising antiserum to the putative amino acid sequence of these clones we have

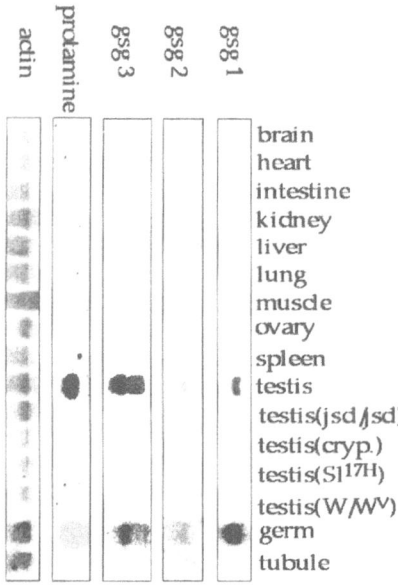

Fig. 4. Northern blot analysis of cloned cDNAs in various tissues, mutant testes, and testicular germ cell fractions. Total RNAs were prepared from various tissues; 10 μg of each sample was electrophoresed, transferred to a nylon membrane, and hybridized with the cloned cDNA probes. After autoradiography the same filter was rehybridized with actin and protamine cDNA. (From Tanaka et al. 1994)

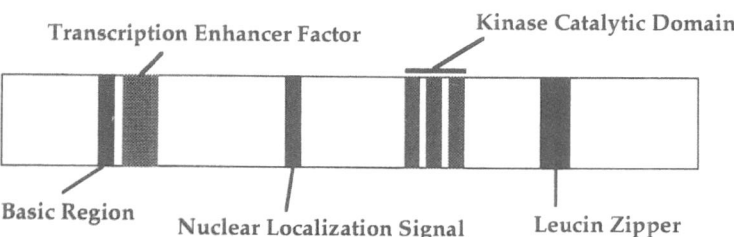

Fig. 5. Identification of consensus motifs and homologous regions in germ cell specific gene, Hhaspin

characterized the biochemical function and the role of these proteins. The germ cell specific genes that we have isolated are not sufficient to explain all of the mechanisms of germ cell differentiation. Further studies are now in progress to isolate more cDNAs and to characterize the cDNA clones coding for germ cell specific protein.

12.3 Structure of the Genome
Specifically Expressed in Testicular Germ Cells

It has been reported that the sequence of some genes specifically expressed in testicular haploid-germ cells have no TATA or CAAT box but a cAMP-responsive element in their promoters (Sun and Means 1996; Monaco et al. 1996). Furthermore, the germ cell specific PGK gene is intronless and differs from the somatic type PGK gene (Boer et al. 1987). There is an interesting genome construction in testis-specific genes. The isolation and characterization of the genome specifically expressed in testicular germ cells are also in progress in our laboratory.

12.4 Analysis of the Function of Testis-Specific cDNAs

12.4.1 Proteins Encoded by Isolated cDNAs

As mentioned above, many testis-specific genes have been cloned. For characterizing the gene products in vitro a culture system is useful especially for further investigation of gene regulation and the function of gene products. However, we still lack efficient culture cell lines and in vitro cultivation systems to investigate the function of germ cell specific genes. In certain cases, however, some culture cell lines could be useful, such as embryonic stem, embryonic germ, and embryonic carcinoma (Doetschman et al. 1985; Matsui et al. 1992; Martin and Evans 1974). Some of the germ cell specific genes are expressed in these cell lines, and the mechanism of specific expression of the gene can be studied. Cocultivation of testicular germ cells with Sertoli cell lines can induce differentiation of the germ cells proceeding to the meiotic prophase and then the production of haploid germ cells (Rassoulzadegan et al. 1993). The use of such transformed Sertoli cell lines may be effective in analyzing the regulation of germ cell specific genes. However, this system does not induce complete germ cell differentiation and is not sufficient for further analysis. Thus we must develop a new cultivation system or culture cell lines of testicular germ cells in order to analyze the mechanism of the expression of germ cell specific genes.

12.4.2 Regulation of Gene Expression in Transgenic Animals

As discussed above, in vitro cultivation of germ cells is technically premature for studying the regulation of gene expression. To overcome the problem of premature in vitro cultivation systems, transgenic animals can be used. DNA is introduced exogenously into fertilized eggs with the DNA having a 5' noncoding sequence of a specific gene fused with a reporter gene such as that for chloramphenicol acetyltransferase or enhanced green fluorescent protein (EGFP). If specific expression of the reporter gene with an appropriate sequence of 5' noncoding region is observed, information can be obtained both on the *cis*-element of germ cell specific and on differentiation-specific expression. Using this technique we identified the meiosis-specific transcription element of the calmegin gene in testicular germ cells (Watanabe et al. 1995; Fig. 6).

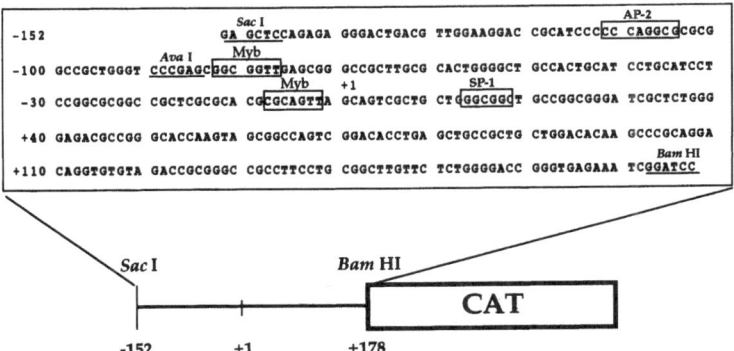

Fig. 6. The 5' flanking DNA sequence of the genomic calmegin gene and a construction used for generating transgenic mice. Nucleotides were numbered from the first nucleotide of the transcription initiation site (+1). *Underlined*, restriction enzyme sites; *boxes*, putative binding sites for nuclear factors (AP2, SP1, Myb). (From Watanabe et al. 1995)

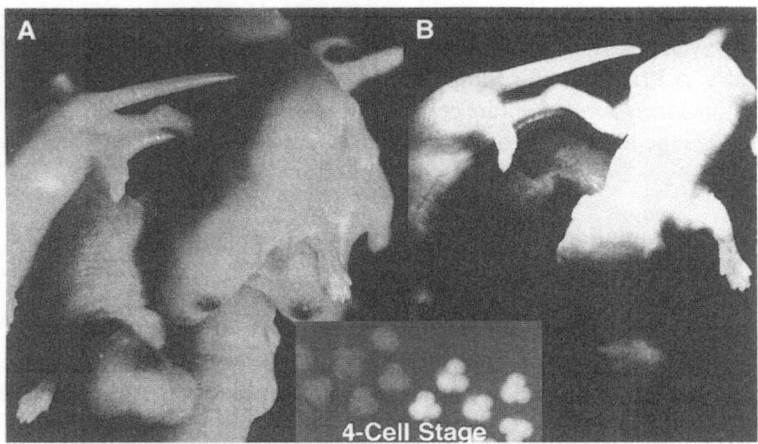

Fig. 7A,B. Green mice produced by injection of the EGFP gene. Photomicrographs of green mice under visual light (**A**) and ultraviolet light (**B**). (From Okabe et al. 1997)

The promoter region of the calmegin gene contained a number of GC-rich sequences and lacked a canonical TATA or CCAAT box in the typical location upstream of the transcriptional starting site.

We have also demonstrated that *trans*-factors binding to this 330-bp DNA fragment exist only in the nuclear extract of testis. This DNA sequence is useful for gaining an understanding of germ cell specific gene expression. Recently we have shown that EGFP is detectable without fixation or substrate addition in the cell of transgenic animals (Okabe et al. 1997; Fig. 7). EGFP could be a useful new marker for gene expression and analysis of protein localization. The regulation of exogenous gene expression does not always reflect the regulation of physiological gene expression. Expression of the gene is also affected by the copy number, sequence character, especially 3' or 5' flanking region of a transgene, and its integration sites (Palmiter et al. 1993; Lee et al. 1996; Gu and Hecht 1997; Miyagawa et al. 1997). Therefore it is necessary to raise many lines of transgenic mice before being able to draw conclusions from the results (Zambrowicz et al. 1993).

12.4.3 Gene Targeting to Elucidate the Function of Isolated Genes

It is often difficult to clarify the physiological role of protein products encoded by the cDNA by biochemical analysis. Although we have successfully identified the biochemical functions of certain specific proteins in vitro, we do not necessarily understand the true role of the gene products in vivo. Analyses of a functional defect resulting from mutations have led us to an understanding of the physiological role of the gene product. Thus it would be useful to generate artificial mutant animals. The development of ES cell lines having excellent germ cell transmission rate has made gene targeting a powerful technique.

The calmegin gene has been cloned and analyzed in our laboratory. Calmegin protein is expressed specifically in meiosis and functions as a molecular chaperone. The physiological role of this molecule in germ cell differentiation was studied by targeted disruption of the gene. The calmegin knockout male mouse showed infertility due to the loss of sperm adhesion to the egg, indicating that calmegin functions as a chaperone for sperm surface proteins to mediate sperm-egg interactions (Table 1; Ikawa et al. 1997).

Many genes are targeted, but some are embryo-lethal in homozygous situations, and it is therefore difficult to identify the function of knocked-out genes. Even in this case conditional knockout of the gene could be effective. Development of the cre-loxP recombination system facilitates study of the effect of gene targeting under specific conditions (Barinaga et al. 1994). Various options are available regarding the question of where and when to knockout the gene. This technique allows the isolation and analysis of the knockout mouse even when it is embryo-lethal.

Table 1. Fecundity of calmegin knockout mice

Genotype	No. of males tested	No. of plugs observed	No. of pups/plug
+/+	5	20	7.6±2.8
+/–	4	15	7.7±2.7
–/–	17	150[a]	0.05±0.03

Each male was mated with three females for 1–3 months.
[a] 36 plugs were counted for 6 males; for the other 11 males the number of plugs was estimated from the counted value.

12.5 Future Prospects

All multicellular organisms consist of two types of cells, somatic cells and germ cells. The former functions to maintain the individual and the latter to maintain the species. A number of biological mechanisms must differ between these two. However, we are not yet able to comprehend fully how primordial germ cells are derived, what comprises the difference between germ cells and somatic cells, or how germ cell differentiation progresses and is maintained. Further analysis of the precise role of molecules specifically expressed in germ cell differentiation and development and advances in new techniques can help us to understand the basic biological rules which exist in germ cells. Detailed knowledge of germ cell proliferation and differentiation will in turn facilitate the development of new techniques in reproduction biology and even of new clinical applications that will control the complex processes of the germ cell differentiation.

References

Anakwe OO, Gerton GL (1990) Acrosome biogenesis begins during meiosis: evidence from the synthesis and distribution of an acrosomal glycoprotein, acrogranin, during guinea pig spermatogenesis. Biol Reprod 42:317–328

Barinaga M (1994) Knockout mice: round two. Science 265:26–28

Boer PH, Adra CN, Lau Y-FC, McBurney MW (1987) The testis-specific phosphoglycerate kinase gene pgk-2 is a recruited retroposon. Mol Cell Biol 7:3107–3112

Doetschman TC, Eistetter H, Katz M, Schmidt W, Kemler R (1985) The in vitro development of blastocyst-derived embryonic stem cell lines: formation of visceral yolk sac, blood islands and myocardium. J Embryol Exp Morphol 87:27–45

Enders GC, May JJ II (1994) Developmentally regulated expression of a mouse germ cell nuclear antigen examined from embryonic day 11 to adult in male and female mice. Develop Biol 163:331–340

Escalier D, Gallo JM, Albert M, Meduri G, Bermudez D, David G, Schrevel J (1991) Human acrosome biogenesis: immunodetection of proacrosin in primary spermatocytes and of its partitioning pattern during meiosis. Development 113:779–788

Fenderson BA, O'Brien DA, Millete CF, Eddy EM (1984) Stage-specific expression of three cell surface carbohydrate antigens during murine spermatogenesis detected with monoclonal antibodies. Develop Biol 103:117–128

Gu W, Hecht NB (1996) Translational of a testis-specific Cu/Zn superoxide dismutase (SOD-1) mRNA is regulated by a 65-kilodalton protein which bind to its 5' untranslated region. Mol cell Biol 16:4335–4543

Head JR, Kresge CK (1985) Reaction the chromatoid body with a monoclonal antibody to a rat histocompatibility antigen. Biol Reprod 33:1001–1008

Ikawa M, Wada I, Kominami K, Watanabe D, Toshimori K, Nishimune Y, Okabe M (1997) The putative chaperone calmegin is required for sperm fertility. Nature 387:607- 611

Kallajoki M, Parvinen M, Suominen JJO (1986) Expression of acrosin during mouse spermatogenesis: a biochemical and immunocytochemical analysis by a monoclonal antibody C 11 H. Biol Reprod 35:157–165

Kondoh N, Nishina Y, Tsuchida J, Koga M, Tanaka H, Uchida K, Inazawa J, Taketo M, Nozaki N, Nojima H, Matsumiya K, Namiki M, Okuyama A, Nishimune Y (1997) Assignment of synaptosomal complex protein 1 (SCP1) to human choromosome 1p13 by fluorscence in situ hybridization and its expression in the testis. Cytogenet Cellgenet 78:103–104

Koshimizu U, Watanabe D, Sawada K, Nishimune Y (1993) A novel stage-specific differentiation antigen is expressed on mouse testicular germ cells during early meiotic prophase. Biol Reprod 49:875–884

Koshimizu U, Nishioka H, Watanabe D, Dohmae K, Nishimune Y (1995) Characterization of a novel spematogenic cell antigen specific for early stage of germ cells in mouse testis. Mol Reprod Dev 40:221–227

Lee K, Fajardo MA, Braun RE (1996) A testis cytoplasmic RNA-binding protein that has the properties of a translational repressor. Mol Cell Biol 16:3023–3034

Maekawa M, Nishimune Y (1985) Separation of germ cells from somatic cells in mouse testis by affinity for a lectin, peanut agglutinin. Biol Reprod 32:419–425

Matsui Y, Zsebo K, Hogan BL (1992) Derivation of pluripotential embryonic stem cells from murine primordial germ cells in culture. Cell 70:841–847

Martin GR, Evans MJ (1974) The morphology and growth of a pluripotent teratocarcinoma cell line and its derivatives in tissue culture. Cell 2:163–172

Millette CF (1979) Cell surface antigens during mammalian spermatogenesis. Curr Top Dev Biol 1:1–29

Millette CF, Bellve AR (1977) Temporal expression of membrane antigens during mouse spermatogenesis. J Cell Biol 74:86–97

Millette CF, Moulding CT (1981) Cell surface marker proteins during mouse spermatogenesis: two-dimensional electrophoretic analysis. J Cell Sci 48:367–382

Millete CF, Scott BK (1984) Identification of spermatogenic cell plasma membrane glycoproteins by two-dimensional electrophoresis and lectin blotting. J Cell Sci 65:233–248

Miyagawa S, Mikata S, Tanaka H, Ikawa M, Kominami K, Seya T, Nishimune Y, Shirakura R, Okabe M (1997) The regulation of membrane cofactor protein (CD46) expression by the 3' untranslated region in transgenic mice. Biochem Biophys Res Commun 233:829–833

Monaco L, Nantel F, Foulkes NS, Sassone-Corsi P (1996) A transcriptional master switch governing the cAMP response in the testis. In: Hansson V, Levy FO, Tasken K (eds) Signal transduction in testicular cells. Springer, Berlin Heidelberg New York, p 71

O'Brien DA, Millette CF (1984) Identification and immunochemical characterization of spermatogenic cell surface antigens that appear during early meiotic prophase. Dev Biol 101:307–317

O'Brien DA, Gerton GL, Eddy EM (1988) Acrosomal constituents identified with a monoclonal antibody are modified during late spermiogenesis in the mouse. Biol Reprod 38:955–967

Ohsako S, Kurohmaru M, Nishida T, Hayashi H (1991) Analysis of various antigens in golden hamster testis by monoclonal antibodies. J Vet Med Sci. 53:969–974

Ohsako S, Bunick D, Hess RA, Nishida T, Kurohmaru M, Hayashi Y (1994) Characterization of a testis specific protein localized to endoplasmic reticulum of spermatogenic cells. Anat Rec 238:335–348

Okabe M, Ikawa M, Kominami K, Nakanishi T, Yoshitake N (1997) "Green mice" as a source of ubiquitous green cells. FEBS Lett 407:313–319

Palmiter RD, Sandgren EP, Koeller DM, Brinster RL (1993) Distal regulatory elements from the mouse metallothionein locus stimulate gene expression in transgenic mice. Mol Cell Biol 13:5266–5275

Pereira AVDL, Tanaka H, Nagata Y, Sawada K, Mori H, Chimelli L, Nishimune Y (1998) Characterization and expression of a stage specific antigen by monoclonal antibody TRA 54 in testicular germ cells. Int J Androl (in press)

Rassoulzadegan M, Paquis-Flucklinger V, Bertino B, Sage J, Jasin M, Miyagawa K, van-Heyningen V, Besmer P, Cuzin F (1993) Transmeiotic differentiation of male germ cells in culture. Cell 75:997–1006

Schopperle WM, Armant DR, Dewolf WC (1992) Purification of a tumor-specific RNA- binding glycoprotein, gp200, from a human embryonal carcinoma cell line. Arch Biochem Biophys 298:538–543

Sun Z, Means AR (1996) A role for cAMP-response element motifs in transcriptional regulation of postmeiotic male germ cell-specific genes. In: Hansson V, Levy FO, Tasken K (eds) Signal transduction in testicular cells. Springer, Berlin Heidelberg New York, p 29

Tanaka H, Yoshimura Y, Nishina Y, Nozaki M, Nojima H, Nishimune Y (1994) Isolation and characterization of cDNA clones specifically expressed in testicular germ cells. FEBS Lett 355:4–10

Tanaka H, Pereira AVDL, Nozaki M, Tsuchida J, Sawada K, Mori H, Nishimune Y (1998a) A germ cell-specific nuclear antigen recognized by monoclonal antibody raised against mouse testicular germ cells. Int J Androl (in press)

Tanaka H; Yoshimua Y, Nozaki M, Tsuchida J, Yomogida K, Habu T, Tosaka Y, Periera AVDP, Nojima H, Nishimune Y (1998b) Identification and characterization of haploid germ cell specific phophoprotein (Haspin) in spermatid nuclei. (Submitted)

Tanii I, Toshimori K, Araki S, Oura C (1992) Appearance of an intra-acrosomal antigen during the terminal step of spermiogenesis in the rat. Cell Tissue Res 267:203–208

Tanii I, Araki S, Toshimori K (1994) Intra-acrosomal organization of a 90-kilodalton antigen during spermiogenesis in the rat. Cell Tissue Res 277:61–67

Toshimori K, Tanii I, Araki S (1995) Intra-acrosomal 155,000 dalton protein increases the antigenicity during mouse sperm maturation in the epididymidis: a study using a monoclonal antibody MC101. Mol Reprod Develop 42:72–79

Tsuchida J, Nishina Y, Akamatsu T, Nishimune Y (1995) Characterization of development-specific, cell type-specific mouse testicular antigens using testis-specific polyclonal antibodies. Int J Androl 18:208–212

Watanabe D, Sawada K, Koshimizu U, Kagawa T, Nishimune Y (1992) Characterization of male meiotic germ cell-specific antigen (Meg 1) by monoclonal antibody TRA369 in mice. Mol Reprod Dev 33:307–312

Watanabe D, Yamada K, Nishina Y, Tajima Y, Koshimizu U, Nagata A, Nishimune Y (1994) Molecular cloning of a novel Ca(2+)-binding protein (calmegin) specifically expressed during male meiotic germ cell development. J Biol Chem 269:7744-7749

Watanabe D, Okabe M, Hamajima N, Morita T, Nishina Y, Nishimune Y (1995) Characterization of the testis-specific gene 'calmegin' promoter sequence and its activity defined by transgenic mouse experiments. FEBS Lett 365:509–512

Welber JE, Turner TT, Tung KSK, Russell LD (1988) Efferct of cytochalasin D on the integrity of the Sertoli cell (blood-testis) barrier. Am J Anat 182:130–147

Zambrowicz BP, Harendza CJ, Zimmermann JW, Brinster RL, Palmiter RD (1993) Analysis of the mouse protamine 1 promoter in transgenic mice. Proc Natl Acad Sci USA 90:5071–5075

13 Role of c-kit in Egg Activation

P. Rossi, C. Sette, A. Bevilacqua, F. Mangia, and R. Geremia

13.1 Introduction

In many species a series of Ca^{2+} oscillations is the first event triggered by egg-sperm fusion (Whitaker and Swann 1993). It is widely accepted that this series of increases in intracellular free Ca^{2+} is responsible for the following egg activation; however, the molecular mechanisms underlying such Ca^{2+} mobilization within the egg are not fully understood (Kline and Kline 1992; Whitaker and Swann 1993; Homa et al. 1993; Berridge 1996).

Two main mechanisms have been proposed (Yanagimachi 1994). According to the first, sperm-egg fusion induces activation of an egg-membrane receptor and subsequent phospholipase C (PLC) activation by either G proteins or protein tyrosine kinases. The consequence of PLC activation is phosphatidylinositol 4,5 biphosphate (PIP_2) hydrolysis and production of diacylglycerol (DAG) and inositol 1,4,5-triphosphate ($InsP_3$). DAG is a powerful stimulator of some protein kinase C (PKC) isoforms whereas $InsP_3$ binds to specific receptors which are coupled to channels responsible for the release of Ca^{2+} from intracellular stores (Berridge 1993) through a mechanism known as $InsP_3$-induced calcium release (IICR). The second hypothesis proposes that a soluble sperm factor enters the egg at fertilization and elicits Ca^{2+} oscillations. In agreement with the sperm factor hypothesis, it has been shown that intracytoplasmic injection of soluble sperm extracts into metaphase II (MII) arrested oocytes induces a series of Ca^{2+} spikes and complete egg activation in several mammalian species (Swann 1990; Stice and Robl 1990; Wu et al. 1997), including humans (Homa and Swann 1994; Dozortsev et al. 1995). Microinjection of soluble extracts from spermatozoa of sea urchin (Dale et al. 1985) and nemertean worms (Stricker 1997) can also activate eggs of the same species. The hypothesis that a soluble sperm protein is responsible for the onset of these Ca^{2+} transients and the consequent egg activation after introduction into the egg cytoplasm has been strengthened in recent years by the success of intracytoplasmatic sperm injection as the most promising technique for assisted fertilization (Tesarik et al. 1994; Palermo et al. 1997).

However, the identity of the sperm protein required for egg activation is still uncertain (Wilding and Dale 1997). A possible candidate is a glucosamine 6-phosphate isomerase, termed oscillin, which has been purified from hamster sperm (Parrington et al. 1996). Although the purified fraction induces Ca^{2+} oscillations when microinjected into mouse eggs, it has not been shown that oscillin itself is the only component of this fraction, and it is not clear whether microinjection of the product of the cloned gene is sufficient to elicit the full complement of events associated with egg activation, which include cortical granule exocytosis, completion of the second meiotic division, with second polar body extrusion, formation of the female pronucleus, and progression through cleavage stages. It has been hypothesized that the sperm factor sensitizes calcium-induced calcium release (CICR) within eggs, thus generating the classical Ca^{2+} oscillations observed at fertilization (Whitaker and Swann 1993).

However, it is not clear how after sperm-egg fusion eggs can achieve the initial calcium release, which depends the generation of $InsP_3$, whose essential role at fertilization has been firmly established (Miyazaki et al. 1992; Xu et al. 1994). It has been proposed that two independent sperm-derived factors cooperate in generating calcium oscillations at fertilization: one activates IICR through $InsP_3$ production, and the other sensitizes CICR within the egg cytoplasm (Wilding and Dale 1997). However, it is known that $InsP_3$ by itself can elicit Ca^{2+} oscillations of variable frequency, depending on its intracellular concentration, since Ca^{2+} released through IICR can generate CICR in mammalian eggs (Miyazaki et al. 1993; Berridge 1996). Alternatively, it has been proposed that the putative soluble sperm factor which activate eggs at fertilization is a kinase or a modulator of a kinase activity (Yanagimachi 1994). The sperm factor could trigger $[Ca^{2+}]_i$ elevation within the mouse egg, again, through activation of PLC activity, with consequent production of $InsP_3$ (Berridge 1996). The essential role of $InsP_3$ produced by PLC in mammalian fertilization has been further strengthened by the recent observation that specific PLC inhibitors can block the sperm-induced Ca^{2+} spiking at fertilization in mouse eggs (Dupont et al. 1996). PLCγ1, which is normally activated by tyrosine kinase dependent pathways, is the most readily detectable PLC isoform present in mouse eggs (Dupont et al. 1996). Very recent data indicate that PLCγ1 plays an essential role in Ca^{2+} rise during fertilization of starfish eggs (Carroll et al. 1997). PLCγ1 is probably essential for Ca^{2+} oscillations also in mouse eggs since these oscillations are impaired by inhibitors of tyrosine kinase activity (Dupont et al. 1996).

The Ca^{2+} rise at fertilization is probably essential for cortical granule exocytosis, an early sign of oocyte activation that is observed in natural fertilization and is considered essential for the hardening of the zona pellucida and the block of polyspermy (Yanagimachi 1994). The Ca^{2+} rise is probably also important for resumption of meiosis in ovulated mammalian oocytes which are arrested in the metaphase of the second meiotic division. The mechanism responsible for the developmental arrest of mouse oocytes at MII depends on cytoplasmic conditions that cause chromosome condensation to the metaphase state (Clarke et al. 1988). It is widely accepted that a dephosphorylation-dependent decrease in mitogen-activated protein (MAP) kinase activity rather than a decrease in the Ca^{2+}-sensitive maturation promoting factor (MPF, i.e., the cdc2/cyclin B complex with histone H1 kinase activity) is required for modifications of spindle-associated microtubules at anaphase, chromosome decondensation, and reconstitution of a nuclear envelope (Verlhac et al. 1993, 1994, 1996; Moos et al. 1995, 1996).

In mouse eggs MAP kinase activity is stimulated by the product of the c-*mos* proto-oncogene (Verlhac et al. 1996). C-mos is essential both in *Xenopus* (Sagata et al. 1989) and in the mouse (Colledge et al. 1994; Hashimoto et al. 1994) to maintain MII arrest in the egg (Vande Woude 1994). Studies on *Xenopus* egg extracts suggest that the Ca^{2+}-induced release from metaphase arrest, which is mediated by activation of calmodulin-dependent protein kinase II (Lorca et al. 1993), involves inhibition of a complex positive feedback loop between the serine-threonine kinases MPF, c-mos, and MAP kinase (Minshull et al. 1994), and that MAP kinase has intrinsic cytostatic factor (CSF) activity (Haccard et al. 1993). Therefore MAP kinase must be considered the ultimate component of the CSF system in vertebrate eggs. It is not known whether the Ca^{2+} rise at fertilization is directly related to the inhibition of MAP kinase activity and the consequent formation of the female pronucleus, which is a relatively later event of egg activation.

13.2 Tr-kit, an Alternative c-kit Gene Product Expressed in Late Spermiogenesis, Is a Truncated Tyrosine Kinase

The 150-kDa c-kit tyrosine kinase transmembrane receptor (Qiu et al. 1988) is expressed in primordial germ cells in the embryonal gonad, and its ligand, stem cell factor (SCF), promotes survival of these cells in vitro (Dolci et al. 1991). After birth c-kit is expressed in the mitotic stages of spermatogenesis (Sorrentino et al. 1991; Yoshinaga et al. 1991), and SCF, produced by the surrounding Sertoli cells (Rossi et al. 1991) under follicle-stimulating hormone stimulation, promotes proliferation of type A spermatogonia in culture (Rossi et al. 1993). SCF has also been proposed as a survival factor for type A spermatogonia in the postnatal testis (Packer et al. 1995). Experiments with spermatogonial transplantation also support an important in vivo role for the c-kit receptor in mitotic germ cells of the postnatal testis (reviewed by Dym

1994). Expression of c-kit also occurs in postnatal oocytes (Manova et al. 1990; Horie et al. 1991; Yoshinaga et al. 1991) and SCF produced by the surrounding granulosa cells promotes oocyte growth (Packer et al. 1994) and may be involved in the negative control of meiotic progression of oocytes (Ismail et al. 1996; 1997).

The c-kit receptor mRNA can still be detected, at lower levels, in the meiotic stages of mouse spermatogenesis, and its expression ceases completely in the haploid phase, when an alternative form of c-kit mRNA is present (Sorrentino et al. 1991). An alternative c-kit transcript of similar size is also expressed in spermatids of adult rat testis (Orth et al. 1996). The alternative mouse c-kit mRNA is transcribed under the control of a cell-specific intronic promoter, which specifically drives the expression of a reporter *lacZ* gene in late spermiogenesis in transgenic mice (Albanesi et al. 1996). An anti-c-kit immunoreactive 24-kDa protein (tr-kit), corresponding to the size predicted by the open reading frame (ORF) of the mouse spermatid-specific c-kit cDNA, is actually accumulated during late spermiogenesis (Albanesi et al. 1996). Tr-kit consists of 202 amino acids, corresponding to 12 hydrophobic residues encoded by intronic sequences, followed by the 190 carboxyterminal amino acids of the c-kit ORF (Rossi et al. 1992). Tr-kit contains the phosphotransferase catalytic domain of the c-kit cytoplasmic portion but not the ATP binding site. It also lacks the interkinase domain, including the phosphotyrosine docking site for the interaction with the 85-kDa subunit of inositol 3-phosphate kinase (Serve et al. 1994), but contains the carboxyterminal region relevant for c-kit interaction with PLCγ1 (Herbst et al. 1995).

13.3 Tr-kit Is Present in the Residual Cytoplasm of Mature Spermatozoa

In agreement with the activation of the c-kit intronic promoter in the haploid phase of spermatogenesis are the results of western blot analysis using an antibody directed against the 13 carboxyterminal amino acids encoded by the mouse c-kit ORF, which revealed the presence of a 24-kDa anti-c-kit immunoreactive band in round spermatids, and its accumulation in elongating spermatids and in epididymal spermatozoa (Albanesi et al. 1996). In the mature sperm the intracellular distribution of the tr-kit protein is mainly restricted to the midpiece of the flagellum (Sette et al. 1997), which together with the mitochondrial sheath contains most of the residual sperm cytoplasm. A weaker positivity to the c-kit antibody is also detected in the postacrosomal region at the basis of the sperm head and in the principal piece of the tail, but not in the acrosomal region, the connecting piece, or terminal tail segment (Sette et al. 1997). In immature sperms tr-kit accumulates mainly in the cytoplasmic droplet of the midpiece. The presence of tr-kit in the residual bodies of the spermatids (Albanesi et al. 1996) and in the midpiece of mature sperm indicates that this protein accumulates essentially in the residual sperm cytoplasm.

It is known that, together with the sperm head which provides paternal chromosomes, the sperm midpiece also penetrates the mammalian egg, and supplies centrosome components responsible for aster formation after fertilization (Yanagimachi 1994). Therefore the localization of tr-kit is compatible with its entry into the egg and with a possible action inside the oocyte after sperm-egg fusion.

13.4 Microinjection of Recombinant tr-kit into MII-Arrested Oocytes Causes Complete Parthenogenetic Activation of Mouse Eggs

The potential action of tr-kit in the egg cytoplasm was investigated by microinjection of a recombinant tr-kit protein expressed in COS cells into mouse oocytes arrested in metaphase II.

Microinjection of extracts from COS cells expressing tr-kit reproducibly causes complete parthenogenetic activation of 70% of the oocytes (Sette et al. 1997). Activation of MII oocytes triggered by extracts of tr-kit expressing transfected COS cells is coupled to exocytosis of cortical granules; moreover, the emission of the second polar body occurs, indicating MII-anaphase transition and completion of the second meiotic division. Activated oocytes also proceed through the first mitotic cycle. Pronuclei appear between 4 and 7 h after microinjection, a time approximating that observed during natural fertilization (Hogan et al. 1994), and most of the activated eggs reach the two-blastomere stage after 24 h in culture. Furthermore, many of the activated eggs develop to morula stages when cultured for 2–4 days. Microinjection of the extracts from mock-transfected COS cells does not induce any of the activation events triggered by tr-kit, indicating that the presence of the truncated c-kit protein in extracts from transfected COS cells is necessary for egg activation.

To determine whether tr-kit is also sufficient to induce the set of events observed after its microinjection into MII oocytes we synthesized tr-kit ORF RNA in vitro and performed similar microinjection experiments. Synthetic tr-kit RNA reproducibly induced pronuclear formation in 60% of the oocytes between 4 and 7 h after microinjection, whereas microinjection of control RNAs did not trigger activation above background levels observed in noninjected oocytes (Sette et al. 1997). Again, cortical granule exocytosis and second meiotic division preceded pronuclear formation.

We conclude that the microinjected tr-kit protein is directly responsible for MII-arrested oocyte activation, and that posttranslational modifications possibly achieved in a eukaryotic expression environment can be achieved in the MII oocyte cytoplasm after translation of tr-kit RNA. We did not see an appreciable delay in the timing of egg activation when we injected tr-kit RNA with respect to the timing of egg activation after injection of cell extracts expressing the recombinant tr-kit protein, suggesting that only a very small amount of tr-kit is needed to trigger egg activation, and that as soon as the RNA is translated in the egg cytoplasm tr-kit elicits its action.

13.5 Tr-kit Dependent Egg Activation Requires Calcium Ions, and Is Associated with a Decrease in MAP Kinase Activity

Intracellular Ca^{2+} mobilization is associated with sperm-induced egg activation at fertilization (Yanagimachi 1994). The rise in intracellular Ca^{2+} is responsible for the onset of cortical granules exocytosis and for the destruction of MPF activity necessary for the completion of meiosis. The possibility that tr-kit induced egg activation also depends at least in part on oocyte intracellular calcium ions was investigated. Intracellular Ca^{2+} was chelated by preincubation with the membrane permeable compound BAPTA-AM before microinjection of extracts from COS cells expressing tr-kit. BAPTA-AM completely blocked both second

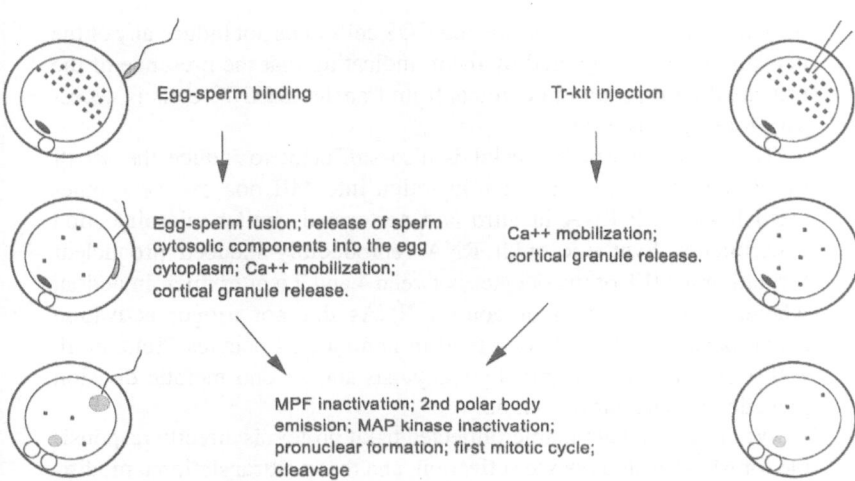

Fig. 1. Microinjection of recombinant sperm-carried tr-kit faithfully reproduces the events of egg activation occurring at natural fertilization. Schematic
representation of the ordered series of events which occur after the contact of
the sperm and the egg plasma membranes (*left*) and after the microinjection of
extracts from transfected COS cells expressing the tr-kit protein, or of in vitro
synthesized tr-kit RNA (*right*). In both cases exocytosis of cortical granules,
meiotic resumption with MII-anaphase transition, and extrusion of the second
polar body, pronuclear formation (and subsequent mitotic cycles of the new
formed zygote or of the parthenogenote) follow each other with similar time
courses

polar body extrusion and pronuclear formation (Sette et al. 1997),
indicating that egg activation by tr-kit requires calcium ions, and that it
could involve intracellular Ca^{2+} mobilization. This last hypothesis is
also supported by the evidence that tr-kit is able to trigger cortical
granule exocytosis with a pattern similar to that observed in natural
fertilization.

Inhibition of egg MAP kinase activity is observed at fertilization in
mouse eggs and is essential for formation of a female pronucleus (Moos
et al. 1995). We found that tr-kit RNA microinjection in MII oocytes is
associated with a dramatic decrease in MAP kinase activity coupled to
a shift to a slightly higher electrophoretic mobility of p42 MAP kinase
(ERK2) due to inactivating dephosphorylation (Sette et al. 1997). This

effect could be the consequence of the putative tr-kit induced increase in intracellular Ca^{2+} concentration, but effects of tr-kit microinjection on other components of the CSF system cannot be ruled out yet.

As a whole these data demonstrate that tr-kit microinjection into mouse eggs faithfully reproduces many events associated with egg activation occurring after sperm-egg fusion in natural fertilization (Fig. 1).

13.6 Tr-kit Mediated Egg Activation Is Blocked by Inhibition of PLC Activity

The recent finding that PLC inhibitors suppress Ca^{2+} oscillations at fertilization (Dupont et al. 1996) suggests that sperm-egg fusion induces the activation of a PLC isoform which in turn is responsible for $InsP_3$ production and Ca^{2+} release from the intracellular stores. To investigate whether tr-kit action inside the egg also involves PLC activation we tested the effect of preincubation of mouse eggs with specific PLC inhibitors before microinjection experiments. Indeed, tr-kit-induced pronuclear formation proved to be completely suppressed by incubation of eggs with the specific PLC inhibitor U73122 but not by incubation with its inactive analog U73433 (Sette et al. 1997). These results indicate that egg PLC activity is essential for tr-kit mediated MII oocyte activation, and they suggest that tr-kit mediated Ca^{2+} mobilization inside the egg is mediated through PLC activation. This observation reinforces the hypothesis that sperm-derived tr-kit could play a physiological role in natural egg activation at fertilization.

13.7 PLCγ1 Is the Most Likely Candidate PLC Isoform Mediating tr-kit Action Inside the Egg

PLCγ1 is activated by ligand-stimulated tyrosine kinase receptors or by cytoplasmic src-related tyrosine kinases (Rhee and Choi 1992; Valius and Kazlauskas 1993). Both physical interaction with the activated receptors and tyrosine phosphorylation of the enzyme seem to be important for PLCγ1 activation by tyrosine kinase receptors and consequent stimulation of PIP_2 hydrolysis, which gives rise to DAG and $InsP_3$

production (Kim et al. 1991; Rhee and Lee 1995). In addition to domains which are essential for catalytic activity, PLCγ1 contains several regulatory domains that mediate its interaction with upstream and downstream effectors, and in particular src-homology 2 (SH2), src-homology 3 (SH3), and pleckstrin-homology domains (Cohen et al. 1995; Pawson 1995).

We propose that PLCγ1 is the most likely candidate isoform required for sperm-carried tr-kit action within the egg cytoplasm, since: (a) PLCγ1 is the most readily detectable PLC isoenzyme in ovulated mouse oocytes (Dupont et al. 1996); (b) as previously discussed, PLCγ1 is activated by interaction with tyrosine kinase receptors or with src-related tyrosine kinases; (c) PLCγ1 interacts with c-kit after its stimulation by SCF, the physiological ligand, in several cellular systems, and c-kit-PLCγ1 physical interaction requires the c-kit carboxyterminal portion (Herbst et al. 1995), which is also present in tr-kit (Rossi et al. 1992).

The precise docking site for PLCγ1 has not been identified yet in the c-kit protein, however, mutation of a tyrosine residue (Y936) present in the carboxyterminal portion of human c-kit strongly impairs PLCγ1 association with the activated receptor in vitro (Herbst et al. 1995). The equivalent tyrosine residue is also present in the mouse c-kit receptor (Y934) and in tr-kit (Y161). As mentioned in the introduction to this chapter, the full-length c-kit receptor is present in ovulated oocytes (Manova et al. 1990; Horie et al. 1991; Yoshinaga et al. 1991). Although tr-kit lacks an ATP binding site, and thus it should lack intrinsic tyrosine kinase activity (Rossi et al. 1992), we speculate (Fig. 2) that it might be transphosphorylated by the c-kit receptor or by other tyrosine kinase activities expressed in MII-arrested oocytes. As a consequence, tr-kit would bind and activate soluble PLCγ1, and provoke its translocation to the particulate fraction, in which PIP_2 hydrolysis occurs (Bar-Sagi et al. 1993; Yang et al. 1994). Alternatively, tr-kit might compete for interaction of PLCγ1 with the SCF-activated c-kit receptor expressed in MII oocytes. The SCF-c-kit interaction in ovulated eggs is probably unproductive, because SCF does not induce egg activation (Sette et al. 1997). Indeed, SCF stimulation promotes binding of PLCγ1 to the c-kit receptor, but subsequent PLCγ1 tyrosine-phosphorylation and activation of PIP_2 hydrolysis has not been unambiguously demonstrated (Reith et al. 1991; Rottapel et al. 1991; Lev et al. 1991; Herbst et al. 1991; Hallek et al. 1992; Koike et al. 1993; Blume-Jensen et al. 1994). As shown in the

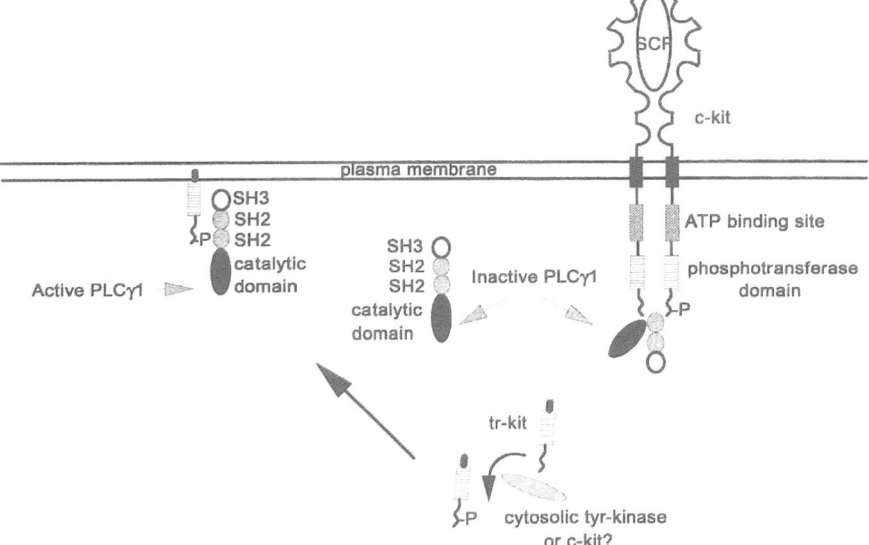

Fig. 2. Possible models for the mechanism of tr-kit induced egg activation. The carboxyterminal phosphotyrosine 934 of the c-kit receptor is important for binding PLCγ1 (Herbst et al. 1995), probably through the SH2 domain of this PLC isoenzyme. The equivalent residue (tyrosine 161) is present in the tr-kit carboxyterminal portion. Tr-kit contains the phosphotransferase portion of the tyrosine kinase, but it lacks the ATP binding site. However, once transphosphorylated by the c-kit receptor itself or by a soluble src-related kinase active within the MII-arrested oocyte, tr-kit injected by the sperm in the egg cytoplasm might bind to soluble PLCγ1. As a consequence PLCγ1 would be activated and allowed to interact (probably through its SH3 domain) with its targets in the particulate fraction, where PIP$_2$ hydrolysis must occur (Bar-Sagi et al. 1993; Yang et al. 1994). Alternatively, tr-kit might compete for interaction of PLCγ1 with the SCF-activated c-kit receptor expressed in MII oocytes. The c-kit PLCγ1 interaction is probably unproductive because SCF does not induce egg activation (Sette et al. 1997), and PLCγ1 is in an inactive state after its interaction with the c-kit receptor in other cellular systems (Lev et al. 1991; Koike et al. 1993; Blume-Jensen et al. 1994)

case of the closely related PDGFβ receptor (Valius et al. 1995), silencing of PLCγ1 might be due to contemporaneous binding of a particular blend of other signal transduction molecules to other domains of the cytoplasmic portion of the c-kit receptor.

The hypothesis that PLCγ1 mediates tr-kit effects on egg activation is being tested by coinjection into mouse eggs of cell extracts from COS cells transiently expressing a recombinant tr-kit protein, together with GST-fusion proteins containing the entire Src-homology region of PLCγ1, or its fragments, or antibodies directed against these domains. The Src homology region is known to mediate interaction of PLCγ1 with upstream and/or downstream effectors. Therefore, we expect that injection of the Src-homology region should compete for binding of effectors to the endogenous PLCγ1, and prevent its activation.

13.8 Is tr-kit the Sperm Factor that Naturally Activates Mammalian Eggs at Fertilization?

On the basis of the results described above, tr-kit seems a good candidate as the sperm factor which naturally activates mouse eggs. This is supported by the following: (a) We have shown that tr-kit-induced egg activation is suppressed by preincubation with either chelators of intracellular calcium or with specific PLC inhibitors which also block sperm-induced Ca^{2+} spiking at fertilization. (b) As discussed above, tr-kit might conceivably interact with PLCF"Symbol"g1, which can bind to the full-length c-kit receptor through a domain also present in tr-kit, and PLCγ1 has been shown to be responsible for Ca^{2+} mobilization at fertilization in echinoderms (Carroll et al. 1997). (c) The consequence of PLC activation is PIP_2 hydrolysis and production of DAG (powerful stimulator of some PKC isoforms) and $InsP_3$ (responsible for the release of Ca^{2+} from intracellular stores), and it is widely accepted that both DAG (Colonna et al. 1997) and $InsP_3$ (Miyazaki et al. 1993; Xu et al. 1994) are essential for activation of mammalian eggs at fertilization. (d) Tr-kit also elicits a decrease in egg MAP kinase activity, a c-mos dependent component of CSF, and a similar decrease in MAP kinase activity occurs in natural fertilization. (e) The observation that intracytoplasmic injection of round spermatids fails to activate mouse eggs without additional artificial stimulation, whereas testicular spermatozoa are successful (Kimura and Yanagimachi 1995), indicates that an oocyte activating factor must be accumulated during the elongation steps of spermiogenesis, and this is exactly the case for tr-kit (Albanesi et al. 1996).

The evidence that tr-kit actually functions during natural egg activation could come through studies in genetically modified mice. We are planning to knock-out the intronic promoter which drives its specific expression in late spermiogenesis. This approach might reveal whether tr-kit plays a role also in the differentiative events of mouse spermiogenesis (e.g., the transition to round spermatids of secondary spermatocytes going through the second meiotic division, or the process of spermatid elongation). The demonstration that tr-kit is present in spermatozoa of other mammalian and/or vertebrate species, including humans, and that it is eventually able to activate the eggs in the same species, will be important. Further elucidation of its mechanism of action inside the oocyte cytoplasm will also help to demonstrate its potential role during natural egg activation. For this purpose we will test whether tr-kit elicits the same spectrum of sperm-induced Ca^{2+} oscillations that are observed during natural fertilization, and whether it does in fact act through stimulation of PLCγ1. Finally, the possible interaction with the full-length c-kit receptor or with other tyrosine kinase activities expressed in mouse eggs, and the consequent putative activation of PLCγ1 (Fig. 2), will be tested through biochemical studies in transfected cell lines.

Acknowledgements. We thank Drs. Cristina Albanesi, Andrea Bianchini, Susanna Dolci, and Maria Teresa Fiorenza for their help and/or advice. This work was supported by the WHO special project for Research Development, and Research Training in Human Reproduction, by the CNR strategic project "Cell Cycle and Apoptosis" (ST/74), by MURST, and by the Fondazione Istituto Pasteur-Cenci Bolognetti.

References

Albanesi C, Geremia R, Giorgio M, Dolci S, Sette C, Rossi P (1996) A cell- and developmental stage-specific promoter drives the expression of a truncated c-kit protein during mouse spermatid elongation. Development 122:1291–1302

Bar-Sagi D, Rotin D, Batzer A, Mandiyan V, Schlessinger J (1993) SH3 domains direct cellular localization of signaling molecules. Cell 74:83–91

Berridge MJ (1993) Inositol triphosphate and calcium signaling. Nature 361:315–325

Berridge MJ (1996) Regulation of calcium spiking in mammalian oocytes through a combination of inositol triphosphate-dependent entry and release. Mol Hum Reprod 2:386–388

Blume-Jensen P, Ronnstrand L, Gout I, Waterfield MD, Heldin CH (1994) Modulation of Kit/stem cell factor receptor-induced signaling by protein kinase C. J Biol Chem 269:21793–21802

Carroll DJ, Ramarao CS, Mehlmann LM, Roche S, Terasaki M, Jaffe LA (1997) Calcium release at fertilization in starfish eggs is mediated by phospholipase Cγ. J Cell Biol 138:1303–1311

Clarke HJ, Rossant J, Masui Y (1988) Suppression of chromosome condensation during meiotic maturation induces parthenogenetic development of mouse oocytes. Development 104:97–103

Cohen GB, Ren R, Baltimore D (1995) Modular binding domains in signal transduction proteins Cell 80:237–248

Colledge WH, Carlton MBL, Udy GB, Evans MJ (1994) Disruption of c-mos causes parthenogenetic development of unfertilized mouse eggs. Nature 370:65–68

Colonna R, Tatone C, Francione A, Rosati F, Callaini G, Corda D, Di Francesco L (1997) Protein kinase C is required for the disappearence of MPF upon artificial activation in mouse eggs. Mol Reprod Dev 48:292–299

Dale B, De Felice LJ, Ehrenstein G (1985) Injection of a soluble sperm fraction into sea-urchin eggs triggers the cortical reaction. Experientia 41:1068–1070

Dolci S, Williams DE, Ernst MK, Resnick JL, Brannan CI, Lock LF, Lyman SD, Boswell HS, Donovan PJ (1991) Requirement for mast cell growth factor for primordial germ cell survival in culture. Nature 352:809–811

Dozortsev D, Rybouchkin A, De Sutter P, Qian C, Dhont M (1995) Human oocyte activation following intracytoplasmic injection: the role of the sperm cell. Hum Reprod 10:403–407

Dupont G, McGuinness OM, Johnson MH, Berridge MJ, Borgese F (1996) Phospholipase C in mouse oocytes: characterization of β and γ isoforms and their possible involvement in sperm-induced Ca^{2+} spiking. Biochem J 316:53–591

Dym M (1994) Spermatogonial stem cells of the testis. Proc Natl Acad Sci USA 91:11287–11289

Haccard O, Sarcevic B, Lewellyn A, Hartley R, Roy L, Izumi T, Erikson E, Maller JL (1993) Induction of metaphase arrest in cleaving Xenopus embryos by MAP kinase. Science 262:1262–1265

Hallek M, Druker B, Lepisto EM, Wood KW, Ernst TJ, Griffin JD (1992) Granulocyte-macrophage colony-stimulating factor and steel factor induce phosphorylation of both unique and overlapping signal transduction intermediates in a human factor-dependent hematopoietic cell line. J Cell Physiol 153:176–186

Hashimoto N, Watanabe N, Furuta Y, Tamemoto H, Sagata N, Yokoyama M, Okazaki K, Nagayoshi M, Takeda N, Ikawa Y, Aizawa S (1994) Parthenogenetic activation of oocytes in c-mos-deficient mice. Nature 370:68–71

Herbst R, Lammers R, Schlessinger J, Ullrich A (1991) Substrate phosphorylation specificity of the human c-kit receptor tyrosine kinase. J Biol Chem 266:19908–19916

Herbst R, Shearman MS, Jallal B, Schlessinger J, Ullrich A (1995) Formation of signal transfer complexes between stem cell and platelet-derived growth factor receptors and SH2 domain proteins in vitro. Biochemistry 34:5971–5979

Hogan B, Beddington R, Costantini F, Lacy E (1994) Manipulating the mouse embryo. Cold Spring Harbor Laboratory, Cold Spring Harbor

Homa ST, Swann K (1994) A cytosolic sperm factor triggers calcium oscillations and membrane hyperpolarization in human oocytes. Hum Reprod 9:2356–2361

Homa ST, Carroll J, Swann K (1993) The role of calcium in mammalian oocyte maturation and egg activation. Hum Reprod 8:1274–1281

Horie K, Takakura K, Taii S, Narimoto K, Noda Y, Nishikawa S, Nakayama H, Fujita J, Mori T (1991) The expression of the c-kit protein during oogenesis and early embryonic development. Biol Reprod 45:547–552

Ismail RS, Okawara Y, Fryer JN, Vanderhyden BC (1996) Hormonal regulation of the ligand of c-kit in the rat ovary and its effects on spontaneous oocyte meiotic maturation. Mol Reprod Dev 43:458–469

Ismail RS, Dube M, Vanderhyden BC (1997) Hormonally regulated expression and alternative splicing of kit ligand may regulate kit-induced inhibition of meiosis in rat oocytes. Dev Biol 184:333–342

Kim HK, Kim JW, Zilberstein A, Margolis B, Kim JG, Schlessinger J, Rhee SG (1991) PDGF stimulation of inositol phospholipid hydrolysis requires PLC-γ1 phosphorylation on tyrosine residues 783 and 1254. Cell 65:435–441

Kimura Y, Yanagimachi R (1995) Mouse oocytes injected with testicular spermatozoa or round spermatids can develop into normal offspring. Development 121:2397–2405
Kline D, Kline JT (1992) Repetitive calcium transients and the role of calcium
  in exocytosis and cell cycle activation in the mouse egg. Dev Biol
  149:80–89
Koike T, Hirai K, Morita Y, Nozawa Y (1993) Stem cell factor-induced signal
  transduction in rat mast cells. Activation of phospholipase D but not phos-
  phoinositide-specific phospholipase C in c-kit receptor stimulation. J Immunol 151:359–366
Lev S, Givol D, Yarden Y (1991) A specific combination of substrates is involved in signal transduction by the kit-encoded receptor. EMBO J
  10:647–654
Lorca T, Cruzalegui FH, Fesquet D, Cavadore JC, Mery J, Means A, Doree M
  (1993) Calmodulin-dependent protein kinase II mediates inactivation of
  MPF and CSF upon fertilization of Xenopus eggs. Nature 366:270–273
Manova K, Nocka K, Besmer P, Bachvarova RF (1990) Gonadal expression of
  c-kit encoded at the W locus of the mouse. Development 110:1057–1069
Minshull J, Sun H, Tonks NK, Murray AW (1994) A MAP kinase-dependent
  spindle assembly checkpoint in Xenopus egg extracts. Cell 79:475–486
Miyazaki S, Yuzaki M, Nakada K, Shirakawa H, Nakanishi S, Nakade S, Mik-
  oshiba K (1992) Block of Ca^{2+} wave and Ca^{2+} oscillation by antibody to
  the inositol 1,4,5-triphosphate receptor in fertilized hamster eggs. Science
  257:251–255
Miyazaki S, Shirakawa H, Nakada K, Honda Y (1993) Essential role of the
  inositol 1,4,5-triphosphate receptor/Ca^{2+} release channel in Ca^{2+} waves and
  Ca^{2+} oscillations at fertilization of mammalian eggs. Dev Biol 158:62–78
Moos J, Visconti PE, Moore GD, Schultz RM, Kopf GS (1995) Potential role
  of mitogen-activated protein kinase in pronuclear envelope assembly and
  disassembly following fertilization of mouse eggs. Biol Reprod 53:692–699
Moos J, Xu Z, Schultz RM, Kopf GS (1996) Regulation of nuclear envelope
  assembly/disassembly by MAP kinase. Dev Biol 175:358–361
Orth JM, Jester WF, Qiu J (1996) Gonocytes in testes of neonatal rats express
  the c-kit gene. Mol Reprod Dev 45:123–131
Packer AI, Hsu YC, Besmer P, Bachvarova RF (1994) The ligand of the c-kit
  receptor promotes oocyte growth. Dev Biol 161:194–205
Packer AI, Besmer P, Bachvarova RF (1995) Kit ligand mediates survival of
  type A spermatogonia and dividing spermatocytes in postnatal mouse testes.
  Mol Reprod Dev 42:303–310
Palermo GD, Avrech OM, Colombero LT, Wu H, Wolny YM, Fissore RA,
  Rosenwaks Z (1997) Human sperm cytosolic factor triggers Ca^{2+} oscilla-

tions and overcomes activation failure of mammalian oocytes. Mol Hum Reprod 3:367–374

Parrington J, Swann K, Shevchenko VI, Sesay AK, Lai FA (1996) Calcium oscillations in mammalian eggs triggered by a soluble sperm protein. Nature 379:364–368

Pawson T (1995) Protein modules and signaling networks. Nature 373:573–580

Qiu F, Ray P, Barker PE, Jhanwar S, Ruddle FH, Besmer P (1988) Primary structure of c-kit: relationship with the CSF-1/PDGF receptor kinase family – oncogene activation of v-kit involves deletion of extracellular domain and C terminus. EMBO J 7:1003–1011

Reith AD, Ellis C, Lyman SD, Anderson DM, Williams DE, Bernstein A, Pawson T (1991) Signal transduction by normal isoforms and W mutant variants of the Kit receptor tyrosine kinase. EMBO J 10:2451–2459

Rhee SG, Choi KDP (1992) Regulation of inositol phospholipid-specific phospholipase C isozymes. J Biol Chem 267:12393–12396

Rhee SG, Lee SB (1995) Significance of PIP2 hydrolysis and regulation of phospholipase C isozymes. Curr Opin Cell Biol 7:183–189

Rossi P, Albanesi C, Grimaldi P, Geremia R (1991) Expression of the mRNA for the ligand of c-kit in mouse Sertoli cells. Biochem Biophys Res Commun 176:910–914

Rossi P, Marziali G, Albanesi C, Charlesworth A, Geremia R, Sorrentino V (1992) A novel c-kit transcript, potentially encoding a truncated receptor, originates within a kit gene intron in mouse spermatids. Dev Biol 152:203–207

Rossi P, Dolci S, Albanesi C, Grimaldi P, Ricca R, Geremia R (1993) Follicle-stimulating hormone induction of steel factor (SLF) mRNA in mouse Sertoli cells, and stimulation of DNA synthesis in spermatogonia by soluble SLF. Dev Biol 155:68–74

Rottapel R, Reedijk M, Williams DE, Lyman SD, Anderson DM, Pawson T, Bernstein A (1991) The Steel/W transduction pathway: kit autophosphorylation and its association with a unique subset of cytoplasmic signaling proteins is induced by the Steel factor. Mol Cell Biol 11:3043–3051

Sagata N, Watanabe N, Vande Woude GF, Ikawa Y (1989) The c-mos proto-oncogene product is a cytostatic factor responsible for meiotic arrest in vertebrate eggs. Nature 342:512–518

Serve H, Hsu YC, Besmer P (1994) Tyrosine residue 719 of the c-kit receptor is essential for binding of the P85 subunit of phosphatidylinositol (PI) 3-kinase and for c-kit-associated PI 3-kinase activity in COS-1 cells. J Biol Chem 269:6026–6030

Sette C, Bevilacqua A, Bianchini A, Mangia F, Geremia R, Rossi P (1997) Parthenogenetic activation of mouse eggs by microinjection of a truncated c-kit tyrosine kinase present in spermatozoa. Development 124:2267–2274

Sorrentino V, Giorgi M, Geremia R, Besmer P, Rossi P (1991) Expression of the c-kit proto-oncogene in the murine male germ cells. Oncogene 6:149–151

Stice SL, Robl JM (1990) Activation of mammalian oocytes by a factor obtained from rabbit sperm. Mol Reprod Dev 25:272–280

Stricker SA (1997) Intracellular injections of a soluble sperm factor trigger calcium oscillations and meiotic maturation in unfertilized oocytes of a marine worm. Dev Biol 186:185–201

Swann K (1990) A cytosolic sperm factor stimulates repetitive calcium increases and mimics fertilization in hamster eggs. Development 110:1295–1302

Tesarik J, Sousa M, Testart J (1994) Human oocyte activation after intracytoplasmic sperm injection. Hum Reprod 9:511–518

Valius M, Kazlauskas A (1993) Phospholipase C-γ1 and phosphatidylinositol 3' kinase are the downstream mediators of the PDGF receptor's mitogenic signal. Cell 73:321–334

Valius M, Secrist JP, Kazlauskas A (1995) The GTPase-activating protein of ras suppresses platelet-derived growth factor β receptor signaling by silencing phospholipase C-γ1 Mol Cell Biol 15:3058–3071

Vande Woude GF (1994) On the loss of Mos. Nature 370:20–21

Verlhac M-H, de Pennart H, Maro B, Cobb MH, Clarke HJ (1993) MAP kinase becomes stably activated at metaphase and is associated with microtubule-organizing centers during meiotic maturation of mouse oocytes. Dev Biol 158:330–340

Verlhac M-H, Kubiak JZ, Clarke HJ, Maro B (1994) Microtubule and chromatin behavior follow MAP kinase activity but not MPF activity during meiosis in mouse oocytes. Development 120:1017–1025

Verlhac M-H, Kubiak JZ, Weber M, Geraud G, Colledge WH, Evans MJ, Maro B (1996) Mos is required for MAP kinase activation and is involved in microtubule organization during meiotic maturation in the mouse. Development 122:815–822

Whitaker M, Swann K (1993) Lighting the fuse at fertilization. Development 117:1–12

Wilding M, Dale B (1997) Sperm factor: what is it and what does it do? Mol Hum Reprod 3:269–273

Wu H, He CL, Fissore RA (1997) Injection of a porcine sperm factor triggers calcium oscillations in mouse oocytes and bovine eggs. Mol Reprod Dev 46:176–189

Xu Z, Kopf GS, Schultz RM (1994) Involvment of inositol 1,4,5-triphosphate-mediated Ca2+ release in early and late events of mouse egg activation. Development 120:1851–1859

Yanagimachi R (1994) Mammalian fertilization. In: Knobil E, Neill JD (eds) The physiology of reproduction. Raven, New York, pp 189–317

Yang LJ, Rhee SG, Williamson JR (1994) Epidermal growth factor-induced activation and translocation of phospholipase C-γ1 to the cytoskeleton in rat hepatocytes. J Biol Chem 269:7156–7162

Yoshinaga K, Nishikawa S, Ogawa M, Hayashi S, Kunisada T, Fujimoto T, Nishikawa S-I (1991) Role of c-kit in mouse spermatogenesis: identification of spermatogonia as a specific site of c-kit expression and function. Development 113:689–699

14 Spermatogenesis-Specific Genes Deleted in Infertile Men: DAZ/DAZH Clinical Aspects and Animal Models

J. Gromoll, M. Simoni, G.F. Weinbauer, and E. Nieschlag

14.1 Introduction

The XY sex chromosomes are found in a multitude of species through-out the animal kingdom. During evolution the Y-chromosome, as the X-chromosome, evolved from an autosomal chromosome. In the human it represents only 2% of the haploid genome and is the smallest among the 24 chromosomes. It can be divided into pseudoautosomal regions and the nonrecombining region (NRY). The pseudoautosomal regions exist on both X- and Y-chromosomes and therefore can easily recombine. NRY can be divided into a euchromatic and heterochromatic half. NRY is the only haploid compartment of the human genome, and since it does not recombine, rearrangements (i.e., inversions, duplications) within this region are fully transmitted through meiosis (Lahn and Page 1997). Consequently, repetitive sequences in shuffled arrangements can accumulate. Genes found so far in the repetitive sequences TSPY (Arnemann et al. 1991) and RBM (Ma et al. 1993) are themselves repeated. Of the genes previously cloned from the NRY the most prominent one is the SRY (sex determining region on the Y-chromosome) which is crucial for testis formation (Sinclair et al. 1990). Whereas all the genes described until now derive from the euchromatic region, no gene has been found in the heterochromatic region.

The existence of a gene or a group of genes on the Y-chromosome, important for human spermatogenesis, was first postulated by the studies of Tiepolo and Zuffardi (1976), who described microscopically detectable deletions of the distal part of the long arm of the Y-chromosome Yq11 in azoospermic men. These hypothetical genes have been collectively designated as the azoospermia factor (AZF). Using high-resolution molecular DNA techniques, nearly two decades later several investigators described various types of terminal and interstitial microdeletions of Yq11 in patients with normal karyotype and azoospermia or severe oligozoospermia, thus supporting the hypothesis that specific genes on the Y-chromosome are required for male gamete maturation (Vogt et al. 1992; Ma et al. 1993). With the delineation of Y-chromosomal maps based on molecular markers (Foote et al. 1992; Vollrath et al. 1992) large deletions are now detected routinely either by hybridization markers or more commonly by sequence-tagged sites (STS) based polymerase chain reaction (PCR) markers. These techniques also allow the detection of smaller, interstitial deletions of the Y-chromosome that are undetectable by microscopy. A recent multicenter study identified several loci on the Y-chromosome which, when deleted, cause severely impaired spermatogenesis. (Vogt et al. 1996). The nomenclature for these three loci is AZFa, AZFb, and AZFc (comprising deleted in azoospermia, DAZ).

14.2 Identification and Characterization of DAZ

In a recent survey Reijo et al. (1995) screened 89 azoospermic men using over 80 Y-specific STSs. With this set of Y-DNA markers a common deletion in interval 6 of the long arm of the Y-chromosome was found in 12 men. By sophisticated methods such as exon trapping a gene could be confined to this region which, as expected, was absent in the 12 azoospermic patients but was present in normal fertile males. Upon screening a testis cDNA library using the trapped exons as a probe, a cDNA was identified encoding a protein of 366 amino acids with a predicted molecular weight of 41 kDa. Inspection of the predicted amino acid sequence revealed the presence of an RNA recognition motif (RRM) in the N-terminal domain of the protein. Such a domain has been found in a variety of proteins involved in RNA processing, transport, and metabolism (Nagai 1996). The domain consists of two short, highly conserved ribonucleoprotein sequence motifs called RNP-1 (RNP octamer) and RNP-2 (RNP hexamer) within a weakly conserved motif of 85 residues, when compared to other RNA binding proteins. Crystallographic analysis of the RRM from other RNA binding proteins indicates a three-dimensional structure in which antiparallel β sheets encoded by RNP1 and RNP2 are flanked by α-helices, a structure crucial for the interaction with RNA (Siomi and Dreyfuss 1997).

A repeat structure is characteristic for the remaining part of the protein. In this repeat sequence a 72-nucleotide unit encoding 24 amino acids is tandemly repeated (Reijo et al. 1995). Both the repeats and the C-terminal part of the protein are characterized by a high concentration of proline, glutamine, and tyrosine residues, as is typical of many RRM proteins (Siomi and Dreyfuss 1997). Since the function of the gene is unknown, but as it is deleted in certain azoospermic patients, it was named deleted in azoospermia (DAZ).

14.3 DAZ Homologues

Soon after the first description of the Y-chromosomal DAZ, several studies appeared describing an autosomal version of DAZ. Until now homologues have been described for the human (DAZH, Saxena et al. 1996; DAZLA, Yen et al. 1996; SPYGLA, Shan et al. 1996; DAZLA,

```
                                                          RNP-2
CYNDAZLA   MSAANPETPNSTISREASTQSSSAAASQGYVLPEGKIMPNTVFVGGIDVR    50
DAZH       MSTANPETPNSTISREASTQSSSAATSQGYILPEGKIMPNTVFVGGIDAR    50
DAZLA      MSATTSEAPNSAVSREASTQSSSATTSQGYVLPEGKIMPNTVFVGGIDVR    50
BOULE      MHKIAAAPPPSAT---PGGGLETPLAAPKY----GTLIPNRIFVGGISGD    43
           *      *  **.  **********  ***.**** *..*.*****. *

                                                  RNP-1
CYNDAZLA   MDETEIRSFFARYGSVKEVKIITDRTGVSKGYGFVSFFNDVDVQKIVESQ   100
DAZH       MDETEIRSFFARYGSVKEVKIITDRTGVSKGYGFVSFFNDVDVQKIVESQ   100
DAZLA      MDETEIRSFFARYGSVKEVKIITDRTGVSKGYGFVSFYNDVDVQKIVESQ   100
BOULE      TTEADLTRVFSAYGTVKSTKIIVDRAGVSKGYGFVTFETEQEAQRLQADG    93
           **.******.**.*.**..**.**.**.*.*****.* *****.******

CYNDAZLA   --INFHGKKLKLGPAIRKQNLCAYHVQPRPLVFNHPPPPQFQNVWTNPNT   148
DAZH       --INFHGKKLKLGPAIRKQNLCAYHVQPRPLVFNHPPPPQFQNVWTNPNT   148
DAZLA      --INFHGKKLKLGPAIRKQNLCTYHVQPRPLIFNPPPPPQFQSVWSSPNA   148
BOULE      ECVVLRDRKLNIAPAIKK--------QPNPL-----------QSI-VATNG   124
           ******.***.*.*.***.* ***.***.** ******* .** *.

                                 DAZ repeat motif
CYNDAZLA   ETYMQPPTTMNPITQYVQAYPTYPNSPVQVITGYQLPVYNYQMPPQWPVG   198
DAZH       ETYMQPPTTMNPITQYVQAYPTYPNSPVQVITGYQLPVYNYQMPPQWPVG   198
DAZLA      ETYMQPPTMMNPITQYVQAYPPYPSSPVQVITGYQLPVYNYQMPPQVPAG   198
BOULE      AVY--------------YTTTPPAPISNIPMDQFAAAVYPPAAGVPA-    157
           **.***  *  ********** **.*.* *.  ******..* . *

CYNDAZLA   EQRSYVVPPAYSAVNYHCNEVDPGAFVVPNECSVHEATPPSGNGPQKKSV   248
DAZH       EQRSYVVPPAYSAVNYHCNEVDPGAEVVPNECSVHEATPPSGNGPQKKSV...248
DAZLA      EQRSYVIPPAYTTVNYHCSEVDPGADILPNECSVHDAAPASGNGPQKKSV   248
BOULE      IYPPSAMQYQPFYQYYSVPMNVPTIWPQNYQEMHSPLLHSPTSNPHSPHS   207
           ******  ****  **.**.***.*    *******  * *  ***.******

CYNDAZLA   DRSIQTVVSCLFNPENRLRNTVVTQDDYFKDKRVHHFRRSRAMLKSV   295
DAZH       DRSIQTVVSCLFNPENRLRNSVVTQDDYFKDKRVHHFRRSRAMLKSV   295
DAZLA      DRSIQTVVSCLFNPENRLRNSLVTQDDYFKDKRVHHFRRSRAVLKSDHLC   298
BOULE      QSHPQSPCWSIEDLRDTLPRV   228
           **** .*********.*.**   ******************** ***
```

Fig. 1. Amino acid sequence comparison of CYNDAZLA, DAZH, DAZLA, and BOULE. *Asterisks*, identical amino acids in the monkey, human, and mouse DAZ homologues; *closed circles*, identical amino acids in monkey, human, mouse, and fly; *shaded boxes*, RNA recognition motifs (*RNP-1*, *RNP-2*); *open box*, the 24 amino acid repeat motif

Seboun et al. 1997; according to the new nomenclature all human DAZ homologues are designated DAZH), the Old World monkey (cyn-DAZLA, Carani et al. 1997), mouse (Dazh, Reijo et al. 1996; Dazla, Cooke et al. 1996), and interestingly in a species which in evolutionary terms is very old, the fruitfly *Drosophila* (boule, Eberhart et al. 1996; Fig. 1). In the human DAZH can be mapped to chromosome 3p25, whereas in the mouse it is allocated to chromosome 17. Protein analysis and sequence comparisons reveal a high homology between the Y-chromosomal DAZ and the autosomal DAZH in the RRM region (Saxena et al. 1996; Cooke and Elliott 1997), but while the human Y-encoded DAZ includes several tandemly arranged repeats, the human, monkey, mouse, and fly DAZH proteins contain only one such unit. Furthermore, in the C-termini of DAZ and DAZH the observed low homology is due to amino acid changes and deletions.

Structural analysis of the genomic organization of the autosomal DAZH reveals that the protein is encoded by 11 exons, where exon 1 encodes only the initiation codon, exons 2–6 bear the information for the RRM domain, exon 7 displays the single repeat unit, and exons 8–11 encode the C-terminus (Saxena et al. 1996; Chai et al. 1997). A similar genomic organization in the 5' region encoding exons 1–6 was observed for DAZ (Seboun et al. 1997; Vereb et al. 1997). Exons 7 and 8 are located within a genomic 2.4-kb unit which is tandemly repeated. The last two exons, 10 and 11, are located 3' of the tandem array (Saxena et al. 1996). The relatively high amino acid sequence homology between the autosomal DAZH and the Y-chromosomal DAZ, also resulting in similar structural characteristics such as the RRM domain and the repeat unit, indicates the possibility that DAZH is the ancestor of the development of DAZ.

14.4 Evolution of DAZ

Intensive studies on the structure and evolution of the human DAZ gene family then gave rise to the current model of events leading to the generation of the Y-chromosomal DAZ (Fig. 2).

During evolution in a first step a complete copy of DAZH was transposed to the Y-chromosome. Within the newly transposed gene, a 2.4-kb genomic segment encoding exons 7 and 8 was tandemly repeated. In most of the repeats one, generally exon 8, or both exons degenerated or were deleted, resulting in the present form of DAZ with a repeat structure encoded by several copies of exon 7 and the fact that presumably only the last repeat contains a preserved repeat structure of exons 7 and 8. Exon 9 of DAZH degenerated without any amplification and is lacking in DAZ.

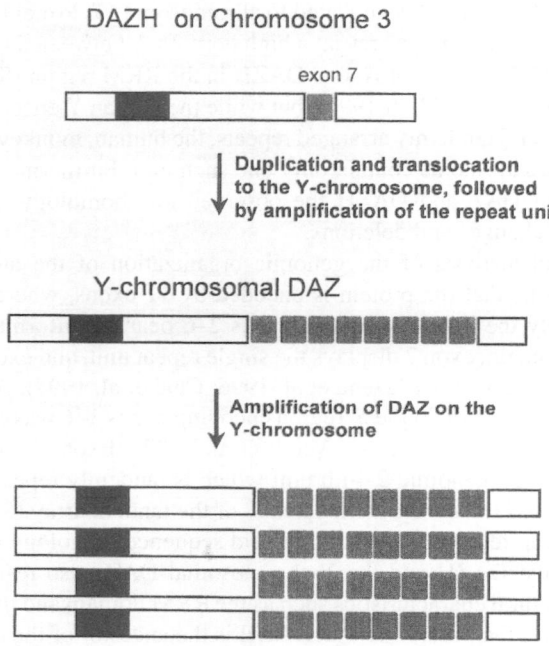

Fig. 2. Schematic representation of DAZ/DAZH protein structure and the evolutionary events leading to Y encoded DAZ. *Open box*, the protein; *black box*, RRM domain; *gray box*, repeat unit. The autosomal DAZH is located on chromosome 3; during evolution it was first duplicated and then translocated to the Y-chromosome. In addition to the translocation, a genomic fragment encoding exons 7 and 8 was amplified, giving rise to the first copy of DAZ. Finally, the whole gene itself was amplified and is present on the Y-chromosome in at least three copies

Finally, the whole DAZ gene itself was amplified, giving rise to at least three copies (Yen et al. 1997). The sequence similarity between the different copies reaches 99%. All copies are in close proximity in the AZF region of the Y-chromosome. Recent data show that multiple DAZ genes with varying numbers of DAZ repeats are present in each male, and that the copy number of the DAZ repeats are polymorphic in the population. Moreover, at the mRNA level several transcripts are detectable, deriving not only from alternative splicing of the primary transcript, since the arrangement of DAZ repeats are different. These results indicate a variable amplification event of the repeat unit, encoded by exons 7 and 8, within the different gene copies and the transcription of more than one DAZ gene (Yen et al. 1997).

Although the DAZ genes have undergone a series of structural transformations, the general protein sequence is maintained. This conservation of an open reading frame is generally believed to be a crucial parameter for a functional gene.

Southern blotting experiments of female and male genomic DNA using DAZ DNA probes in a variety of species ranging from marsupials to humans have revealed hybridization signals common to both sexes, presumably conferring to the autosomal DAZH (Cooke et al. 1996; Shan et al. 1996; Seboun et al. 1997; Delbridge et al. 1997). Male-specific hybridization signals, however, have been detected only in certain primates species such as the Old World monkey and in humans and were absent in mice and other mammals. This is in agreement with the localization of the mouse Dazla gene on chromosome 3 and the absence of any cross-hybridization to the Y-chromosome (Cooke et al. 1996; Reijo et al. 1996). Studies on the evolution of the Y-linked DAZ reveal the presence of DAZ in Old World monkeys, apes, and humans, whereas it is absent in New World Monkeys and all other species. This distribution of DAZ suggests a translocation of a copy of the autosomal DAZ on the primate Y-chromosome sometime after the splitting of the New World/Old World monkey lineages. This evolutionary event would also indicate that DAZ is a relatively young acquisition of the Y-chromosome, since the splitting of the two monkey lineages occurred 35–40 million years ago. This view is also supported by the close proximity of the different DAZ copies, while other genes such as TSPY and RBM, also present in several copies on the Y-chromosome, are much more dispersed throughout the chromosome, thereby indicating that these genes have been translocated to the Y-chromosome well in advance of the translocation of DAZ (Glaser et al. 1997; Delbridge et al. 1997). This acquisition of putative autosomal fertility genes is considered an important process in the human Y-chromosome but has recently been shown for a gene in *Drosophila*, suggesting that such a translocation is a general mechanism in the Y-chromosome evolution in eukaryotes (Kalmykova et al. 1997).

14.5 DAZ/DAZH Expression

DAZ and DAZH are expressed exclusively in the germ cells of female and male gonads of various species (Reijo et al. 1995, 1996; Cooke et al. 1996; Carani et al. 1997). Northern blot experiments revealed the presence of a 3.5-kb transcript expressed predominantly in the adult testis, with other transcripts being present at a lower transcript size (Shan et al. 1997). The origin of the smaller transcripts is not yet known, but they may be due to alternative splicing of the primary transcript. In situ hybridization of human testis sections has shown that DAZ is expressed in spermatogonia and in early spermatocytes (Menke et al. 1997). A similar picture has been obtained for DAZH expression (Niederberger et al. 1997). In the mouse DAZH expression can be confined to B-spermatogonia, dividing to form preleptotene spermatocytes and to enter the meiotic pathway (Reijo et al. 1996; Niederberger et al. 1997). Studies on male germ cell development in mice showed the expression of DAZH to be detectable as early as day 1 after birth, when only prespermatogonia are present in the testis. Expression increases steadily as spermatogonial stem cells appear and plateaus as the first wave of spermatogenic cells enters meiosis and is maintained at a similar level in the adult testis (Reijo et al. 1996). Recent studies on the protein expression of DAZH in the mouse indicate a cytoplasmatic localization of the protein in B-spermatogonia, early spermatocytes, and highest expression in pachytene spermatocytes (Ruggiu et al. 1997). In contrast to the nuclear localization of the RBM protein (Elliott et al. 1997), DAZH protein is detectable mainly in the cytosol, indicating different functions of the two RNA binding proteins.

Further studies on the expression of DAZ/DAZH during spermatogenesis have shown the presence of the protein in mature spermatozoa and in the tail of elongated spermatozoa. This suggests that DAZ/DAZH is constitutively expressed during germ cell maturation, an expression pattern which may be related to a role for DAZ/DAZH in addition to the suspected function during meiosis.

14.6 Clinical Aspects

The first description of DAZ, together with the fact that in about 13% of men with nonobstructive azoospermia this gene is deleted (Reijo et al. 1995), was the starting point for a worldwide search for microdeletions in infertile men. Molecular diagnosis of the Y-chromosome is now widely used in human genetics and in the andrological patient workup. Since 1995 several publications on microdeletions of the Y-chromosome in infertile men and candidates for intracytoplasmic sperm injection have been published, but using different experimental designs and methodological approaches. The variety of incidence of microdeletions detected in infertile men is remarkable, ranging from 1% (Van der Ven et al. 1997) to 29% (Foresta et al. 1997). An overview of recent literature shows that patient selection criteria is probably the crucial factor influencing this parameter, and that the overall frequency of microdeletions for men with azoospermia is about 12%, and with severe oligozoospermia 3% (sperm concentration less than 5×10^6/ml; Table 1). About four-fifths of all microdeletions involve DAZ, whereas in only one-fifth of the cases is the infertile phenotype associated with a microdeletion in the AZFa and/or AZFb regions and not extended to AZFc (Simoni et al. 1998).

Our own experience to date is based on PCR diagnosis of microdeletions in more than 700 patients consulting our infertility clinic. We have identified nine patients with DAZ deletions, one with a microdeletion limited to AZFa, and one with a microdeletion involving only AZFb. Two patients with DAZ deletion had a sperm concentration below 1×10^6/ml; the others were azoospermic. This corresponds to a microdeletion frequency of 4.5% of azoospermic and 1.8% of severely oligozoospermic men. The clinical characteristics of these patients showed that testicular volume is generally reduced, and that serum follicle-stimulating hormone levels were usually but not always elevated – features compatible with a primary spermatogenic failure. Varicocele and/or a history of testicular maldescent were present in seven patients, indicating that the occurrence of such clinical conditions should not exclude patients from analysis. Finally, among patients with Sertoli-cell-only syndrome, microdeletions seem to be more frequent (approx. 10%).

282   J. Gromoll et al.

Table 1. Summary of the literature on Y-chromosomal microdeletions (1995–1997): number of subjects analyzed and deletions

Reference	Infertile men			Controls (proven fathers)	
	n	n	%	n	Deletions
Reijo et al. (1995)	89	12	13.5	90	0
Nakahori et al. (1996)	153	20	13.1	0	0
Qureshi et al. (1996)	100	8	8	80	0
Stuppia et al. (1996)	33	6	18.2	10	0
Reijo et al. (1996)	35	2	5.7	0	0
Vogt et al. (1996)	370	13	3.5	200	0
Najmabadi et al. (1996)	60	11	18.3	16	0
Kent-First et al. (1996)	32	1	3.1	200	0
Pryor et al. (1997)	200	14	7	200	0
Foresta et al. (1997)	38	11	28.9	10	0
Vereb et al. (1997)	168	5	3	55	0
Kremer et al. (1997)	164	7	4.3	100	0
Mulhall et al. (1997)	83	8	9.1	0	0
Simoni et al. (1997)	168	5	3	86	0
van der Ven et al. (1997)	204	2	1	50	0
In't Veld et al. (1997)	58	3	5.2	0	0
Total	1995	128	6.4 (Av.)	1097	0

Although the causal role of DAZ deletion in azoospermia still awaits formal confirmation, as no small intragenic deletions or point mutations have yet been described, the data obtained so far support the idea that DAZ is involved in the control of male fertility. In fact, microdeletions of DAZ are not found in the large group of confirmed fathers analyzed to date (Table 1).

It is clear, however, that deletions of DAZ are sometimes compatible with some degree of ongoing spermatogenesis. In fact, DAZ deletions have been found in fathers of infertile men (Vogt et al. 1996; Pryor et al. 1997) and in severely oligozoospermic men (Reijo et al. 1996; Simoni et al. 1997). Previous paternity and/or oligozoospermia has been reported in some cases of azoospermic men with deletions (Simoni et al. 1997; Pryor et al. 1997). These clinical data suggest a possible progression from oligozoospermia to azoospermia at least in some cases (Vogt 1995).

Apart from the few cases of inherited deletions described above, the large majority of deletions are clearly de novo events. It is speculated that deletions originate mainly in the germ cells of the father (Edwards and Bishop 1997). Primary spermatocytes in meiotic prophase are the most likely source of deletions during chromosome alignment, pairing, and crossing-over. Deletions are then limited only to germ cells deriving from this affected spermatocyte, leaving the other germ cells intact. This would explain the puzzling finding that microdeletions in the brothers of patients with deletions are absent. Concerning the frequency of deletions in men, only speculative estimations can be made, i.e., that several thousand spermatozoa with deletions may be present among millions of normal spermatozoa (Edwards and Bishop 1997). Mosaicisms are possible but practically impossible to demonstrate with conventional PCR techniques. Alternatively, microdeletions could originate de novo in the fertilized eggs or embryos, preventing the formation of spermatogonia. If this is the case, the possibility of mosaicism in infertile men (DAZ present in leukocytes, deleted in the germ cells) exists and should be analyzed in the future.

Recent studies by Saxena et al. (1996) and Yen et al. (1997) have demonstrated that DAZ is a multicopy gene. The diagnostic technique currently used worldwide for screening of DAZ deletions allows only the detection of DAZ or its absence, independently of the copy number. Therefore no estimations can be made whether a reduced number of DAZ genes results in disturbed spermatogenesis. More sophisticated techniques are required to determine whether a gene dose effect such as that described for DAZH is also true for DAZ. For this purpose, assays must be developed which enable the detection of the copy number of DAZ, for example quantitative PCR. A putative correlation between DAZ copy number and spermatogenesis can be evaluated by these methods.

In summary, based on the actual knowledge of the clinical characteristics of patients with deletions, showing varying sperm concentrations and hormonal parameters, molecular analysis of the three azoospermic loci should be performed in all men with sperm concentration below 5×10^6/ml (Meschede et al. 1997) Moreover, analysis of microdeletions should be performed in all patients who are candidates for microassisted fertilization techniques, in view of the high risk of producing an infertile son. The present state of molecular analysis for microdeletions reveals the highest frequency by far in the AZFc region, comprising DAZ. However, the various laboratories listed in Table 1 used differing numbers of primers, ranging from 5 to 118, in varying locations on the Y-chromosome. At present there is no consensus about the number and type of STS primers that should be used for diagnostic purposes. An international quality assessment scheme for Y-chromosomal microdeletions was recently initiated by our institute and should enable the formulation of standardized diagnostic protocols, which definitely will improve the quality of molecular analysis, crucial for the diagnosis of infertility.

14.7 Animal Models

Understanding the functional role of DAZ/DAZH requires detailed analysis of the structural components of the protein, followed by biochemical studies in which putative characteristics are further investigated. In the case of DAZ/DAZH, resembling RNA binding proteins, this approach is very difficult to undertake. Until now a specific interaction with mRNAs has been shown only for a few RNA binding proteins (for review see Siomi and Dreyfuss 1997; Hecht 1996). The challenge is therefore to isolate the target mRNAs among the numerous newly synthesized mRNAs during germ cell maturation. The different repeat structure between the autosomal DAZH and DAZ may participate in different RNA binding characteristics, which would implement a different specific function for both proteins. Furthermore, interactions of DAZ/DAZH with hormones and/or other factors controlling their expression or activity must be identified.

A more straightforward approach is offered by the use of animal models in which the gene can be inactivated to study the consequences of loss of DAZ/DAZH function.

14.7.1 The *Drosophila* Model

Soon after the identification and characterization of the human Y-chromosomal DAZ an initial study appeared that provided insights into the putative function of the protein. In the fruitfly *Drosophila,* during screening for transposon-induced male-sterile mutations, the autosomal homologue of human DAZ, boule, was identified. This shares high homology in the RRM domain to DAZ/DAZH and displays only one repeat unit (Eberhart et al. 1996). Boule expression is limited to males and is testis specific. Male flies deficient in boule are azoospermic, and detailed analysis of the affected homozygous males has revealed a failure of germ cells to undergo meiosis. This is probably due to the fact that the transition to metaphase does not occur. Partial spermatogenesis was recovered again when the boule cDNA was introduced in boule mutant flies.

The accessibility of spermatogenesis and the variety of mutations affecting spermatogenesis at nearly every step of germ cell maturation makes the fruitfly one of the preferred animal models to study the possible function of DAZH (Hackstein 1991; Castrillon et al. 1993). For example, in another *Drosophila* mutant, named twine, a close similarity to the boule-mutant males was observed in respect to the stage at which spermatogenic arrest occurs (Eberhart et al. 1996). The twine locus encodes a meiosis-specific homologue of CDC25 phosphatase, which is crucial for the cell cycle. Based on the findings in boule-deficient flies, and by analogy to the twine mutants, one can presume a function for DAZH in the control of meiotic cell divisions. By searching for mutant flies with genes mutated acting either before the time of function for DAZH or shortly thereafter, the exact role of DAZH, for example the interactions with other proteins, could be clarified further.

However, this approach of using fruitflies as a model for DAZ/DAZH function is somewhat limited in relevance for the human. While some genetic processes during spermatogenesis may be similar, differences such as the architecture of spermatogenesis and the absence of a Y-encoded DAZ make it difficult to predict the causes for spermatogenic failure in humans.

14.7.2 The Mouse Model

The mouse is an animal model widely used for the study of spermatogenesis. Although the hormonal regulation of spermatogenesis is different from that in the human, its overall validity as a suitable model is generally accepted. Cooke's group has recently generated Dazla knockout mice in which exons 5–11 of the gene were replaced by a neomycin-resistance marker leaving the RRM domain intact (Ruggiu et al. 1997). The disruption of Dazla leads to nearly complete absence of germ cells beyond the spermatogonial stage. The markedly decreased numbers of spermatogonia indicate a reduced proliferation of gonocytes, the pro-genitors of spermatogonia in the fetus, or a loss of germ cells after proliferation. Immunohistochemical methods confined Dazla expres-sion in wild-type adult mice mainly to primary spermatocytes, stages which do not correspond directly to the effects of gene disruption seen in the knockout mice. This suggests that Dazla has different functions in embryonic and adult gonads. In this context it is noteworthy that other studies demonstrate expression of the autosomal DAZ from gonocytes to mature sperm (R. Reijo, personal communication). This constitutive expression pattern suggests that Dazla has a different function through germ cell maturation and acts as a kind of a differentiation factor. The loss of Dazla then consequently leads to a loss of germ cells.

Heterozygous Dazla knockout mice show reduced sperm counts and, most strikingly, a high percentage of abnormal sperm, characterized by abnormal head and tail formations (Ruggiu et al. 1997). In this respect it is also noteworthy that Habermann et al. (1997) have recently publish-ed data of DAZ expression in the tail of human sperm. The expression of DAZ in the tail of sperm and the abnormal tail formation found in heterozygous Dazla knockout mice strongly suggest a crucial function for the morphogenesis of mature sperm. Together with the observation of reduced spermatogenesis in heterozygous boule mutants, the pres-ence of a gene dose effect of Dazla is evident, where a certain threshold of expression is required for quantitative and qualitative normal sperma-togenesis.

14.7.3 The Non-human Primate Model

Southern blots of genomic DNA from male primates hybridized to human DAZ DNA probes display clear hybridization signals common to male and female monkeys, but in addition male-specific signals can also be observed (Shan et al. 1996; Seboun et al. 1997). This first indirect observation was recently confirmed when human DAZ specific primers were used to amplify a specific DAZ fragment from genomic

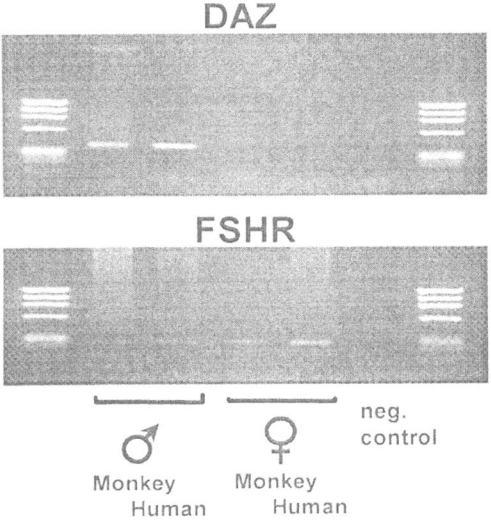

Fig. 3. Evidence for a Y-encoded DAZ in the Old World monkey. Genomic DNA was isolated from blood samples of a female and male cynomolgus monkey and human. Using the primer pair sY254 amplifying Y-specific human DAZ sequences, a DNA fragment was obtained in the male monkey and human, whereas no fragment was detected in the female monkey or human. As a positive control, the autosomal follicle-stimulating hormone receptor (*FSHR*) was amplified from all genomic DNAs used in this experiment

DNA of the Old World monkey. The fact that only male monkey genomic DNA gives rise to a fragment of the Y-chromosomal DAZ is strong evidence for the presence of a Y-encoded DAZ (Fig. 3). However, a male-specific DAZ signal was obtained only in Old World monkeys such as the macaques, not in New World monkeys such as the marmosets (Fig. 4).

The Old World monkey *Macaca fascicularis* has been used as an animal model for many years in studies on male contraception and in studies on the efficacy and hormonal regulation of spermatogenesis (Weinbauer and Nieschlag 1993). All data obtained so far clearly show that this animal model, unlike other animal models, is particularly suitable for preclinical studies on human spermatogenesis. The fact that

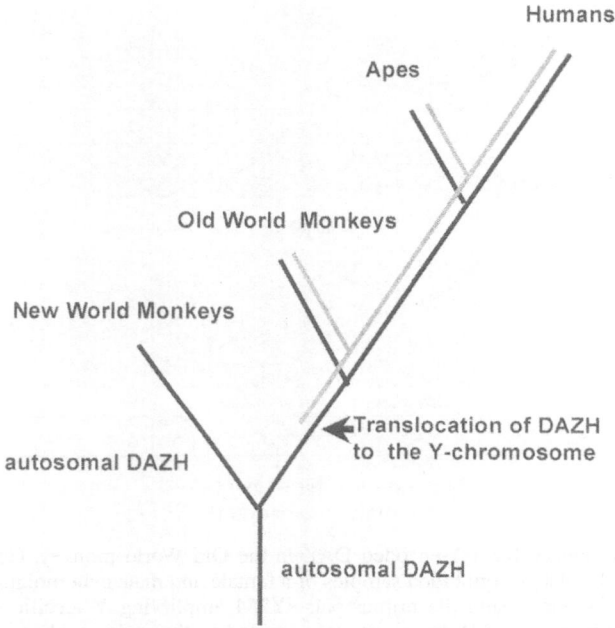

Fig. 4. Hypothetical model for the translocation of the ancestor of DAZ during primate evolution. While the autosomal DAZH (*black line*) is present in all primates, DAZ (*gray line*) is present only in the Old World monkeys, apes, and humans. The translocation therefore must have taken place after the splitting of the two primate lineages 30–40 million years ago

the monkey possesses a Y-encoded DAZ which is absent in other classical animal models makes it the ideal, possibly the only animal model suitable for functional analysis of the protein.

Following this line, we therefore isolated the corresponding DAZH gene of the cynomolgus monkey *M. fascicularis* by reverse-transcription PCR from testis mRNA. The monkey DAZ homologue cynDAZLA has an open reading frame of 888 bp and encodes 295 amino acids. Comparison of the cynDAZLA sequence to autosomal DAZ homologues from human, mouse, and fly shows the presence of an RRM consisting of an RNP-1 and RNP-2 motif and only one DAZ consensus repeat, compared with several repeats found in the human DAZ gene on the Y-chromosome. The homology of the cynDAZLA cDNA is 97% to human DAZH and 87% to mouse Dazla (Fig. 1). Hybridization of labeled cDNA to RNA isolated from various tissues has revealed a transcript of 3.5 kb which is expressed only in the testis (Carani et al. 1997).

The limitation of our first approach in isolating the DAZH cDNA by reverse-transcription PCR is, however, that only the coding region is amplified, and no data can be obtained for the 3' and 5' regions of that gene. In an extension of our studies on the isolation of DAZH from the cynomolgus monkey we therefore screened a recently generated testis cDNA library with human or monkey DAZH probes. A positive clone was isolated bearing the full length cDNA of the monkey DAZH. The cDNA is approximately 3.2 kb and contains an open reading frame and amino acid sequence as previously published (Carani et al. 1997; Fig. 1). The large 3' untranslated region displayed a high homology (89%) to the human DAZH.

The isolation of the Y-encoded DAZ from the monkey will be most interesting, and work on this is currently in progress. Detailed sequence comparisons of translated and untranslated regions of the DAZ and DAZH genes from the human and the monkey should yield further insights into the evolution of DAZ, for example which parts have been acquired or deleted during the past 30 million years, what is the repeat structure in the monkey, and whether DAZ is also a multicopy gene in the monkey. Another important point to be investigated in this animal model is the onset and regulation of expression of DAZ/DAZH during prepubertal, pubertal, and adult development of the testis. Specific DNA probes or specific antibodies must be used to clarify where and when DAZ/DAZH is expressed, and possible differences in the expressive pattern of the two proteins.

14.8 Conclusions

The fact that animals such as marsupials, mice, and fruitflies possess only an autosomal DAZ homologue and have normal spermatogenesis indicates, if extrapolated to the human situation, that DAZH is crucial for spermatogenesis, and suggests that the Y-encoded DAZ is a vestigial gene acquired and accumulated on the Y-chromosome. Conversely, even if the Y-encoded DAZ has only a minor positive impact on spermato-genesis, this would have a strong selective advantage during evolution. Different expression patterns of DAZ and DAZH during spermatogene-sis might indicate a diverging function of the two genes; the repeat structure in DAZ might possibly lead to other or to better binding characteristics to target mRNA. To this purpose the Old World monkey closely resembles the human in respect to general endocrine regulation of spermatogenesis, structural architecture and morphology of the testis, and very importantly in respect to gene content.

Acknowledgements. The work was supported by the German Research Founda-tion in the Confocal Research Group "The Male Gamete." The authors thank N. Terwort, L. Pekel, and B. Schuhmann for their excellent technical assis-tance. The language editing of S. Nieschlag is gratefully acknowledged.

References

Arnemann J, Jakubiczka S, Thuring S, Schmidtke J (1991) Cloning and se-quence analysis of a human Y-chromosome derived, testicular cDNA, TSPY. Genomics 11:108–114

Carani C, Gromoll J, Brinkworth MH, Simoni M, Weinbauer GF, Nieschlag E (1997) cynDAZLA: a cynomolgus homologue of the human autosomal DAZ gene. Mol Hum Reprod 3:479–483

Castrillon DH, Gonczy P, Alexander S, Rawson R, Eberhart CG, Viswanathan S, Di Nardo S, Wasserman SA (1993) Toward a molecular genetic analysis of spermatogenesis in *Drosophila melanogaster*: characterization of male-sterile mutants generated by single P element mutagenesis. Genetics 135:489–505

Chai NN, Salido EC, Yen PH (1997) Multiple functional copies of the RBM gene family, a spermatogenesis candidate on the human Y-chromosome. Genomics 45:355–361

Cooke HJ, Elliott DJ (1997) RNA-binding proteins and human infertility. Trends Genet 3:87–89

Cooke HJ, Lee M, Kerr S, Ruggiu M (1996) A murine homologue of the hu-man DAZ gene is autosomal and expressed only in male and female go-nads. Hum Mol Genet 5:513–516

Delbridge ML, Harry JL, Toder R, Waugh O'Neill RJ, Ma K, Chandley AC, Marshall Graves AM (1997) A human candidate spermatogenesis gene, RBM1, is conserved and amplified on marsupial Y chromosome. Nat Genet 15:131–136

Eberhart CG, Maines JZ, Wasserman SA (1996) Meiotic cell cycle requirement for a fly homologue of human deleted in azoospermia. Nature
381:783–785

Edwards RG, Bishop CE (1997) On the origin and frequency of Y chromosome deletions responsible for severe male infertility. Mol Hum Reprod
3:549–554

Elliott DJ, Millar MR, Oghene K, Ross A, Kiesewetter F, Pryor J, McIntyre M,
Hargreave TB, Saunders PTK, Vogt PH, Chandley AC, Cooke H (1997) Expression of RBM in the nuclei of human germ cells is dependent on a critical region of the Y chromosome long arm. Proc Natl Acad Sci USA
94:3848–3853

Foote S, Vollrath D, Hilton A, Page D (1992) The human Y chromosome: overlapping DNA clones spanning the euchromatic region. Science 258:60–66

Foresta C, Ferlin A, Garolla A, Rossato M, Barbaux S, De Bortoli A (1997) Y-
chromosome deletions in idiopathic severe testiculopathies. J Clin Endocrinol Metab 82:1975–1080

Glaser B, Hierl T, Taylor K, Schiebel K, Zeitler S, Papadopoulos K, Rappold
G, Schempp W (1997) High-resolution fluoresence in situ hybridization of
human Y-linked genes on released chromatin. Chromosom Res 5:23–30

Habermann B, Kiesewetter F, Mi H, Krause W, Vogt PH (1997) Lokalisation
eines SPGY-Gen-Produkts in Hodengewebe und ejakulierten Spermato-
zoen. 9th Annual Meeting of the Deutsche Gesellschaft für Andrologie,
Lübeck (abstract)

Hackstein JHP (1991) Spermatogenesis in Drosophila. A genetic approach to
cellular and subcellular differentiation. Eur J Cell Biol 56:151–169

Hecht NB (1996) Posttranscriptional regulation of postmeiotic gene expression. In: Hansson V, Levy FO, Tasken K (eds) Signal transduction in testicular cells. Springer, Berlin Heidelberg New York, pp 123–140

In't Veld PA, Halley DJJ, van Hemel JO, Niermeijer MF, Dohle G, Weber RFA
(1997) Genetic counseling before intracytoplasmic sperm injection. Lancet
350:490

Kalmykova AI, Shevelyov YY, Dobritsa AA, Gvozdev VA (1997) Acquisition
and amplification of a testis-expressed autosomal gene, SSL, by the Drosophila Y chromosome. Proc Natl Acad Sci 94:6297–6302

Karsch-Mizrachi I, Haynes SR (1993) The RB97D gene encodes a potential
RNA-binding protein required for spermatogenesis in Drosophilia. Nucl
Acids Res 21:2229–2235

Kent-First MG, Kol S, Muallem A, Ofir R, Manor D, Blazer S, First N,
Itskovitz-Eldor J (1996) The incidence and possible relevance of Y-linked
microdeletions in babies born after intracytoplasmic sperm injection and
their infertile fathers. Mol Hum Reprod 2:943–959

Kremer JAM, Tuerlings JH AM, Meuleman EJH, Schoute F, Mariman E, Smeets DFCM, Hoefsloot LH, Braat DDM, Merkus HMWM (1997) Microdeletions of the Y-chromosome and intracytoplasmic sperm injection: from gene to clinic. Hum Reprod 12:687–691

Lahn B and Page DC (1997) Functional coherence of the human Y chromosome. Science 278:675–680

Ma K, Inglis JD, Sharkey A, Bickmore WA, Hill RE, Prosser EJ, Speed RM, Thomson EJ, Jobling M, Taylor K, Wolfe J, Kooke HJ, Hargreave TB, Chandley AC (1993) A Y chromosome gene family with RNA-binding protein homology: candidates for the azoospermia factor AZF controlling human spermatogensis. Cell 75:1287–1295

Menke DB, Mutter GL, Page DC (1997) Expression of DAZ, an azoospermia factor candidate, in human spermatogonia. Am J Hum Genet 60:237–241

Meschede D, Nieschlag E, Horst J (1997) Assisted reproduction for infertile couples at high genetic risk: an ethical consideration. Biomed Ethics 2:4–6

Mulhall JP, Reijo R, Alagappan R, Brown L, Page D, Carson R and Oates RD (1997) Azoospermic men with deletion of the DAZ gene cluster are capable of completing spermatogenesis: fertilization, normal embryonic development and pregnancy occur when retrieved testicular spermatozoa are used for intracytoplasmatic sperm injection. Hum Reprod 12:503–508

Nagai K (1996) RNA-protein complexes. Curr Opin Struct Biol 6:53–61

Najmabadi H, Huang V, Yen P, Subbaru MN, Bhasin D, Banaag L, Naseeruddin S, De Kretser DM, Baker HWG, McLachlan RI, Loveland KA, Bhasin S (1996) Substantial prevalence of microdeletions of the Y-chromosome in infertile men with idiopathic azoospermia and oligozoospermia detected using a sequence-tagged site-based mapping strategy. J Clin Endocrinol Metab 81:1347–1352

Nakahori Y, Kuroki Y, Komaki R, Kondoh N, Namiki M, Iwamoto T, Toda T, Kobayashi K (1996) The Y chromosome region essential for spermatogenesis. Horm Res 46 [Suppl 1]:20–23

Niederberger C, Agulnik AI, Cho Y, Lamb D, Bishop CE (1997) In situ hybridization shows that Dazla expression in mouse testis is restricted to premeiotic stages IV–VI of spermatogenesis. Mamm Genome 8:277–278

Pryor JL, Kent-First M, Muallem A, Van Bergen AH, Nolten WE, Meisner L, Roberts KP (1997) Microdeletion of the Y chromosome of infertile men. New Engl J Med 336:534–539

Qureshi SJ, Ross AR, Ma K, Cooke HJ, McIntyre MA, Chandley AC and Hargreave TB (1996) Polymerase chain reaction screening for Y chromosome microdeletions: a first step towards the diagnosis of genetically-determined spermatogenic failure in men. Mol Hum Reprod 2:775–779

Reijo R, Lee TY, Salo P, Alagappan R, Brown LG, Rosenberg M, Rozen S, Jaffe T, Straus D, Hovatta O, De la Chapelle A, Silber S, Page DC (1995)

Diverse spermatogenic defects in humans caused by Y chromosome deletions encompassing a novel RNA-binding protein gene. Nat Genet 10:383–393

Reijo R, Alagappan RK, Patrizio P, Page DC (1996a) Severe oligozoospermia resulting from deletions of azoospermia factor gene on Y chromosome. Lancet 347:1290–1293

Reijo R, Seligman J, Dinulos MB, Jaffe T, Brown LG, Disteche CM, Page DC (1996b) Mouse autosomal homolog of DAZ, a candidate male sterility gene in humans, is expresssed in male germ cells before and after puberty. Genomics 35:346–352

Ruggiu M, Speed R, Taggart M, McKay SJ, Kilanowski F, Saunders P, Dorin J, Cooke HJ (1997) The mouse Dazla gene encodes a cytoplasmic protein essential for gametogenesis. Nature 389:73–77

Saxena R, Brown LG, Hawkins T, Alagappan RK, Skaletsky H, Reeve MP, Reijo R, Rozen S, Dinulos MB, Disteche CM, Page DC (1996) The DAZ gene cluster on the human Y chromosome arose from an autosomal gene that was transposed, repeatedly amplified and pruned. Nat Genet 14:292–299

Seboun E, Barbaux S, Bourgeron T, Nishi S, Algonik A, Egashira M, Nikkawa N, Bishop C, Fellous M, McElreavy K, Kasahara M (1997) Gene sequence, localization, and evolutionary conservation of DAZLA, a candidate male sterility gene. Genomics 41:227–235

Shan Z, Hirschmann P, Seebacher T, Edelmann A, Jauch A, Morell J, Urbitsch P, Vogt HP (1996) A SPGY copy homologous to the mouse gene Dazla and the Drosophila gene boule is autosomal and expressed only in human male gonad. Hum Mol Genet 5:2005–2011

Simoni M, Gromoll J, Dworniczak B, Rolf C, Abshagen K, Kamischke A, Carani C, Meschede D, Behre HM, Horst J, Nieschlag E (1997) Screening for deletion of Y chromosome involving the DAZ (deleted in azoospermia) gene in azoospermia and severe oligozoospermia. Fertil Steril 67:542–547

Simoni M, Kamischke A, Nieschlag E (1998) Current status of the molecular diagnosis of Y-chromosomal microdeletions in the workup of male infertility. Hum Reprod (in press)

Siomi H, Dreyfuss G (1997) RNA-binding proteins as regulators of gene expression. Curr Opin Genet Develop 7:345–353

Sinclair AH, Berta P, Palmer MS, Hawkins JR, Griffiths BL, Smith MJ, Foster JW, Frischauf AM, Lovell-Badge R, Goodfellow PN (1990) A gene from the human sex-determining region encodes a protein with homology to a conserved DNA-binding motif. Nature 346:240–244

Stuppia L, Mastroprimiano G, Calabrese G, Peila R, Tenaglia R, Palka G (1996) Microdeletions in interval 6 of the Y chromosome detected by STS-PCR in 6 of 33 patients with idiopathic oligo- or azoospermia. Cytogenet Cell Genet 72:155–158

Tiepolo L, Zuffardi O (1976) Localization of factors controlling spermatogenesis in the non-fluorescent portion of the human y chromosome long
   arm. Hum Genet 34:119–124
Van der Ven K, Montag M, Peschka B, Leygraaf J, Schwanitz G, Haidl G,
   Krebs D, Van der Ven H (1997) Combined cytogenetic and Y chromosome
   microdeletion screening in males undergoing intracytoplasmic sperm injec-
   tion. Mol Hum Reprod 3:699–704
Vereb M, Agulnik AI, Houston JT, Lipschultz LI, Lamb DJ, Bishop CE (1997)
   Absence of DAZ gene mutations in case of non-obstructed azoospermia.
   Mol Hum Reprod 3:55–59
Vogt P, Chandley AC, Hargreave TB, Keil R, Ma K, Sharkey A (1992) Mi-
   crodeletions in interval 6 of the Y chromosome of males with idiopathic ste-
   rility point to disruption of AZF, a human spermatogenesis gene. Hum
   Genet 89:491–496
Vogt P, Edelmann A, Kirsch S, Henegariu O, Hirschmann P, Kiesewetter F,
   Köhn FM, Schill WB, Farah S, Ramos C, Hartmann M, Hartschuh W, Mes-
   chede D, Behre HM, Castel A, Nieschlag E, Weidner W, Gröne HJ, Engel
   W, Haidl G (1996) Human Y chromosome azoospermia factors (AZF)
   mapped to different subregions in Yq11. Hum Mol Genet 5:933–943
Vogt PH (1995) Genetic aspects of artificial fertilization. Hum Reprod 10
   [Suppl 1]:128–137
Vollrath D, Foote S, Hilton A, Brown LG, Beer-Romero P, Bogan JS, Page D
   (1992) The human Y chromosome: a 43-interval map based on naturally oc-
   curing deletions. Science 258:52–59
Weinbauer GF, Nieschlag E (1993) Hormonal regulation of spermatogenesis.
   In: de Kretser D (ed) Molecular biology of the male reproductive system.
   Academic, New York, pp 99–142
Yen PH, Chai NN, Salido EC (1996) The human autosomal gene DAZLA: tes-
   tis specificity and a candidate for male infertility. Hum Mol Genet
   5:2013–2017
Yen PH, Chai NN, Salido EC (1997) The human DAZ genes, a putative male
   infertility factor on the Y chromosome, are highly polymorphic in the DAZ
   repeat regions. Mamm Genome 8:756–759

15 Follicle-Stimulating Hormone Receptor Mutation and Fertility

T. Vaskivuo, K. Aittomäki, I.T. Huhtaniemi, and J.S. Tapanainen

15.1 Introduction

Recent studies on the molecular pathogenesis of diseases have shown that even infertility can be hereditary. This contrasts with the general opinion that infertility cannot by nature be an inherited condition. Rapid progress in the field of molecular biology has enabled the identification and detailed characterization of mutations and polymorphisms causing impaired fertility. Although the ultimate cause of such disorders cannot be treated today, affected individuals suffering from these conditions can be effectively helped with the new assisted reproductive techniques.

Many of the recognized causes of infertility have been found to affect the function of the pituitary-gonadal axis. Mutations of the gonadotropin genes, i.e., the common α-subunit and the follicle-stimulating hormone (FSH) or luteinizing hormone (LH) β-subunits, are rare. On the other hand, a number gonadotropin receptor mutations, explaining certain pathologies of gonadal function, have been recently discovered. Most of these reports describe mutations in the LH receptor (LHR) gene, and only recently three mutations in the FSH receptor (FSHR) gene have been documented.

This review focuses on the FSHR. First, the FSHR function and structure are briefly summarized, and then the currently known FSHR mutations and the phenotypic alterations that they cause are described in more detail.

15.2 Physiological Functions of Gonadotropins

FSH is a member of the glycoprotein hormone family that includes, in addition, LH, thyroid-stimulating hormone (TSH) and human chorionic gonadotropin (hCG). FSH, LH, and TSH are synthesized in the anterior pituitary gland, whereas hCG is synthesized by the placenta. Ovarian and testicular differentiation and function are controlled by FSH and LH. In females FSH is required for normal ovarian development and follicle maturation while LH regulates theca cell androgen production, induces ovulation, and regulates the corpus luteum function. FSH binds to its receptor, exclusively present in ovarian granulosa cells (Richards 1994), stimulates their growth, and activates the production of estrogens initiating a normal menstrual cycle. Although FSH is essential for the last stages of follicular maturation, the initiation of ovarian follicular growth is thought to be independent of FSH. This is supported by persistent follicular growth in gonadotropin-deficient mice (Halpin et al. 1986). Furthermore, follicular growth also occurs in the perinatal rat ovary before the appearance of gonadotropin receptors (Sokka and Huhtaniemi 1990; Rannikko et al. 1995). At the time of puberty the interrupted process of follicular growth is overcome when serum FSH levels increase, and cyclic ovarian function starts.

In the testis FSH binds to its receptors in Sertoli cells, stimulating their differentiation, growth and various steps of metabolism. FSH is generally considered essential for the prepubertal phase of Sertoli cell proliferation, the pubertal initiation of spermatogenesis, and later for quantitatively normal sperm production (Knobil 1980). Androgens secreted by Leydig cells in response to LH have synergistic effect with FSH on spermatogenesis (Sharpe et al. 1994) and maintain the male sexual functions.

15.3 Structure of Gonadotropin Receptors

The gonadotropin receptors, together with that of TSH, belong to a superfamily of seven transmembrane domain G protein coupled receptors. Other receptors of this gene family include muscarinic, adrenergic, cholinergic, dopamine, and substance-K receptors. The structure of these proteins includes seven transmembrane spanning domains, the extracellular amino-terminus, and the intracellular carboxy-terminus. The transmembrane domains are most homologous between the members of this receptor superfamily. Most of these receptors appear to have a short extracellular amino-terminus. However, a large amino-terminal domain, ranging in size from 333 to 398 amino acids, is typical of glycoprotein hormone receptors. Each of these receptors is specific to its cognate ligand hormone, with the exception of LHR which binds both LH and hCG with roughly similar affinity and triggers similar cellular responses.

The gonadotropin receptor genes have been cloned from several species, including the human (Minegishi et al. 1990; Minegishi et al. 1991; Rousseau-Merck et al. 1990; Koo et al. 1991). The FSHR gene is located in chromosome 2 p21. The gonadotropin receptors are coded by long genes (>84 and 64 kb for FSHR and LHR, respectively). Although the size of the genes varies, the similarities between FSHR and LHR genes are striking. The number of exons in the gonadotropin receptor genes differs; the FSHR gene has 10 and the LHR gene 11. However, in both of them, the last exon encodes the whole transmembrane and intracellular part, which is about 50% of the size of the receptor protein. These exons share a 62% similarity at the nucleotide level (Heckert et al. 1992).

15.4 Mutations in Gonadotropins and Their Receptors

Mutations of gonadotropin genes are very rare; they have been described in the β-subunit genes, but not in that of the common α-subunit. An inactivating mutation of the LHβ gene described in a hypogonadal man was shown to cause a complete loss of LH bioactivity, expressed as total absence of Leydig cells and infertility (Weiss et al. 1992). This single base substitution changed codon 54 from Glu to Arg. A polymorphic variant of the LH β-subunit gene containing two missense mutations (Trp 8 Arg and Ile 15 Thr) has been reported from Finland (Pettersson et al. 1992; Haavisto et al. 1995) and Japan (Furui et al. 1994). The variant LH has increased in vitro bioactivity but reduced circulatory half-life. Although it has been related with a number of conditions with altered LH action (e.g., puberty, polycystic ovary syndrome), its final pathophysiological significance is still unknown.

Genetic defects in the gonadotropin receptors can be divided into activating (i.e., gain of function) and inactivating (i.e., loss of function) mutations. Usually in the case of activating mutations only heterozygosity is required for the phenotypic alteration (e.g., a constitutively activated receptor). On the other hand, the inactivating mutations more often demand homozygosity for the changed phenotype. Most LHR mutations have been discovered in or next to the sixth transmembrane helix, which is an important region for the binding of G proteins (Kremer et al. 1993, 1995; Laue et al. 1996; Tsigos et al. 1997; Toledo et al. 1996).

Females with inactivating LHR mutations have normal sexual differentiation and apparently normal pubertal development. The same would probably be the phenotype with inactivating LH mutations, but such cases have not yet been reported in the female. However, after puberty, the lack of normal LH action causes, as expected, amenorrhea and infertility (Kremer et al. 1995; Toledo et al. 1996). Males with impaired LH action have been shown to have Leydig cell hypoplasia, diverted masculinization, pseudohermaphroditism, and spermatogenic failure (Kremer et al. 1995; Laue et al. 1995; Latronico et al. 1996). Activating mutations of the LHR gene cause precocious puberty in boys (Shenker et al. 1993; Yano et al. 1996), but no phenotype has so far been detected in females.

Table 1. List of mutations of FSH receptor with the presenting phenotype

Amino acid change	Female phenotype	Male phenotype	Reference
Inactivating			
Ala 189 Val	Ovarian dysgenesis		Aittomäki et al.1995
		Suppressed spermatogenesis	Tapanainen et al. 1997
Phe 591 Ser	Ovarian sex cord tumors		Kotlar et al. 1997
Activating			
Asp 567 Gly		Gonadtropin independent spermatogenesis	Gromoll et al. 1996

The first mutation in the FSH β-subunit was discovered in a woman with primary amenorrhea and infertility (Matthews et al. 1993). Analysis revealed a two-nucleotide frameshift deletion in codon 70 of the FSH β-subunit gene. The subject's fertility was restored by the administration of FSH. Recently, compound heterozygous mutations of FSHβ gene were discovered in a female with primary amenorrhea (Layman et al. 1997). DNA sequencing revealed a 2-bp deletion at codon 61 (Val 61 X) and a missense mutation at codon 51 (Cys 51 Gly). Each of these mutations prevented efficient combination of the α- and β-subunits to form intact FSH. No mutation of FSHβ gene has been discovered in males so far. However, the clinical findings on such cases would obviously be analogous to the presentation of inactivating FSHR mutation (see Sect. 15.5.1).

15.5 Mutations in the FSH Receptor Genes

Although several LHR mutations have been discovered, only two inactivating and one activating mutation of FSHR have so far been found. The phenotype of the inactivating mutation have been described in both men and women, and the activating mutation has been characterized in a male with gonadotropin deficiency (Table 1).

15.5.1 Inactivating Mutations of the FSH Receptor

The first mutation of FSHR was discovered in six Finnish families with two or more women suffering from hypergonadotropic ovarian dysgenesis (ODG). A total of 75 patients with ODG were identified (Aittomäki 1994), and they all showed primary or early-onset secondary amenorrhea and infertility. The arrest of ovarian maturation at puberty was found to be caused by the lack of ovarian response to FSH, leading to missing gonadal negative feedback and elevated serum FSH levels. In a systematic search for linkage in the affected families, the ODG locus was mapped to chromosome 2p where both of the gonadotropin receptor genes are located. Due to the critical role of FSH in the early follicular development, and to the fact that no pseudohermaphoriditism was apparent in the affected families, an FSHR mutation seemed more likely. It turned out that 22 of these 75 females had an inactivating point mutation in the FSHR gene.

Unlike the LHR mutations which are mostly located in the transmembrane domain of the receptor, the inactivating FSHR mutation is found in the extracellular ligand binding domain of the protein. A C566 T transition in exon 7 of FSHR predicting an Ala to Val substitution at residue 189 has been found to cause ODG (Fig. 1). Functional testing in transfected MSC-1 cells demonstrated a dramatic reduction in binding capacity and signal transduction, but apparently normal ligand binding affinity by the mutated FSHR (Aittomäki et al. 1995). The mutation was located in a highly conserved region when compared with the FSHR of the monkey, sheep, and rat. This emphasizes the functional importance of the location. In addition, it belongs to a sequence of five amino acids that are identical in the FSHR, LHR, and TSHR and contain a consensus N-linked glycosylation site. The high conservation of this region in the three glycoprotein hormone receptors suggests that it is not the site of ligand recognition. It more likely participates in the nonspecific aspects of ligand binding or plays a role in transfer of the receptor to the plasma membrane, or in its turnover. The normal affinity of the low number of mutated receptors that can be detected in transfected cells supports this (Aittomäki et al. 1995).

The 22 females with the inactivating FSHR mutation came from 13 families and had 25 male sibs. Blood samples of 15 brothers were obtained for testing of the FSHR mutation, and 5 of the men tested

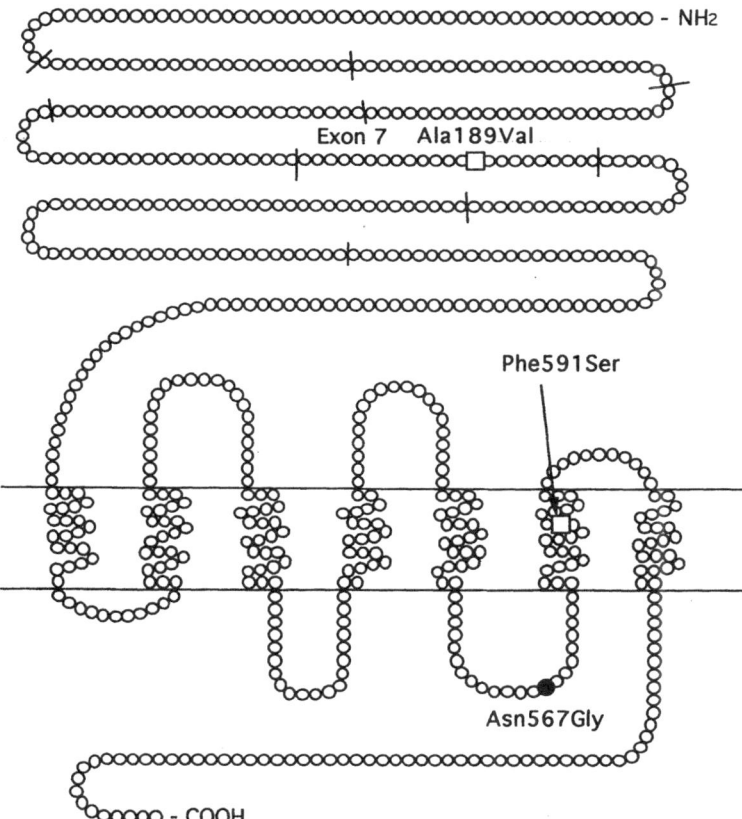

Fig. 1. The structure of FSH receptor and the locations of two inactivating mutations (*open squares*) and the activating mutation (*black circle*) so far detected. *Short lines* across the amino acid chain separate the 10 exons

proved homozygotes for the FSHR mutation. All of them had normal serum testosterone levels and were normally masculinized. Although the affected men had low-normal to clearly low testicular volume, sperm was found in the semen of all of them. However, none of them had fully normal sperm parameters. Three of the men had severe and one had moderate oligozoospermia. The fifth man had normal sperm

Table 2. Clinical and hormonal data of the men homozygous for the C566 T (Ala 189 Val) FSH receptor mutation

Pat. no. (years)	Age (years)	Testis size (ml)	Sperm analysis Count/ml	Norm. morph.	FSH (IU/l)	LH (IU/l)	T (nmol/l)
1	45	4.0/4.0	$.1\times10^6$	–	23.5	16.3	14.5
2	47	15.0/13.8	5.6×10^6	2%	12.5	5.6	8.8
3	55	13.5/15.8	$.1\times10^6$	–1	5.1	4.2	15.8
4	42	8.0/8.0	$.0\times10^6$	16%	20.6	16.2	26.2
5	29	8.6/6.0	42×10^6	16%	39.6	11.1	14.7
Ref. range	≥15		$≥20\times10^6$	≥40%	1–10.5	1–8.4	8.2–34.6

concentration but low volume and teratozoospermia. In addition, two of the men were fertile (Table 2). While all women with the inactivating C566 T mutation are infertile, the same FSHR mutation does not seem to cause absolute infertility in men. The FSHR mutation suppresses spermatogenesis to a variable degree but does not totally disable it. This suggests that FSH is not an absolute requirement for spermatogenesis as it is for ovarian follicle maturation (Tapanainen et al. 1997).

Previous studies have indicated that FSH together with testosterone is needed for the pubertal initiation of spermatogenesis. However, it is known that in adult men FSH is not necessary for the reinitiation of spermatogenesis (Bremner et al. 1981). The study on men with inactivating FSHR mutation shows that, in contrast to earlier views, FSH is not required for the pubertal initiation of spermatogenesis. Recent studies with FSHβ knockout mice support this fact. FSH-deficient female mice are infertile due to a block in folliculogenesis prior to antral follicle formation. FSH-deficient male mice have smaller testes than wild type males and suppressed spermatogenesis, but they are fertile (Kumar et al. 1997). The smaller testicular volume in affected men and in FSHβ knockout mice supports the notion that FSH induces Sertoli cell proliferation in immature testes and thus has an important role in determining the final testicular size.

Recently a heterozygous point mutation of FSHR was discovered in patients with ovarian sex cord tumors (Kotlar et al. 1997). This mutation, T1777 C, converts Phe to Ser at residue 591 (Fig. 1). Transfection studies on COS-7 cells demonstrated that the mutation eliminated FSH-stimulated cAMP production. The role of this inhibiting FSHR mutation in the development of ovarian sex tumors is unclear, and it is likely that it is only one of several genetic abnormalities in these tumors.

15.5.2 Activating FSH Receptor Mutation

One case of activating FSHR mutation has been reported. A hypophysectomized 28-year-old man was unexpectedly found to be fertile despite gonadotropin deficiency. A point mutation a was found in exon 10 of the FSHR gene. This A1700G mutation, predicting an Asp to Gly transition in amino acid 567, was located in the third transmembrane loop of the receptor protein (Fig. 1). In functional studies on COS-7 cells transfected with the mutant FSHR, a 1.5-fold increase in basal cAMP production over wild type receptor, was found in the absence of FSH. The wild type and mutated FSHR reacted to increasing concentrations of FSH with a similar dose-dependent stimulation of cAMP production (Gromoll et al. 1995). These findings suggested that the activating mutation of the FSHR autonomously sustains spermatogenesis in the absence of gonadotropins.

15.6 Summary

Recently discovered mutations of the FSHR gene have markedly expanded our knowledge on the role of FSH in reproduction. Inactivating mutation of the FSHR leads to amenorrhea and absolute infertility in females, but in males spermatogenesis and fertility are only partially affected despite lacking FSH action, suggesting that FSH is more important for female than male fertility. Thus it seems that female reproductive tract is predominantly FSH dependent and accommodating changes in LH. On the other hand, male reproductive organs are sensitive to changes in LH activity and are relatively resistant to changes in FSH activity.

It has been suggested that the inhibition of FSH action would be an optimal method for male contraception. The only lowered fertility in males with inactivating FSHR mutation and in FSHβ knockout mice demonstrates, however, that spermatogenesis can start and be maintained without FSH. This suggests that the blockade of FSH action, for example using anti-FSH vaccines, FSH antagonists or inhibin, is unlikely to be a successful method of male contraception.

References

Aittomäki K (1994) The genetics of XX gonadal dysgenesis. Am J Hum Genet 54:844–851

Aittomäki K, Dieguez Lucena JL, Pakarinen P, Sistonen P, Tapanainen J, Gromoll J, Kaskikari R, Sankila E-M, Lehväslaiho H, Engel AR, Nieschlag E, Huhtaniemi I, de la Chapelle A (1995) Mutation in the follicle-stimulating hormone receptor gene causes hereditary hypergonadotropic ovarian failure. Cell 82:956–968

Bremner WR, Matsumoto AM, Sussman AM, Paulsen CA (1981) Follicle-stimulating hormone and human spermatogenesis. J Clin Invest 68:1044–1052

Furui K, Suganuma N, Tsukahara S, Asada Y, Kikkawa F, Tanaka M, Ozawa T, Tomoda Y (1994) Identification of two point mutations in the gene coding luteinizing hormone (LH) β-subunit, associated with immunologically anomalous LH variants. J Clin Endocrinol Metab 78:107–113

Gromoll J, Simoni M, Nieschlag E (1995) An activating mutation of the follicle-stimulating hormone receptor autonomously sustains spermatogenesis in a hypophysectomised man. J Clin Endocrinol Metab 81:1367–1370

Haavisto A-M, Petterson K, Bergendahl M, Virkamäki A, Huhtaniemi I (1995) Occurrence and biological properties of a common genetic variant of luteinizing hormone. J Clin Endocrinol Metab 80:1257–1263

Halpin DM, Charlton HM, Faddy MJ (1986) Effects of gonadotrophin deficiency on follicular development in hypogonald (hpg) mice. J Reprod Fertil 78:119–125

Heckert LL, Daley IJ, Griswold MD (1992) Structural organization of the follicle-stimulating hormone receptor gene. Mol Endorcinol 6:70–80

Knobil E (1980) The neuroendocrine control of the menstrual cycle. Recent Progr Horm Res 1980:53–88

Koo YB, Ji I, Slaughter RG, Ji TH (1991) Structure of the luteinizing hormone receptor gene and multiple exons of the coding sequence. Endocrinology 128:2297–2308

Kotlar TJ, Young RH, Albanese C, Crowley WF, Scully RE, Jameson JL (1997) A mutation in the follicle-stimulating hormone receptor occurs frequently in human ovarian sex cord tumors. J Clin Endocrinol Metab 82:1020–1026

Kremer H, Mariman E, Otten BJ, Moll GW Jr, Stoelinga GB, Wit JM, Jansen M, Drop SL, Faas B, Ropers HH, Brunner HG (1993) Cosegregation of missense mutations of the luteinizing hormone receptor gene with familial male-limited precocious puberty. Hum Mol Genet 2:1779–1783

Kremer H, Kraaij R, Toledo SPA, Post M, Fridman JB, Hayashida CY, van Reen M, Milgrom E, Ropers HH, Mariman E, Themmen APN, Brunner HG (1995) Male pseudohermaphroditism due to a homozygous missense mutation of the luteinizing hormone receptor gene. Nat Genet 9:160–164

Kumar TR, Wang Y, Lu N, Matzuk MM (1997) Follicle stimulating hormone is required for ovarian follicle maturation but not male fertility. Nat Genet 15:201–204

Latronico AC, Anasti J, Arnhold IJ, Rapaport R, Mendonca BB, Bloise W, Castro M, Tsigos C, Chrousos GP (1996) Testicular and ovarian resistance to luteinizing hormone caused by inactivating mutations of the luteinizing hormone receptor gene. N Engl J Med 344:507–512

Laue L, Wu SM, Kudo M, Hsueh AJW, Cutler GB Jr, Chan WY (1995) Missense mutations in exons 10 and 11 of the human luteinizing hormone receptor gene are associated with Leydig cell hypoplasia. Am J Hum Genet 57 [Suppl 1253]

Laue LL, Wu SM, Kudo M, Bourdony CJ, Cutler GB Jr, Hsueh AJ, Chan WY (1996) Compound heterozygous mutations of the luteinizing hormone receptor gene in Leydig cell hypoplasia. Mol Endocrinol 10:987–997

Layman LC, Shelley ME, Huey LO, Wall SW, Tho SP, McDonough PG (1993) Follicle-stimulating hormone beta gene structure in premature ovarian failure. Fertil Steril 60:852–857

Matthews CH, Borgato S, Beck-Peccoz P, Adams M, Tone Y, Gambino G, Casagrande S, Tedeschini G, Benedetti A, Chatterjee VK (1993) Primary amennorrhoea and infertility due to a mutation in the betasubunit of follicle-stimulating hormone. Nat Genet 5:83–86

Minegishi T, Nakamura K, Takakura Y, Miyamoto K, Hasegawa Y, Ibuki Y, Igarishi M (1990) Cloning and sequencing of human LH/hCG receptor cDNA. Biochem Biophys Res Commun 172:1049–1054

Minegishi T, Nakamura K, Takakura Y, Ibuki Y, Igarishi M (1991) Cloning and sequencing of human FSH receptor cDNA. Biochem Biophys Res Commun 175:1125–1130

Pettersson K, Ding Y-Q, Huhtaniemi I (1992) An immunologically anomalous luteinizing hormone variant in a healthy woman. J Clin Endocrinol Metab 74:164–171

Rannikko AS, Zhang FP, Huhtaniemi I (1995) Ontogeny of folliclestimulating hormone receptor gene expression in the rat testis and ovary. Mol Cell Endocrinol 107:196–208

Richards JS (1994) Hormonal control of gene expression in the ovary. Endocr Rev 15:725–751

Rousseau-Merck MF, Misrahi M, Atger M, Loosfelt H, Milgrom E, Berger R (1990) Localization of the human luteinizing hormone/ receptor gene (LHCGR) to chromosome 2p21. Cytogenet Cell Genet 54:77–79

Sharpe RM, Kerr JB, McKinnell C, Miller M (1994) Temporal relationship between androgen-dependent changes in the volume of seminiferous tubule fluid, lumen size and seminiferous tubule protein secretion in rats. J Reprod Fertil 101:193–198

Shenker A, Laue L, Kosugi S, Meredino JJ Jr, Minegishi T, Cutler GB Jr (1993) A constitutively activating mutation of the luteinizing hormone receptor in familial male precocious puberty. Nature 365:652–654

Sokka T and Huhtaniemi I (1990) Ontogeny of gonadotrophin receptors and gonadotrophin stimulated cAMP production in the neonatal rat ovary. J Endocrinol 127:297–303

Tapanainen JS, Aittomäki K, Min J, Vaskivuo T, Huhtaniemi I (1997) Men homozygous for an inactivating mutation of the follicle stimulating hormone (FSH) receptor gene present variable suppression of spermatogenesis and fertility. Nat Genet 15:205–206

Toledo SP, Brunner HG, Kraaij R, Post M, Dahia PL, Hayashida CY, Kremer H, Themmen AP (1996) An inactivating mutation of the luteinizing hormone receptor causes amenorrhea in a 46,XX female. J Clin Endocrinol Metab 81:3850–3854

Tsigos C, Latronico C, Chrousos GP (1997) Luteinizing hormone resistance syndromes. Ann NY Acad Sci 816:263–273

Weiss J, Axelrod L, Whitcomb RW, Harris PE, Crowley WF, Jameson JL (1992) Hypogonadism caused by a single amino acid substitution in the beta subunit of luteinizing hormone. N Engl J Med 326:179–183

Yano K, Kohn LD, Saji M, Kataoka N, Okuno A, Cutler GB Jr (1996) A case of male-limited precocious puberty caused by a point mutation in the second transmembrane domain of the luteinizing hormone choriongonadotrophin gene. Biochem Biophys Res Commun 220:1036–1042

Subject Index

metaphase II (MII) arrested oocytes
   254
mHR6A   87
mHR6B   89
mHR6B knockout   92
microassisted fertilization   283
microdeletions   274, 281
microinjection   44, 254, 258
midpiece   258
MII-anaphase transition   258
mitochondria   179
mitochondrial derivative   62
mitogen-activated protein (MAP)
   kinase   256
MLN64   197
monoclonal antibodies   236, 237
mouse embryo   24
multicopy gene   283
multigene family   2, 9, 14
muscarinic acetylcholine receptors
   (AChR)   143
mutations   295, 298

N-terminal truncations   196
neuroblastoma   140
neurosecretory PC12   141
New World Monkeys   279, 287
NGD⁺   140
nicotinamide   141
nicotinic acid adenine dinucleotide
   phosphate   134
nitric oxide   141
nonrecombining region   273
nuclear localization signal   242
nude mice   44

Old World monkeys   279, 287
oligo-astheno-teratozoospermia   96
oligozoospermia   301
oligozoospermic   281
ovarian dysgenesis   299, 300
ovary   180, 214

parthenogenetic activation   258
Pdha-1   87
permeability   4, 12
Pgk-1   87
phospholipase C (PLC)   254
phosphorylation   5, 11, 192
phosphotransferase   257
pituitary adenylate cyclase
   activating peptides   33
placenta   184, 214
PLC inhibitors   255
PLC isoforms   255, 261
PLCγ1   255
point mutation   300
polyclonal antibodies   236, 240
post-transcriptional regulation   222
postacrosomal region   258
postmeiotic expression   86
postmeiotic spermatid
   differentiation   63
postreplication DNA repair   92
postreplication repair   93
primary spermatocytes   61, 63, 72
primordial germ cells (PGC)   23,
   30, 32, 34, 36, 84
– adhesion   33
– apoptosis   29
– development   26, 36
– migration   27, 36
– proliferation   31, 33
– purification of   24
processed genes   229
pronucleus   96, 254, 256
prospermatogonia   23, 34, 35
protamines   90
proteasome   87
protein turnover   77
purinergic receptors   143

race   111
radioimmunoassay   143
rat to mouse transplantation   46, 49

Ernst Schering Research Foundation Workshop

Editors: Günter Stock
            Ursula-F. Habenicht